HEALTHY HEALING
AN ALTERNATIVE HEALING REFERENCE

by LINDA G. RECTOR-PAGE, N.D., Ph. D.

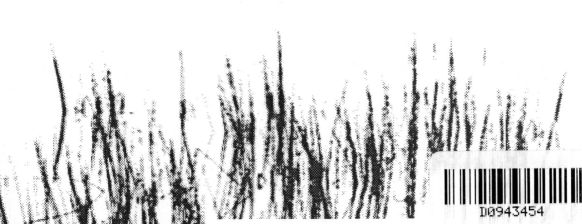

Printed by Griffin Printing

To Everyone who is striving for a more natural
drug-free, financially responsible way of healing

❧   ❧   ❧   ❧

NEITHER DRUGS NOR HERBS NOR VITAMINS ARE A CURE
FOR ANYTHING. THE BODY HEALS ITSELF. THE HUMAN
BODY IS INCREDIBLY INTELLIGENT. IT USUALLY
RESPONDS TO INTELLIGENT THERAPIES. THE HEALING
PROFESSIONAL CAN HELP THIS PROCESS ALONG BY
OFFERING INTELLIGENT CHOICES.

🐢   🐢   🐢

EVEN <u>ONE</u> MIRACLE CURE CAN SHOW THE VALUE OF A THERAPY
WITH THE BODY'S OWN HEALING POWERS. IF THE THERAPY IS NATURAL,
NON-INVASIVE, AND DOES NO HARM, IT CAN BE TRIED WITH
CONFIDENCE AS A VALID CHOICE.

First Printing, June 1985. Copywrite req. Nov. 1985.
Second Printing, January 1986.
Third printing, Revised Edition, September 1986.
Fourth Printing, Revised/Updated, May 1987.
Fifth Printing, November 1987
Sixth Printing, Newly Revised/Updated, June 1988.
Seventh Printing, Revised/Update, Jan. 1989, Sept. 1989, March 1990.

Eighth Printing, Revised/Updated/Expanded, July 1990.

ABOUT THE AUTHOR

Linda Rector-Page has been working with natural and herbal medicinals for the last twelve years in the Sierra foothills, as a self-taught and now certified Doctor of Naturopathy and Ph.D. Her experience has been extensive in formulating and testing herbal combinations.

She has owned and operated The Rainbow Kitchen, a natural foods restaurant, worked as an employee and now half owner of The Country Store Natural Foods store, and is developer/owner of Crystal Star Herbs.

The circumstance of active involvement in both wholesale and retail operations has been very beneficial in writing "HEALTHY HEALING". The Country Store sees over 200 customers a day, and much of the learning experience and concrete successes have come from them. These have then been translated into Crystal Star Products, and recorded in "HEALTHY HEALING" every year. The book is now in its eighth edition.

"COOKING FOR HEALTHY HEALING" is a companion book and sequel to "HEALTHY HEALING". It too, is a result and synthesis of her background and experience in the natural healing fields, drawing both on the nutritional recipes from The Rainbow Kitchen and the more specific, defined healing diets that have developed with her training since then. It contains 26 full spectrum healing diets, over 750 recipes to support the diets throughout the healing process, and an exercise/bodywork section as a part of healing. Every recipe has been thoroughly tested in each program to insure workability and delicious taste with the highest nutrition. It is a book that can be used every day to help assure health.

Linda is currently working on a new book, "HOW TO BE YOUR OWN HERBAL PHARMACIST" designed for those interested in learning how to formulate and use herbal combinations for their own individual needs.

This reference is to be used for information only.
It is not a claim for cure or mitigation of disease,
but is rather an adjunctive approach - supplying
individual daily nutritional needs that otherwise
might be lacking in today's diet.

TABLE OF CONTENTS

HEALTHY HEALING

A COMPLETE ALTERNATIVE HEALING REFERENCE

HOW TO USE THIS BOOK

The natural healing suggestions in this book work <u>with</u> the body functions, not outside them - so there are no side effects or trauma on the system.

For long-lasting permanent health, the body must do its own work. The natural healing methods described here will help rebalance specific areas of the body, so that it can function normally.

Because each body is very individual, there are several suggestions under each healing category: **FOOD THERAPY, VITAMINS/MINERALS, HERBAL THERAPY, BODYWORK.** All have been used extensively in our experience, and found to be effective. Obviously no one will use everything in any one category, or even use each category - but there is a great deal to choose from, so that each person can put together the best program for themselves.

The **bold print** suggestions within each category are those we have found to be the most helpful for the most people. These emphasized recommendations can often be considered complete programs in themselves, and can be successfully used together.

✦ Where a method has also proven effective for children, a small child's face ☺ will appear at the end of the recommendation.

✦ Where a remedy has proven particularly successful for women, a female symbol ♀ will appear at the end of the recommendation.

✦ Where a remedy has proven particularly for men, a male symbol ♂ will appear at the end of the recommendation.

All recommended doses are daily amounts unless otherwise specified.

HOW HERBAL FORMULAS WORK

Each individual body has its own unique and wondeful mechanism, and each has the ability to bring itself to its own balanced and healthy state.

Herbs simply pave the way for the body to do its own work, by breaking up toxins, cleansing, lubricating, toning and nourishing. They often work through the glands at the deepest levels of the body processes - and as very concentrated plant foods, give the body nutrients it does not always receive, either from a poor diet or environmental deficiencies in the soil and air. Herbs are naturally grown and dried nutrients that nourish and work <u>with</u> the body functions instead of outside them. Herbal combinations are not addictive or habit-forming, even in extract form, and very small doses can be used over a period of time to help build a healthy base for restoring body balance. But they are powerful agents that are cumulative in the body and should be used with care. **When correctly used, herbs promote the elimination of waste matter and toxins from the system by simple natural means. They support nature in the fight against disease.**

With these things in mind, we have found that it is best to take herbal capsule combinations in descending strength: 6 the first day, 5 the second day, 4 the third, 3, 2 and 2 for the first week. Rest on the 7th day. When this healing base is built in the system, decrease to the daily maintenance dose recommended for each particular formula. Most combinations should be taken no more than 6 days in a row to allow the body to regularly restore its own balance.

Other tips on taking herbal combinations:

1) A 24 hour juice fast before starting an herbal formula will often produce greater effectiveness.

2) Take capsules with a warm drink for faster results. (Do not take with citrus juice if the formula contains a Ginseng)

3) Abstain from alcohol, red meat, caffeine and tobacco if possible during use to give the herbs a cleaner environment in which to work.

4) Herbs work best with a natural foods diet. Everyone can benefit from herbal mixtures, but the more you are eating naturally, the more you can expect to receive their advantages.

5) Herbs are concentrated foods, and are identified by the body as such. They are quickly assimilated by digestive enzyme action. With a few exceptions, they should be taken before or with meals.

The body knows how to use herbs. Give them time. They are working.

TEAS ✧ CAPSULES ✧ EXTRACTS ✧ BATHS

HOW TO USE THEM
WHICH FORM IS RIGHT FOR YOU

HERBAL TEAS are the most basic of all natural healing mediums, easily absorbed by the body as hot liquid. They are the least concentrated of all herbal forms, but many herbs are optimally effective when steeped in boiling water. The hot brewing water releases herbal potency and volatile oils, providing a flushing action that is excellent for cleansing toxic wastes that have been loosened and dissolved by the herbs. Teas have milder and more subtle effects than capsules or extracts, but they often work synergistically with both of these stronger forms to boost efficiency and value.

Tips on taking herbal teas:

1) Use 1 <u>packed</u> small teaball to 3 cups of water for medicinal-strength tea.

2) Bring water to a boil, remove from heat, add herbs and steep, covered, off heat: 10-15 minutes for a leaf and flower tea, or 15-25 minutes for a root and bark tea. Keep the lid tightly closed during steeping so the volatile oils will not escape.

3) Use a teapot of glass, ceramic or earthenware, not aluminum. Aluminum can negate the effect of the herbs as the metal dissolves into the hot liquid and gets into the body.

4) Drink teas in small sips throughout the day rather than all at once to allow more absorption of the liquid without passing before it has a chance to work.

5) Use distilled water or pure spring water for increased herbal strength and effectiveness.

HERBAL CAPSULES are four times stronger than teas, more concentrated in form, and convenient. (See HOW HERBAL FORMULAS WORK)

HERBAL EXTRACTS are four to eight times stronger than capsules, and are especially effective when taken as drops and held under the tongue, bypassing the digestive system and its acid/alkaline breakdown of substances. Their strength and ready availability make extracts efficient emergency measures. 10-15 drops under the tongue, held as long as possible, 3-4 times daily are effective for the first week of an acute condition. After this first week, the vital force of the body will often have been sufficiently stimulated in its own healing ability, and the dose may be reduced to allow the system to take its own individual route to balance. **As with other forms of herbal mixtures, most extracts should be taken no more than 6 days in a row with a rest on the seventh day, before resuming, to allow the body to do its own work.** As the body increases its ability to right itself, the amount, frequency and strength of the dosage should be decreased.

Note: Homeopathic formulas in liquid form are <u>not</u> the same as herbal tinctures or extracts, and their use is different (See HOMEOPATHIC REMEDIES in this book)

HERBAL BATHS, SALVES AND COMPRESSES provide a soothing gentle way of absorbing herbal benefits. The skin is, of course, the body's largest organ of ingestion, and these topical herbal mediums can be used frequently for all over relief and support.

Whichever herbal form you choose, it is usually most beneficial to take greater amounts at the beginning of your program, to build a good healing base in the system, and start the body's own vital balancing force more quickly. As the therapeutic agents establish and build in the body, and you begin to notice good response and balance returning, less and less of the large initial doses should be taken, finally reducing the dosage to longer range maintenance and preventive amounts.

However, and this is very important, we have found over and over again that with **Immune Deficient, Opportunistic, and Degenerative Diseases,** that it takes a great deal of time to rebuild a healthy system. Even when a good healing program is working, and obvious improvement is being made, **adding more of the healing agents in an effort to speed progression can often aggravate the symptoms,** and bring about worse results!

The Immune System is a very fragile entity, and can become overwhelmed instead of stimulated. An afflicting virus can even seem to mutate and be nourished by supplementation, instead of arrested by it. **In this type of case, including Candida Albicans, Multiple Sclerosis, Epstein Barr Virus, Lupus. and particularly AIDS and ARC, moderate amounts are excellent, mega-doses are not.** Much better results can be obtained by giving yourself more time and gentler treatment.

When working with herbs and alternative healing methods, choose the elements that will address your worst problem first. One of the bonuses of a natural healing program is the frequent discovery that other conditions were really complications of the first problem, and are often taking care of themselves as the body comes into balance.

All recommendations in this book are for adults.

Child dosage is as follows: 1/2 dose for children 10-14 years
1/3 dose for children 6-10 years
1/4 dose for children 2-6 years
1/8 dose for infants and babies

An electuary, such as honey, juice, peanut butter or a cooky can be used for children if there is taste resistance, or the child has trouble taking pills, etc. Simply open up the capsules or mix the tea or extract into the electuary.

Herbal effectiveness usually goes by body weight. Dose decisions should be based on that reasoning for adults as well as children.

MINERALS & TRACE MINERALS

WHAT THEY ARE ✦ HOW THEY WORK ✦ WHY YOU NEED THEM

Minerals and trace minerals are the building blocks of all life. They are the most basic of nutrients, the bonding agents in and between you and your food. They allow the body to absorb its nutrients. **Minerals** are needed by everybody for good health and an active life. They are especially necessary for athletes and people in active sports, because you must have minerals to run. All the minerals together comprise only about 4% of the body weight, but they are responsible for major areas of human health. **Minerals** keep body pH balanced - alkaline instead of acid. They are essential to bone formation, and to the digestion of food. They regulate the osmosis of cellular fluids, electrical activity in the nervous system, and most metabolic functions. They transport oxygen through the system, govern heart rhythm, help you sleep, and are keys to mental and spiritual balance. **Trace minerals** are only .01% of body weight, but deficiencies in even these micro-nutrients can cause severe depression, paranoia, P.M.S. and other menstrual disorders, hyperactivity in children, sugar imbalances such as hypoglycemia and diabetes, nerve and emotional problems, heart disease, high blood pressure, osteoporosis, premature aging of the skin and hair, memory loss and the inability to heal quickly.

Minerals are important. Hardly any of us get enough.

Minerals cannot be synthesized by the body, and must be regularly obtained through our food, drink, or mineral baths. **Minerals from plants and herbs** are higher quality and more absorbable than from other sources. They work optimally with the body's enzyme production for assimilation and strength. Red meats, refined foods (especially white flour and sugar), caffeine, and excess acid foods inhibit mineral absorption. Modern life styles with high stress, tobacco, alcohol, steroid and anti-biotic abuse also contribute to mineral depletion. Unfortunately, many minerals and trace minerals are no longer sufficiently present in our fruits and vegetables. They have been leached from the soil by the chemicals and fertilizers used in commercial farming today, and the sprays and pesticides used on the produce itself. Even foods that still show measureable amounts of mineral composition have less quantitiy and quality than we are led to believe, because most testing was done decades ago when sprays, pesticides and chemical use was not as prolific as it is now. Organically grown, unsprayed produce is difficult to obtain on a regular, high quality basis today.

Plant minerals from herbal sources have become the easiest, most reliable way to assure yourself of their valuable benefits. Herbal minerals are balanced whole foods that the body easily recognizes and uses. Because of their concentrated nature herbs can be used as healing agents, as well as maintaining nutrients in the body. Unlike partitioned or chemically formed supplements, the minerals and other beneficial substances in herbs are cumulative in the body forming a strong, solid base.

Minerals can really give your body a boost.
For mineral strength, eat organically grown produce whenever possible, and take a high quality herbal source mineral supplement

THE MOST ESSENTIAL MINERALS & TRACE MINERALS

☐ **BORON** - an important trace mineral catalyst that enhances Calcium use and uptake by the bones. A significant nutritional deterrent to the onset of osteoporosis.

☐ **CALCIUM** - the most abundant mineral in the body, needs Vitamin D for good absorption. Calcium works with phosphorus to build sound teeth and bones, and with magnesium for cardiovascular health. It helps the blood to clot, lowers blood pressure, prevents abnormal muscle cramping, maintains nervous system health, controls anxiety and depression, and insures high quality rest and sleep. Adequate supply helps prevent colon cancer and osteoporosis. **Effective food sources: green vegetables, milk and milk products, molasses, shellfish.**

☐ **CHLORINE** - <u>naturally occuring</u>, stimulates Liver activity, and smooth joint and tendon operation.

☐ **COPPER** - helps in control of arthritis/bursitis symptoms, aids in iron absorption , protein metabolism, and red blood cell production. Helps prevent hair from losing its color. Deficiencies result in high cholesterol and heart arrhythmias; excess copper sometimes results in mental depression. **Effective food sources: molasses, raisins, seafoods.**

☐ **CHROMIUM** - an essential mineral for glucose tolerance and sugar regulation. A deficiency means high cholesterol, heart trouble diabetes or hypoglycemia, and premature aging. **Effective food sources: brewer's yeast, clams, honey, whole grains, corn oil, grapes, raisins.**

☐ **FLUORINE** - as <u>calcium fluoride</u>, (not sodium fluoride as is added to drinking water), increases bone strength, reduces carbohydrate-caused acidity in the mouth, and the incidence of tooth decay.

☐ **GERMANIUM** - a potent oxygen stimulus to interferon in the body for immune strength and healing, germanium facilitates oxygen uptake and blocks free radicals. **Effective food sources: Chlorella , onions, garlic, greens.**

☐ **IODINE** - a major component of good thyroid function and proper metabolism. Deficiency results in goiter, confused thinking, and menstrual difficulties. Necessary for skin, hair, and nail health, and correct wound healing, iodine also prevents toxicity from radiation. **Effective: seafoods and sea vegetables.**

☐ **IRON** - combines with proteins and copper to produce hemoglobin which carries oxygen throughout the body. Sufficient iron prevents fatigue, muscle weakness and anemic conditions, and strengthens immunity. It keeps hair color young, eyes bright, the body strong and lively. **Effective food sources: Molasses, cherries, dried fruits, eggs, fish.**

☐ **MAGNESIUM** - is necessary for good nerve and muscle function, endurance and exercise capacity. It plays an important part in heart and kidney health, restful sleep and proper metabolic activity. Magnesium counteracts stress, nerves, emotional instability and depression. It calms and helps relieve twitching in hyperactive children. It enhances the absorption and body use of other minerals. **Effective food sources: dark green vegetables, seafood, whole grains.**

☐ **MANGANESE** - nourishes brain, and nerve centers, aids in digestion, sugar and fat metabolism, and is necessary for reproduction. Manganese helps eliminate fatigue, nerve irritability and lower back pain. It reduces seizures in epileptics. **Effective foods sources: eggs, green vegetables, legumes, nuts, pineapple, whole grains.**

☐ **MOLYBDENUM** - is essentially a metabolic mineral, found in all tissue, and necessary for mobilization of certain enzymes. Its presence is completely dependent on good soil content.

☐ **PHOSPHORUS** - the second most abundant mineral in the body, occurs in a ratio balance with calcium. It is necessary for skeletal structure, cell division and reproduction, oxygen to the brain, and assimilation of most vitamin nutrients. Deficiencies occur when using large amounts of antacids. **Effective food sources: eggs, fish, legumes., poultry.**

☐ **POTASSIUM** - balances the acid/alkaline system, and works with sodium to regulate the body's water balance. It is necessary for heart health, normal muscle function, energy, nerve stability, enzyme and hormone production. Potassium helps oxygenate the brain and control allergic reactions. Stress, hypoglycemia, diarrhea and acute mental anxiety all cause potassium deficiency. Potassium is an electrolyte, transmitting electrical signals between cells. **Effective food sources: dried fruits, lean poultry and fish, sunflower seeds, vegetables, whole grains.**

☐ **SELENIUM** - is an powerful anti-oxidant, anti-cancer and immune stimulant factor. It works with Vitamin E to prevent serum fat and cholesterol accumulations in the bloodstream, and protects against heart weakness and degenerative diseases. Selenium enhances elasticity of skin and body tissue. **Effective food sources: bran, brewer's yeast, sesame seeds, tuna, wheat germ, herring and whole grains.**

☐ **SILICON** - is responsible for connective tissue growth and health. It is necessary for collagen production, and all healing and rebuilding processes, especially those of the body's infrastructure.

☐ **SODIUM** - is an electrolyte that helps regulate kidney, and body fluid function. It is necessary for the osmosis of fluid nutrients throughout the cells. It is involved with high blood pressure <u>only</u> when calcium and phosphous are deficient in the body. **Beneficial food sources: celery,seafoods, sea vegetables.**

☐ **SULPHUR** - the beauty mineral for smooth skin, glossy hair, hard nails and collagen synthesis. It is critical to protein absorption, and part of many amino acids. **Effective food sources: eggs, fish, onions, garlic, hot peppers.**

☐ **ZINC** - is essential for protein synthesis, the formation of insulin, strong immunity, glandular health and sexual function. It helps prevent birth defects, and enhances sensory perceptions. It is a brain food, helps control mental disorders such as schizophrenia, and promotes mental alertness. **Effective food sources: brewer's yeast, eggs, mushrooms, soy products, wheat germ, sunflower seeds, pumpkin seeds.**

VITAMINS

Vitamins are organic micro-nutrients that act like spark plugs in the body, keeping it "tuned up", and functioning at high performance. As catalysts, they work on the cellular level, often as co-enzymes, regulating body metabolic processes through enzyme activity, to convert proteins and carbohydrates to tissue and energy. Notwithstanding their minute size and amount in the body, **vitamins** are absolutely necessary for growth, vitality resistance to disease, and healthy aging. Even small deficiencies can endanger the whole body. Unfortunately, it takes weeks or months for signs of some deficiencies to appear as the body uses up its supply, and even then a problem is often hard to pinpoint, because the cells usually continue to function at less and less efficiency until they receive proper nourishment or die.

Vitamin therapy and supplementation do not produce results overnight. **Vitamins** are at the deepest levels of the body processes, and regenerative changes in body chemistry usually require as much time to rebuild as they did to decline.

Even though it is impossible to sustain life without them, **most vitamins cannot be synthesized by the body,** and must be supplied from foods or supplementation. Excess amounts are excreted through the urine, or stored by the body until needed. Consequently, we have found that after a short period of higher dosage in which to build a solid foundation, a program of moderate amounts over a longer period of time brings about better body balance and more permanent results.

Vitamin RDAs were established by the National Academy years ago as a guideline for the amounts of vitamins and minerals needed **to prevent only the most severe deficiency diseases.** Today, because of poor eating habits, over-processed foods, and agri-business practices, most health professionals recognize that increased amounts are needed to achieve optimal nutrition and health.

Remember: vitamins are micro-nutrients, not pep pills or substitutes for food. They are not the components of body structure and have no inherent caloric value.

THE MOST ESSENTIAL VITAMINS

☐ **VITAMIN A** - is fat soluble, requiring fats as well as minerals and enzymes for absorption. It counteracts night blindness, weak eyesight, and strengthens the optical system. It is an anti-infective, builds resistance, is a prime component of strong immunity, and a major factor in the health of skin, hair, teeth and gums. **Effective food sources: vegetables, greens, yams, sweet potatoes, watermelon, fruits, eggs.**

☐ **BETA CAROTENE** - is a pro-vitamin A, converting to A as the body needs it. Beta carotene is highly valuable as an anti-infective, for immune health, allergy control, and as a key in preventing some kinds of Cancer.

☐ **VITAMIN B$_1$ - Thiamine** - is known as the "morale vitamin" because of its beneficial effects on the nervous system and mental attitude. Thiamine promotes proper growth in children, aids digestion, and supports all stress conditions. It helps control motion sickness and wards off mosquitos and stinging insects. Pregnancy and lactation, smoking, sugar consumption and alcohol all deplete Thiamine. **Effective food sources: asparagus, brewer's yeast, brown rice and whole grains, beans, nuts and seeds, wheat germ.**

☐ **VITAMIN B$_2$ - Riboflavin** - is commonly deficient in the American diet. It helps prevent cataracts, and benefits vision generally. It promotes healthy skin, hair and nails. Pregancy and lactation, red meat and dairy consumption, prolonged stress, hypothyroidism, diabetes, ulcers, all deplete Riboflavin. **Effective food sources: almonds, brewer's yeast, broccoli, brie cheese, wild rice, ricotta cheese, swiss cheese, yogurt.**

☐ **VITAMIN B$_3$ - Niacin** - A deficiency brings about negative personality behavior and sometimes high blood pressure, but because it opens up and stimulates circulation, (a niacin flush is evidence of this), niacin can act quickly to reverse deficiencies and disorders. It relieves acne, diarrhea and other gastrointestinal disorders, migraine headaches and vertigo attacks. It helps reduce serum blood fats and cholesterol. **Effective food sources: almonds, avocados, brewer's yeast, poultry, beans, peanut butter, soy products, sunflower seeds, whole grains.**

❑ **VITAMIN B5 - Pantothenic Acid** - is vital for proper adrenal function as a precursor to cortisone production, and is important in control and prevention of arthritis. It fights infection by building antibodies, and defends against stress and fatigue and nerve disorders. After surgery, Pantothenic acid can be a key to overcoming postoperative shock, and drug side effects. It also inhibits hair color loss. **Effective food sources: brewer's yeast, brown rice, poultry, yams, whole grains, mushrooms, broccoli, legumes.**

❑ **VITAMIN B6 - Pyridoxine** - protects all aspects of nerve health including epilepsy and convulsions, and carpal tunnel syndrome. It works as an effective natural diuretic, especially during pre-menstrual days, controls acne, promotes beautiful skin, alleviates morning sickness, and is a key to anti-aging factors in the body. **Effective food sources: bananas, brewer's yeast, buckwheat, salmon, tuna, sunflower seeds, chicken and turkey, nuts and beans.**

❑ **VITAMIN B12 - Cobalamin** - works with calcium for proper absorption. Supplied largely from dairy and meat sources, this essential nutrient is often deficient for vegetarians, and may take five or more years to appear after body stores have been depleted, leaving the body open to anemia, lack of new cell growth and osteoarthritis. B12 acts to energize, relieve fatigue, hangover, the inability to concentrate and depression. **Effective food sources: cheddar cheese, poultry, swiss cheese, tuna, yogurt, eggs, cottage cheese, haddock and halibut.**

❑ **VITAMIN B15 - Pangamic Acid** - is an effective anti-oxidant and energy stimulant. It has been used successfully to improve Down's Syndrome and mental retardation cases, and to curb craving in alcohol addiction. Notable results have also been obtained with atherosclerosis, rheumatic fever, rheumatism, emphysema and liver cirrhosis .

❑ **BIOTIN** - a member of the B Complex family, biotin has shown good results with dermatitis, dandruff and seborrheic scalp problems, eczema, and controlling hair loss. **Effective food sources: poultry, raspberries, grapefruit, tomatoes, tuna, turkey, whole wheat, salmon, eggs, cheddar cheese.**

❑ **CHOLINE** - a B Complex member and lipotropic, it works with inositol to emulsify fats. Choline is a brain nutrient, a neurotransmitter that aids memory, controls dizziness, and is effective against Alzheimers disease. It helps lower cholesterol, and supports liver cleansing and function. **Effective food sources: organ meats, eggs, fish, soy products.**

❑ **FOLIC ACID - Folacin** - a B Complex member, Folic acid is essential for division and growth of new cells, so is an excellent supplement to take during pregnancy to guard against spinal bifida and other neural tube defects. Prevents anemia, helps control Leukemia and pernicious anemia, and is effective against alcoholism. **Effective food sources: beets, peas, brewer's yeast, broccoli, cantaloupe, orange juice.**

❑ **INOSITOL** - a B Complex member and lipotropic, it works with biotin and choline to control male pattern baldness, hypertension and arteriosclerosis, and metabolize serum blood fats. An "inositol cocktail" may be taken as a spring tonic to revive a sluggish system. Inositol helps reduce breast and ovarian cancer risk, and controls estrogen-related pre-menstrual symptoms. It is effective against insomnia. **Effective food sources: almonds, beans, onions, oranges, peanut butter, oats, peas, tomatoes, zucchini.**

❑ **PABA** - a B Complex member, PABA has sun-screening properties, is effective against sun and other burns, and is used in treating vertiligo, (depigmentation of the skin). It is successful with Molasses, Pantothenic acid and Folic acid in restoring lost hair color. **Effective food sources: brewer's yeast, eggs, molasses, wheat germ.**

❑ **VITAMIN C - Ascorbic Acid** - a major component and key to immune strength and maintenance, vitamin C offers protection against Cancer, viral and bacterial infections, and allergies. It is effective in accelerating healing after surgery, is essential to formation of collagen tissue, in controlling alcohol craving, preventing constipation, and lowering cholesterol. It helps control arthritic and rheumatic symptoms, and blood clots in the veins. **Effective food sources: citrus fruits and berries, green peppers, papaya, tomatoes, kiwi, potatoes, greens, cauliflower, broccoli..**

❑ **BIOFLAVONOIDS** - are part of and necessary to the proper function of Vitamin C. Bioflavs increase capillary and vein strength, and connective tissue health. They help control bruising and internal bleeding.

❑ **VITAMIN D** - a fat soluble "sunlight vitamin", it works with vitamin A to utilize calcium and phosphorus in building bone structure and healthy teeth. Helps in all eye problems including spots, conjunctivitis and glaucoma. Air pollution and lack of sunlight deplete Vitamin D. **Effective food sources: cod liver oil, herring halibut, salmon, tuna.**

❑ **VITAMIN E** - an active anti-oxidant and important immune stimulant, vitamin E is an effective anticoagulant and vasodilator against blood clots and heart disease. It retards cellular and mental aging, alleviates fatigue and provides tissue oxygen to accelerate healing of wounds and burns. E neutralizes "free radical" that promote aging and cancer. It improves skin problems and texture, and helps control baldness and dandruff. **Effective food sources: almonds, corn, safflower and peanut oil, salmon, soy products, wheat germ and wheat germ oil, pecans, peanut butter, lobster.**

❑ **UFA - Unsaturated Fatty Acids** - are beneficial in treating many skin disorders, such as eczema, psoriasis, tooth and gum disease and leg ulcers.

❑ **VITAMIN K** - a fat soluble vitamin necessary for blood clotting, it reduces excessive menstruation and hemorrhage in the eye. It improves cirrhosis and jaundice in the liver, and acts as an anti-parasitic for intestinal worms. **Effective food sources: seafoods, sea vegetables, sprouts.**

AMINO ACIDS

WHAT THEY ARE ✦ HOW THEY WORK ✦ WHY YOU NEED THEM

Amino acids are the protein building blocks in the body, valuable sources of energy, and vital buffering agents for proper acid/alkaline balance.

There are 22 of them comprising <u>over 75%</u> of the body's solid weight. Recent research is showing that the **"essential amino acids"**, (those which the body cannot produce on its own) are often not sufficient in the body to produce the "non-essentials", (those formed by metabolic activity). This can be successfully corrected by protein foods and supplementation. For best absorption, take in food source or pre-digested form. Amino acid therapies are also making great impact in alternative medicine as a way of strengthening the body against disease.

THE MOST ESSENTIAL AMINO ACIDS

❏ ARGININE - a valuable stimulant for growth hormone in the Liver; wonderful for body builders, increasing muscle tone while decreasing fat, but so powerful that the advance of some diseases, such as Herpes virus, and Schizophrenia can be retarded by "starving" them of Arginine foods. Arginine also promotes healing of wounds, increases sperm motility, helps lower cholesterol fats, curbs the appetite, and aids in metabolizing fats for weight loss. **Effective Food Sources** include wheat germ, pork, cheeses, poultry, nuts, and whole grain granolas. Take with cranberry or apple juice for best results.

❏ ASPARTIC ACID - a conditionally essential amino acid used mainly as a sweetener, it is a neuro-transmitter made with ATP, and has been clinically used to counteract depression. **Effective Food Sources** include wheat germ, Cheeses, poultry , pork and game.

❏ BRANCH CHAIN AMINOS - Leucine, Isoleucine, Valine - BCAAs - called the stress amino acids, they are easily converted into ATP and critical to energy and muscle metabolism. They have shown excellent results in rebuilding the body from athletic stress, from anorexia deficiency, and liver restoration after surgical trauma. **Effective Food Sources** include wheat germ, cheese, yogurt, pork, poultry, and whole grain granola.

❏ CARNITINE - helps regulate fat metabolism and provide muscle energy to the heart. It speeds fat oxidation for weight loss, helps reduce excess triglycerides in the blood, and aids prostaglandin metabolism. Because it decreases ketone levels, it is valuable to diabetics. **Effective Food Sources** include beef, fish, whole wheat, poultry and cheese.

❏ CYSTEINE - works with Vitamins C, E and Selenium as an anti-oxidant to protect against radiation and free radical damage. It stimulates the immune system, helps prevent cancer, can play an active role in its treatment, and renders toxic chemicals in the body harmless. Taken with Evening Primrose oil, Cysteine prevents damage from alcohol and tobacco. It has been used successfully in cases of hair loss, psoriasis, and skin tissue disease, bronchial asthma relief through release of mucous plugs, and prevention of dental plaque formation. **Effective Food Sources** include poultry, yogurt, wheat germ and cottage cheese.

❏ CYSTINE - the oxidized form of Cysteine, it builds up in the system, can sometimes be harmful in kidney disfunction, and should generally not be used clinically.

❏ GABA - has shown excellent results in several therapeutic areas involving brain and nerve dysfunctions, such as anxiety, depression, extreme nervous tension, high blood pressure and insomnia, schizophrenia, stroke, Parkinson's disease, Alzheimer's disease and control of Hyperkinesis in children. It works with Glutamine and Tyrosine to overcome alcohol and drug abuse. **Effective Food Sources** include wheat germ, whole grain granola, cheeses, poultry pork and yogurt.

❏ GLUTAMINE - helps improve memory and alertness, and is a nutrient for the brain. Increases mental performance in cases of retardation, senility, epileptic seizures and schizophrenia. Helps curb alcohol and sugar cravings in control of hypoglycemia, and aids in better absorption of minerals. **Effective Food Sources** include wheat germ, oats, cheeses, yogurt, poultry, sausage and wild game.

❒ GLUTATHIONE - works with Cysteine and Glutamine as a glucose tolerance factor and anti-oxidant that can deactivate radiation toxicity and free radicals in the body. It helps detoxify from heavy metal, alcohol and drug (especially PCP) overload, and cleans the blood from the effects of Chemotherapy and liver malfunction. It works with vitamin E to protect against stroke, chronic kidney failure and cataract formation. **Effective Food Sources** include liver and organ meats.

❒ GLYCINE AND DI-METHYL-GLYCINE (B 15) - Glycine releases growth hormone when taken in large doses. Therapeutically it has been effective for myasthenia gravis, gout, and muscular dystrophy. It helps detoxify the Liver, and is a key factor in regulating hypoglycemic sugar drop. DMG is a highly reputed energizer and stimulant whose effects can be attributed to its conversion to Glycine. It has been successfully used as a control for epileptic seizure and immune stimulation. **Effective Food Sources** include pork, poultry, and wheat germ.

❒ HISTIDINE - is called an arthritis fighter, as it synthesizes, glutamic acid and helps copper transport through the joints. It helps prevent cataracts, acts as a vasodilator, and raises histamine levels and therefore libido in both sexes. **Effective Food Sources** include cottage cheese, and poultry.

❒ INOSINE - stimulates ATP energy release. Helps provide endurance and strength when the body's own glycogen reserves run out.

❒ LYSINE - inhibits the growth and harmful effects of several viruses, including the herpes virus, and can be used topically or internally for relief. It is useful in cases of osteoporosis by reducing Calcium loss in the urine. Supplementation is helpful in Parkinson's disease and hypothyroidism. **Effective Food Sources** include wild game, avocados, chicken, and cottage cheese.

❒ METHIONINE - is a major source of organic sulphur that affects liver activity , lymph gland and immune health. It is an effective "lipotropic" that aids in metabolizing fats, and keeping high blood pressure and cholesterol deposits low. Effective against toxemia during pregnancy. **Effective Food Sources** include yogurt, pork and wild game.

❒ ORNITHINE - works in balance with Arginine and the pituitary gland to promote growth hormone, muscle development, tissue repair, and endurance. An excellent aid to fat metabolism through the liver.

❒ PHENALALANINE - works as an anti depressant and thyroid stimulant. It helps curb the appetite by increasing the body's production of CCK. Slowing the growth of cancerous melanomas has been achieved through the dietary reduction of Phenalalanine and Tyrosine. **Effective Food Sources** include poultry, cottage cheese, wheat germ, nuts and milk. Phenylketonurics (with elevated natural phenalalanine levels) should avoid aspartame sweeteners. Those with blood pressure imbalance, skin carcinomas, diabetes or blurred vision should avoid phenalalanine.

❒ DLPA - DL-Phenalalanine - a safe, effective pain reliever and anti-depressant with an endorphin effect for arthritis, back and cerebro-spinal pain. (See Phenalalanine for food sources)

❒ TAURINE - serves as a neurotransmitter in the brain, to control hyperactivity, nervous system imbalance after drug or alcohol abuse, and epilepsy. Supplementation is effective as a brain and nerve nutrient that can help prevent loss of sight, stroke, hypothyroidism, obesity and hypertension. **Effective Food Sources** include fish protein, and organ meats, Supplementation is necessary for therapy.

❒ THREONINE - works with Glycine to aid depression and neurologic dysfunction such as genetic spastic disorders and M.S. It is an immune stimulant and Thymus enhancer. **Effective Food Sources** include meats, poultry, cottage and wheat germ.

❒ TRYPTOPHANE - acts through the production of serotonin as a natural non-addictive tranquilizer for restful sleep. It is used successfully to decrease hyperkinetic,aggressive behavior and schizophrenia, and to counteract compulsive overeating, smoking and alcoholism. It is an effective anti-depressant, raises abnormally low blood sugar, and reduces seizures in petit mal epilepsy. **Effective Food Sources** include milk, wheat germ, dairy foods, yogurt, eggs, fish and turkey.

❒ TYROSINE - is rapidly metabolized throughout the body, and is effective as a source of quick energy for the brain. It helps to reduce appetite in weight loss. It is a safe therapy for depression, hypertension, parkinson's disease, low sex drive, and in control of drug abuse. Tumor and cancerous melanoma growth has been slowedthrough dietary reduction of Tyrosine and Phenalalanine. **Effective Food Sources** include milk,, soy products, pork, game and cottage cheese.

RAW GLANDULAR EXTRACTS

WHAT THEY ARE   ✦   HOW THEY WORK

The organs and glands communicate chemically to the physiological needs of the body with micro-nutrients and polypeptides. Only minute amounts are required to have positive effects. Raw glandular tissues contain intrinsic factors distinct from vitamins, minerals, or enzyme micro-nutrients. Glandular or organo-therapy is based on the premise that **"like cells help like cells"**. A very small amount of glandular tissue from an animal gland can be picked up in the bloodstream to support, augment and balance the corresponding gland or organ in a human being. Current research is showing that **glandular therapy** is valid, and is effective and safe. **Predigested** soluble gland tissue can provide all the benefits of whole fresh glands. Raw liquid glandulars should be taken under the tongue for ready absorption. Freeze-dried, dehydrated concentrates are also available and effective. The highest quality of preservation is obviously essential, since heat processing or salt precipitation render the glands useless.

THE MOST ESSENTIAL GLANDULARS

❑ **RAW ADRENAL** - helps stimulate and nourish exhausted adrenals. Aids in adrenal cortex production to reduce inflammation in arthritis and ulcers, and improves body tone without synthetic hormones. Helps protect against Chronic Fatigue Syndrome and stress syndromes such as Candida Albicans through a normal increase of metabolic rate, and overcomes allergy reactions associated with poor adrenal function. Works with Vitamin C and B Complex to control hypoglycemic reactions and the effects of menopause imbalance.

❑ **RAW BRAIN** - helps prevent memory loss, chronic mental fatigue, and senility onset. Encourages better nerve stability and restful sleep. A valid support during alcoholism recovery.

❑ **RAW FEMALE** - helps regulate the menstrual cycle, and control P.M.S. symptoms. Works with vitamins A and E to increase fertility.

❑ **RAW HEART** - improves heart muscle activity and reduces low density lipoproteins in the blood. Works synergistically with vitamin E.

❑ **RAW KIDNEY** - aids in normalization of kidney/urinary disorders, blood pressure imbalance and hypertension. Works synergistically with vitamin C.

❑ **RAW LIVER** - helps restore the liver from abuse, disease and exhaustion. Aids fat metabolism.. Works synergistically with B Complex to purify the blood, and restore acid/alkaline balance.

❑ **RAW LUNG** - supports the lungs against respiratory dysfunctions such as asthma, emphysema, congestion, bronchitis and pneumonia.

❑ **RAW MALE** - helps normalize the functions of diseased or damaged male organs. Works synergistically with zinc and vitamin E toward this end.

❑ **RAW MAMMARY** - helps in healing mastitis and nipple inflammation, in controlling profuse menstruation, and normalizing too-frequent cycles.

❑ **RAW ORCHIC** helps increase male sexual strength and potency by stimulating testosterone production and building sperm count. Also beneficial against male depression and low blood sugar. Supplementation can bring noticeable improvement in athletic performance.

❐ RAW OVARY - helps correct endometrial misplacement and overgrowth, P.M.S. symptoms and menstrual cramping. Improves hormone balance against hot flashes and menopause pain.

❐ RAW PANCREAS - helps maintain balanced blood glucose levels. Improves fat metabolism, hormone balance and secretions, and circulation. Works synergistically with B Complex and chromium to secrete hormones that keep the intestines free from harmful bacteria such as Candida yeasts.

❐ RAW PITUITARY - helps stimulate overall body growth through electrolyte metabolism in the ovaries, testes and adrenals. Supplementation can help in cases of hypoglycemia, stress and infertility. Pituitary glandular is especially effective for athletes and body builders in controlliing excess body stress, sugar balance and fatigue. Works synergistically with B Complex vitamins and Beta-carotene.

❐ RAW SPLEEN - aids in the building and storage of red blood cells to promote strength and good tissue oxygenation. Increases absorption of calcium and iron. Protects against immune and arterial deficiency. Supplementation has been shown to enhance immune function by increasing white blood cell activity.

❐ RAW THYMUS - stimulates and strengthens the immune system against foreign organisms and toxins. Helps activate the T-Cells in the spleen, lymph nodes and bone marrow. Supplementation is effective in minimizing disease problems with aging, since the Thymus gland normally shrinks with age.

❐ RAW THYROID - aids in regulating metabolism, increasing circulation, and controlling obesity and sluggishness caused by thyroid deficiency. Supplementation can also help where there are reproductive or sexual problems.

❐ RAW UTERUS - helps support the body against menses dysfunctions such as amenorrhea, habitual abortion, infertility and irregular periods. Supplementation can help overcome birth control side effects. Works synergistically with raw ovary for best balance.

HOMEOPATHIC MEDICINES

WHAT THEY ARE ✦ HOW TO USE THEM

Homeopathy is a medical philosophy that recognizes disease as an energy imbalance, a disturbance of the body's "vital force" expressed through disease symptoms. Symptoms are the expression of the body attempting to restore its balance. **Homeopathic remedies** are based on the principle of stimulating and increasing this inherent curative harmony.
Negative side effects and hazards of habituation from drugs are causing many people to turn to the risk-free therapy of **Homeopathy**; a wave of the future in America, that has been practiced in Europe for many years. The remedies are mild and non-toxic. Even the highest potencies do not create the side effects of allopathic drugs. They neither cover up nor destroy disease but stimulate the body's own action to rid itself of the problem. The healing can be quite long lasting in its effect.

Homeopathic medicine is based on three prescription principles:

1) THE LAW OF SIMILARS: "like curing like".

2) THE MINIMUM DOSE PRINCIPLE: the dilution of the "like" substance to a correct strength for the individual; strong enough to stimulate the "vital force" without overpowering it. Dilutions, usually in alcohol, are shaken or succussed, a certain number of times (3, 6, or 12 times in commercial use) to increase therapeutic power through the vibratory effect. Each successive dilution <u>decreases</u> the actual amount of the substance in the remedy. In the strongest dilutions, there is virtually none of the substance remaining, yet potentization is the highest for healing effect.

3) THE SINGLE REMEDY PRINCIPLE, where only one remedy is administered at a time.

Although homeopathic treatments are specific to the individual in private practice, we have found two things to be true about the remedies found in most stores today:

1) They seem to work on the **"antidote"** principle. More is <u>not better</u> in this case. Small amounts over a period of time are far more effective. Frequency of dosage is determined by individual reaction time, increasing as the first improvements are noted. When substantial improvement begins, indicating that the body's healing force has been stimulated, the remedy should be discontinued.
2) They also work on the **"trigger"** principle. A good way to start a healing program is with a Homeopathic medicine. The body's electrical activity stimulated by these remedies can allow for much more rapid response to succeeding therapies. The basic rule for dosage is to repeat the medicines as needed.

Occasionally, aggravation of symptoms may be noted at first as the body restructures and begins to rebuild its defenses, much the same as healing crises occur with other natural cleansing therapies. This effect usually passes in a short period of time.

For maximum effectiveness, take 1/2 dropperful under the tongue at a time, and hold for 30 seconds before swallowing; or dissolve the tiny homeopathic lactose tablets under the tongue. For best absorption, do not eat, drink or smoke for 10 minutes before or after taking. Do not use with chemical medicines, caffeine or alcohol. They overpower homeopathy's subtle stimulus.

The right Homeopathic remedy can restore health on all levels.

HOMEOPATHIC CELL SALTS

What They Are ✦ How To Use Them

Mineral salts in the body can be used as healing agents for particular health problems. Homeopathic doctor, William Schuessler, discoverer of the **12 cell salts**, felt that every form of illness was associated with balance disturbances of one or more of the indispensable mineral salts. As with other homeopathic remedies, corresponding mineral salts are used to stimulate body cell salts toward normal metabolic activity and health restoration. They "retune" the body to return it to a healthy balance.

These medicines are available in tiny lactose-based tablets that are dissolved under the tongue for best results.

❐ **CALCAREA FLUOR - calcium fluoride -** contained in the elastic fibers of the skin, blood vessels and connective tissue, and in the bones and tooth enamel. Used for treatment of dilated or weakened blood vessels as those found in hemorrhoids, varicose veins and hardened arteries and glands.

❐ **CALCAREA PHOS - calcium phosphate -** present in all tissues. When deficient, anemia, emaciation, slow growth, poor digestion and general weakness occur.

❐ **CALCAREA SULPH - calcium sulphate -** promotes continual body cleansing. When deficient, toxic build-up occurs in the form of skin disorders, respiratory clog, boils and ulcerations, and slow healing.

❐ **FERRUM PHOS - iron phosphate -** helps form red blood corpuscles to oxygenate the bloodstream. Useful in treatment of colds, flu and skin inflammation.

❐ **KALI MUR - potassium chloride -** a deficiency forms excess mucous production and discharge. Used for inflammatory arthritic and rheumatic conditions.

❐ **KALI PHOS - potassium phosphate -** found in the nerves, brain and blood. Used to treat mental problems, depression, irritability, neuralgia, dizziness, headaches and nervous stomach.

❐ **KALI SULPH - potassium sulphate-** found in the skin and mucous membranes. A deficiency causes slimy nasal, eye, ear and mouth secretions.

❐ **MAGNESIA PHOS - magnesium phosphate -** a deficiency and imbalance cause sharp darting spasmodic pains and neuralgia.

❐ **NATRUM MUR - sodium chloride -** a deficiency causes profuse, watery secretions from the skin, eyes and mucous membranes, excessive salivation, watery stools and vomiting.

❐ **NATRUM PHOS - sodium phosphate -** regulates the acid/alkaline balance. Imbalance is indicated by a coated tongue, itchy skin, sour stomach, loss of appetite and flatulence.

❐ **NATRUM SULPH - sodium sulphate -** an imbalance produces edema in the tissues, dry skin with watery eruptions, poor bile and pancreas activity, headaches, and gouty symptoms.

❐ **SILICEA - silicic acid -** a deficiency produces catarrh in the respiratory system, pus discharges from the skin, slow wound healing, and offensive body odor.

REFLEXOLOGY ✧ ACUPUNCTURE ✧ ACUPRESSURE

WHAT THEY ARE ✦ WHY YOU SHOULD CONSIDER THEM

Reflexology is a science dealing with the fact that there are reflex points in the hands and feet corresponding to every organ and part of the body. The nerves are very like an electrical system, and contact can be made through the feet and hands with each of the ten electro-mechanical zones in the body, allowing location of the reflex points. Proper stimulation of these points through pressure and/or stroking can relieve circulatory and congestive problems naturally, at the body's deepest levels. Reflex pressure attention to a particular meridian point has a definite effect in bringing about better function in all parts of that zone, no matter how remote the point is from the body part in need of healing. The ten reflexology zone meridians connect all the organs and glands in the body, culminating in the hands and feet (see illustration).

BODY ZONES

15 pounds of force can send a surge of energy to the corresponding body area, to remove obstructive crystals, restore normal circulation, and clear congestion. The nerve reflex point on the foot for the afflicted area will be tender or sore indicating crystailline deposits brought about by poor capillary circulation of fluids. Pressure on the known corresponding foot or hand zone can be used for accurate self-diagnosis and treatment. In addition, the amount of soreness on the foot point can indicate the size of the crystalline deposit, and the amount of time it has been accumulating. Pressure point therapy is effective in removing this obstructive congestion, and in relaxing nerve constriction. Circulation is thus increased, and poisons are removed faster. In our experience, we have found that pressing on the sore point three times for 10 seconds each time is effective. This treatment may be applied for twenty to thirty minute sessions at a time, about twice a week. Sessions more often than this will not give Nature the chance to use the stimulation or do the necessary repair work. Most people notice frequent and easy bowel movement in the first twenty-four hours after zone therapy as the body throws off released inorganic wastes.

The **"foot"** and **"hand"** diagrams on the specific ailment pages of this book will graphically show the pressure points for each area, so that you can use reflexology as it is indicated. In some cases, the points are very tiny, particularly for the glands. They will take practice to pinpoint. The best rule for knowing when you have reached the right spot is that it will usually be very tender, indicating crystalline deposits or congestion in the corresponding organ. However, there is often a feeling of immediate relief in the area as the waste deposit breaks up for removal by the body.

Acupuncture and acupressure are ancient systems of natural healing from the Orient, that are only now reaching their due attention, respect and widespread use in the western world. As we have noted, the human body is made up of a complex of meridians or "energy pathways".. These regulate and coordinate vital functions by distributing "Chi" energy throughout the body. When the balance and flow of this energy is upset or obstructed, illness often follows. Acupuncture and Acupressure are a _painless,_ non-toxic therapy for redirecting and restoring Chi energy.

Acupuncture uses hair thin needles to direct and rechannel the energy.

Acupressure uses pressure on these meridians through less-invasive massage or stroking to restore the energy. (see previous page)

Both methods are safe and effective for many health problems, and are free of toxic or additive side effects. Both are successful in disease prevention care. As with other natural therapies, the aim here is to regulate, balance and normalize so the body can function normally. Surgery and drugs can often be avoided, and there are sometimes immediate spectacular results. In any case these therapies can certainly influence the therapuetic course of even very serious problems, and should be considered as a means of mobilizing your own healing energy and balance.

THE BASICS OF BEGINNING A HEALING PROGRAM

DETOXIFICATION ✦ FASTING ✦ BLOOD CLEANSING

Environmental toxins, secondary smoke inhalation, alcohol, prescription and pleasure drug abuse, "hidden" chemicals and pollutants in many foods that cause allergies and addictions, caffeine overload, and increased daily stress are all becoming more and more a part of our lives. These things greatly deplete the body and immune system. Poor immunity eventually results in debilitating disease, This has become the prime factor in allowing today's "civilization", "opportunistic" diseases, such as Candida, Chronic Fatigue Syndrome (EBV), Lupus, AIDS and ARC, HPV, etc. to take hold.

Indeed all disease, physical and psychological, is created or allowed by the saturation and accumulation of toxic matter in the tissues, and the lack of oxygen and minerals in the vital fluids, throwing defense mechanisms off and vitality out of balance.

In the past, detoxification was used either clinically, for recovering alcoholics and drug addicts, or individually, as a once-a-year mild "spring cleaning" for health maintenance. Today detoxification is becoming necessary not only to health, but for the quality of our lives, since we are surrounded by so much involuntary toxicity. Optimally, one should detoxify two to three times a year to prevent disease and encourage health; in the Spring, Summer or early Fall, when the body can get an extra boost in this effort from sunlight and natural Vitamin D.

A good detoxification program should be in three stages:

◆ CLEANSING ◆ REBUILDING ◆ MAINTAINING

The first step is to cleanse the body of waste deposits, so that it isn't running with a dirty "engine", or driving "with the brakes on". Many years of experience with cleansing programs have convinced me that **a moderate three to seven day juice fast** is the best way to release toxins from the system. Shorter fasts can't get to the root of a chronic or major problem. Longer fasts upset the body equilibrium more than most people are ready to deal with except in a controlled clinical environment.

A well thought out moderate fast can bring great advantages to the body, by cleansing it of excess mucous, old fecal matter, trapped cellular and non-food wastes, and uncirculated systemic sludge such as inorganic mineral deposits.

Fasting works by self-digestion. During a cleanse, the body in its infinite wisdom, will decompose and burn only the substances and tissue that are damaged, diseased, or unneeded, such as abscesses, tumors, fat deposits, and congestive waste. Even a relatively short fast can accelerate elimination from the liver, kidneys, lungs and skin, often causing dramatic changes as masses of accumulated waste are expelled. Live foods and juices literally pick up dead matter from the body and carry it away. You will be very aware of this if you experience the short period of headaches, fatigue, body odor, bad breath, diarrhea or mouth sores that commonly accompany accelerated elimination. However, digestion usually improves right away, as do many gland and nerve functions. Cleansing can also help release hormone secretions that stimulate the immune system, and encourage a disease-preventing environment. In a couple of weeks the body will start rebalancing, energy levels will rise physically, psychologically and sexually, and creativity will begin to expand. You will start feeling like a different person, and of course you are. **Outlook and attitude change because actual cell make-up has changed.**

A few days without solid food can be a refreshing and enlightening experience about your life style. A short fast increases awareness as well as available energy for elimination. Your body will become easier to "hear". It can tell you what foods and diet are right for your needs via legitimate cravings. Like a "**cellular phone call**", this is natural biofeedback.

It took years for the body to get to its present state on a poor, deficient diet, and restoration through good nutrition takes time. But the human body is basically a self-healing organism. Nature works slowly but surely. Healing is allowed to occur through a fast.

Getting clean isn't easy, but a clean strong body is the best defense against disease. Remember that the pattern for inherited health for you, your children, and your grandchildren, is laid down by you.

You really are what you eat.

STAGE 1: CLEANSING THE BODY. Three separate **target fasting diets** are included in this section to focus on whole-body cleansing: **the first** is specifically aimed at cleansing excess mucous from the lung and respiratory system; **the second** is a colon and bowel cleanser aimed at removing toxins from the elimination system; **the third** is a short 24 hour juice fast for beginning a cleanse when time is a factor. All will help the body release trapped, excess waste matter and alkalize the bloodstream, so that more efficient healing can take place.

Cleansing diets may be used before and during any therapeutic program, unless the person is weak and pale, with very low energy, or when immediate emergency measures are indicated. Results are well worth the effort.

◆ Have a small fresh salad the night before beginning a liquid fast, with plenty of intestinal "sweepers and scourers", such as beets, celery, cabbage, broccoli, parsley, carrots, etc. Elimination will begin as soon as the first meal is missed. Whenever possible, use organically grown fruits and vegetables for all juices.

◆ End your fasting period gently, with small simple meals. Have toasted wheat germ or whole grain granola in the morning with yogurt, apple, or pineapple/coconut juice. Take a small fresh salad for lunch with Italian or lemon/oil dressing. Have a fresh fruit smoothie during the day. Fix a baked potato with a little butter and a light soup or salad for dinner. Rebuilding starts right away with the highly nutritious foods and juices you are taking in. **You are on your way with a fresh, clean system.**

MUCOUS CLEANSING: A 3-7 DAY LIQUID DIET

ON RISING: take a glass of Lemon juice and water, using 2 fresh squeezed lemons.

BREAKFAST: take a glass of grapefruit juice if the system is over-acid, or cranberry/apple juice or pineapple juice.

MIDMORNING: take a mucous-cleansing herb tea, such as comfrey, comfrey/fenugreek, or wild cherry bark; or an herbal blend specifically for clearing mucous congestion, such as Crystal Star OPEN UP TEA - an expectorant to aid mucous release, or RESPIRTEA - to aid in oxygen uptake.

LUNCH: take a glass of carrot juice, or a potassium broth or essence (MEDICINAL DRINKS, pg. 33)

MIDAFTERNOON: have a mixed green vegetable juice, or a mixed green drink, such as Crystal Star ENERGY GREEN DRINK MIX, or 1 packet of Chlorella granules in a glass of water.

DINNER: take a glass of apple juice or pineapple/papaya juice.

BEFORE RETIRING: take 1 teasp. of Vegex yeast extract in a cup of hot water for relaxation and strength the next day.

SUPPLEMENTS & HERBAL AIDS BENEFICIAL DURING A MUCOUS CLEANSING DIET:

✤ Take 10,000Mg. of Ascorbate Vitamin C crystals daily for the first three days; dissolve 1/4-1/2t. at a time in water or juice throughout the day, and take until bowel tolerance is reached, and tissues are flushed. Take 5,000Mg. daily til the end of the liquid fast.

✤ Take 1 teasp. 3x daily of Garlic/Onion syrup; mash several garlic cloves and a large slice of onion in a bowl, and stir with 3 Tblsp. honey. Cover and let macerate for 24 hours. Remove garlic and onion and take only the honey syrup infusion.

✤ Drink 6-8 glasses pure water daily **in addition** to the juices to thin mucous secretions and aid elimination.

BODYWORK SUGGESTIONS:

✤ Take a 1 hour brisk walk every day during the fast, breathing deeply to help lungs and chest eliminate mucous.

✤ Apply wet Ginger/Cayenne compresses to the chest to increase circulation, and loosen mucous accretions.

✤ Take a hot sauna followed by a brisk rubdown to stimulate circulation.

❦ COLON & BOWEL CLEANSING: A 3-10 DAY LIQUID DIET

Bowel elimination problems are often chronic, and may require several rounds of cleansing. This fast may be done all at once or in two periods of five days each.

❦ The night before you begin, take a gentle herbal laxative in tea or tablet form, such as HERBALTONE, Crystal Star LAXA-TEA, or FIBER & HERBS COLON CLEANSE capsules.
❦ Soak some dried figs, prunes and raisins in water to cover, add 1 Tblsp. unsulphured molasses, and soak overnight in a covered bowl.

ON RISING: take 1 teasp. Sonné Liquid Bentonite, **or** 2 teasp. psyllium husks in juice.
or 1 heaping teasp. Crystal Star CHO-LO FIBER TONE™ DRINK MIX in water.

BREAKFAST: discard fruits from their soaking water .Take a small glass of the liquid.

MIDMORNING: take a glass of Richlife or Yerba Prima ALOE VERA JUICE WITH HERBS.

LUNCH: take a small glass of potassium broth or essence (MEDICINAL DRINKS, pg. 33)
or a glass of fresh carrot juice.

MIDAFTERNOON: take a large glass of fresh apple juice, **or** an herb tea such as alfalfa, lemon grass or red clover, **or** Crystal Star CLEANSING & FASTING TEA, designed to enhance the elimination process while providing energy.

ABOUT 5 O' CLOCK: take another small glass of potassium broth, **or** carrot juice, **or** a green drink, such as Crystal Star ENERGY GREEN DRINK, or BARLEY GREEN MAGMA.

DINNER: take a large glass of apple juice or papaya juice

BEFORE BED: Repeat the cleansing liquids you took on rising, **and** take a cup of peppermint or spearmint tea, or Crystal Star MEALS END TEA.

❧ SUPPLEMENTS AND HERBAL AIDS BENEFICIAL DURING A BOWEL CLEANSING DIET:

✤ 6-8 glasses of pure water a day are necessary for the success of this cleanse.

✤ Take 4-6 Crystal Star FIBER & HERBS COLON CLEANSE CAPS daily, to increase systol/diastol of the colon, and tone bowel tissue during heavy elimination.

✤ Take a Catnip or diluted chlorophyll enema every other night of this fast to help alkalize and detoxify.

❧ BODYWORK SUGGESTIONS:

✤ Take a daily brisk walk for one hour every day during the fast.

✤ Take a warm relaxing bath. Have a lower body massage, with dry skin brushing.

24 HOUR JUICE CLEANSE:

A short 24 hour liquid cleanse is often enough to start a good healing program.
"Beginning" is usually the hardest part of a fast. You have to set aside a block of time, gather all the ingredients for your diet, alter eating times and patterns; in essence change your life style and that of those you live with for a while. This is very difficult to do for many people, and can delay a needed program. The following 24 hour juice and herb tea fast makes things a lot easier. It is a quick cleanse; not with the depth of vegetable juices or satisfactory for major or chronic problems. But it is often enough, and definitely better than no fast at all.
It will make a difference in the speed of healing.

THE NIGHT BEFORE YOUR FAST: have a small fresh green salad with lemon/oil dressing.

ON RISING: take a glass of lemon juice and water, using 2 fresh squeezed lemons.

MIDMORNING: take a glass of cranberry juice from concentrate.

LUNCH: take a glass of fresh apple juice, **or** apple/alfalfa sprout juice with 1 packet of Chlorella or BARLEY GREEN MAGMA granules dissolved in it.

MIDAFTERNOON: take a cup of Crystal Star **CLEANSING & FASTING TEA** or **MEDITATION TEA.**

DINNER: take a glass of papaya/pineapple juice to enhance enzyme production, or another glass of apple juice with 1 packet Chlorella or Barley Green Magma granules.

BEFORE BED: have a cup of mint tea, **or** 1 teasp. Vegex yeast paste extract in a cup of hot water for relaxation and strength the next day.

Break your fast the next morning with fresh fruits and yogurt. Eat light, raw foods during the day, and have a simply prepared, low fat dinner.

SUPPLEMENTS AND HERBAL AIDS BENEFICIAL FOR THIS FAST:

✤ Drink plenty of pure water throughout the day to flush the system.

BODYWORK SUGGESTIONS:

✤ Take a long walk during the day.

✤ Use a dry skin brush to help release toxins coming out through the skin, and take a long, warm relaxing bath before retiring.

STAGE 2: REBUILDING AND RESTORING THE BODY: A 2 - 6 WEEK PROGRAM:
The second part of a good detoxification program is to rebuild healthy tissue and restore body energy. This is usually undertaken after 3-10 days of toxic waste elimination from the blood and bowels.
This phase allows the body's individual regulating powers to become active with obstacles removed, so that it can rebuild at optimum levels.
The diet during this time should emphasize raw, fresh, and very simply prepared foods. It should be very low in fat, with little dairy, and no fried foods. No alcohol, caffeine, tobacco, salt, or sugars should be taken during this phase, and no meats, except fish and seafoods.

ON RISING: take a vitamin/mineral or protein drink, such as All 1, Nature's Plus Spirutein **or** Crystal Star **MIN-ZYME-MINOS** in apple or other fruit juice;
or 2 lemons squeezed in a glass of water with a little honey;
or apple cider vinegar in water with a little honey.

BREAKFAST: have some fresh citrus fruit; add low fat yogurt or soymilk if desired.
or whole grain cereal with a little apple juice or low fat yogurt;
or a fresh fruit smoothie with a banana.

MIDMORNING: take a glass of carrot juice or a potassium juice (MEDICINAL DRINKS, PG. 33)
or a cup of Siberian Ginseng tea, or Crystal Star **FEEL GREAT TEA;**
or a small bottle of mineral water with a packet of Chlorella or Green Magma granules dissolved in it;
or Crystal Star **ENERGY GREEN DRINK MIX** in water.

LUNCH: have a fresh green salad with Lemon/oil dressing;
or some steamed tofu with fresh greens and dressing;
or steamed vegies, such as broccoli, onions or zucchini with BRAGG'S LIQUID AMINOS;
or miso or other light broth soup with ramen noodles and a small whole grain sandwich.

MIDAFTERNOON: take a green drink (see medicinal drinks) or a cup of herb tea such as peppermint or red clover tea, or Crystal Star **HIGH ENERGY TEA;**
or some raw vegie snacks with kefir cheese and a glass of mineral water.

DINNER: have a baked potato with Bragg's Liquid Aminos or tamari, and a salad;
or some steamed vegies with brown rice and tofu;
or baked or broiled white fish with lemon/oil sauce;
or a whole grain and vegetable casserole, or pasta salad
or a light soup and hearty salad with nuts, seeds, or tofu.

BEFORE BED: have a relaxing cup of herb tea, such as Chamomile, SLEEPYTIME, or Crystal Star **GOOD NIGHT TEA;**
or a cup of Vegex yeast paste broth in hot water.

⌁ SUPPLEMENTS AND HERBAL AIDS FOR THE REBUILDING DIET:

✦ Take a potassium drink at least twice a week (Medicinal Drinks, pg. 33), or Crystal Star **MIN-ZYME-MINOS DRINK.**

✦ Take acidolphilus liquid or capsules with meals to encourage friendly G.I. flora.

✦ Take Vitamin B $_{12}$ either sublingual or internasal for healthy cell development.

28

✣ Take Ascorbate or Ester Vitamin C 3-5000Mg. daily for interstitial tissue/collagen growth.

✣ Take Crystal Star ENERGY GREEN, Chlorella, or Barley Green Magma for blood building.

✣ Take 2 Crystal Star ADRN-ALIVE CAPS <u>with</u> 2 BODY RE-BUILDER CAPS daily for a month, to encourage healthy gland activity and strength. Take ANEMI-GIZE CAPS to help build hemoglobin and increase liver, spleen and lymph function.

✣ Take some Crystal Star FEEL GREAT CAPS & TEA as needed for stamina and endurance; Crystal Star HAWTHORNE EXTRACT- 1/2 dropperful 2x daily as a tonic.

⌒ BODYWORK SUGGESTIONS:

✤ Take some mild exercise every day.

✤ Get some sunlight on the body every day possible. Light builds strength along with food. Eating out of doors is especially beneficial.

⌒ STAGE 3: MAINTAINING A HEALTHY IMMUNE SYSTEM:

The final part of a good cleansing program is keeping the body clean and toxin-free; very important after all the hard work of detoxification. Modifying life style habits to include high quality nutrition from both food and supplement sources is the key to strong immunity.

The foods you choose should rely heavily on fresh fruits and vegetables for cleansing and soluble fiber; cooked vegetables, grains and seeds for strength, endurance and alkalinity; with sea foods, eggs and low fat cheeses as alternate sources of protein; and broiled, baked or stir-fried sea foods and vegetables with a little dinner wine for circulatory health. **Red meats, high in saturated fats, and refined foods, high in sugar and fat, should be avoided.**

This "GOOD PROTECTION TEST" can help you monitor your support-system health on a regular basis. Essentially it is a fiber check; enough soluble fiber in the diet to make the stool float, is the protective level against such diseases as Colitis, Constipation, Hemorrhoids, Diverticulitis, Varicose Veins, and Bowel Cancer.

✤ **The bowel movement should be regular and effortless.**
✤ **The stool should be almost odorless.**
✤ **There should be very little flatulence.**
✤ **The stool should float rather than sink.**

⌒ SUPPLEMENT & HERBAL SUGGESTIONS FOR MAINTENANCE & DISEASE PREVENTION:

✣ Keep the tissue oxygen level of the body high with 1000-3000Mg. Vitamin C and Vitamin E 400-800IU daily, Vitamin B_{12}„ Chlorella or Green Magma, and daily exercise.

✣ Keep a good level of potassium in the body with high potassium foods such as broccoli, leafy greens and bananas; or potassium capsules, Twin Lab LIQUID K PLUS, or a potassium drink such as Crystal Star ENERGY GREEN DRINK, or herbal POTASSIUM SOURCE CAPSULES.

✤ Take Bee Pollen granules, 2 teasp. daily for essential amino acids, and/or high potency Royal Jelly, 2 teasp. daily for natural pantothenic acid.

✤ Daily Immune enhancers should include Bee Propolis liquid extract, Beta-Carotene 25,000IU, COQ 10-10Mg., Zinc 30-50Mg., Raw Thymus extract (during high risk seasons) and Crystal Star HERBAL DEFENSE TEAM EXTRACT, TEA and CAPSULES.

✤ High chlorophyll foods and supplements also fortify immunity, body balance, and alkalinity on a daily basis; CHLORELLA, GREEN MAGMA, Spirulina, Nature's Plus SPIRUTEIN, or Crystal Star ENERGY GREEN DRINK MIX.

✤ Foundation vitamins and minerals should be from food or herbal sources for best absorbency. Some of the best are from Living Source, Mezotrace, New Chapter and Floradix. Crystal Star makes several formulas high in concentrated herbal minerals; HIGHLY ABSORBABLE CALCIUM, IRON, and MINERAL COMPLEX EXTRACTS, IRON SOURCE, CALCIUM SOURCE, and MEGA - MINERAL CAPSULES.

✤ Enzymes and lactobacillus acidolphilus are important for good assimilation, and adequate intesinal flora. The best supplements combine many complex living organisms that can easily unite with the body. Good maintenance products include Solaray MULTIDOLPHILUS, DDS DAIRY FREE ACIDOLPHILUS, and for children, Nature's Plus JUNIOR DOLPHILUS CHEWABLE WAFERS. Crystal Star MIN-ZYME-MINOS DRINK MIX, is a broad spectrum combination, with naturally occuring concentrated minerals, enzyme activity and amino acids.

✤ High soluble daily fiber supplements insure a fully active elimination system, digestive regulation, cholesterol and blood sugar balance. These can include guar gum capsules before meals, psyllium husks, 2 T. in water morning and evening, a soluble fiber blend, or Crystal Star CHO-LO FIBER TONE DRINK MIX.

⌁ BODYWORK SUGGESTIONS:

✤ Remember that daily exercise is one of the most important things you can do for your life. It increases oxygen uptake in the body to improve metabolism, circulation, and respiratory activity. Every walk you take, every series of stretches you do, strengthens and lengthens your life and health.

✤ Get early morning sunlight on the body every day possible for regular Vitamin D.

BODYWORK TECHNIQUES FOR SUCCESSFUL CLEANSING

BATHS ✦ WRAPS ✦ HYDROTHERAPY ✦ ENEMAS ✦ COMPRESSES

✤ HEALING BATHS: Clinics and spas are famous all over the world for their mineral, seaweed and enzyme baths. The skin is a large organ of ingestion, and can assimilate the valuable nutrients from a therapeutic bath in a pleasant, stress-free way. Bathe at least twice daily during a cleanse to remove toxins coming out through the skin. The procedure for taking an effective healing bath is important. In essence, you are soaking in an herbal tea or mineral fluid, and allowing the skin to take in the healing nutrients instead of the mouth and digestive system.

There are two good ways to take a therapeutic bath:

1) Draw very hot bath water. Put the bath herbs, seaweeds, or mineral crystals into an extra large tea ball or muslin bath bag, (add mineral salts directly to the water). Steep til water cools and is aromatic.

2) Make a strong tea infusion in a large teapot, strain and add to bath water.

❧ Soak as long as possible to give the body time to absorb the healing properties. Rub the body with the solids in the muslin bag during the bath for best results.
❧ All over dry skin brushing before the bath for 5 minutes with a natural bristle brush will help remove toxins from the skin and open pores for better assimilation.
❧ After the bath, use a mineral salt rub, such as Crystal Star NATURAL SALT GLOW, a traditional spa "finishing" technique to make your skin feel healthy for hours.

NOTE: FOOD GRADE 35% H_2O_2 may be used for a detoxifying rejuvenation bath, to add tissue oxygen through the skin. Use about 1-2 cups to a full tub of water, and soak at least 1/2 hour. Or, add 1/2 cup H_2O_2, 1/2 cup sea salt, and 1/2 cup baking soda to bath water and soak.

✤ HERBAL WRAPS: The best European and American spas use wraps as restorative body-conditioning procedures. Wraps are also sophisticated cleansing techniques that can be used to elasticize, tone, alkalize and release wastes from the body very quickly. They should be used in conjunction with a short cleansing program, and 6-8 glasses of water a day to flush out fats and waste. Crystal Star makes three wraps for home use: TIGHTENING & TONING to improve muscle, vein and skin tone, ALKALIZING ENZYME to replace and balance important minerals, enhance metabolism and alkalize the system, and DRAWING & SWEATING with "house-cleaning" herbs to increase metabolism, and encourage waste release by sweating.

✤ HOT AND COLD HYDROTHERAPY: This technique helps open and stimulate the body's vital energies toward healing. Alternating hot and cold showers, or hot and cold compresses are very effective in several areas for getting the body started on a positive track toward healing. Spasmodic pain and cramping, circulation stimulation, muscle and sinew tone, bowel and bladder problems, system stability, relaxation, energy and balance, all show improvement with hydrotherapy.

There are many forms of hydrotherapy. The one included here is easy and convenient for in-home use. Follow with a full or partial massage, or a brisk towel rub and mild stretching exercises for best results.

31

❦ Begin with a comfortably hot shower for 3 minutes. Follow with a sudden change to cold water for 2 minutes. Repeat this cycle three times, ending with cold. Rub the skin briskly with a rough towel for 1 minute to bring up circulation.

✤ ENEMAS: Enemas can greatly aid the release of old, encrusted colon waste, and make the whole body cleansing process easier and more thorough.

Herbal Enemas can serve to immediately alkalize the bowel area, help control irritation and inflammation, and provide local healing action for ulcerated tissue.
We recommend three herbs regularly for enemas: Catnip, when stomach and digestive problems are involved, and for childhood disease. Use 2 cups of very strong brewed tea to 1 qt. of water. Pau de Arco, when the acid/alkaline system is imbalanced, as in chronic yeast and fungal infections. Use 2 cups strong brewed tea to 1 qt. water. Spirulina, when both blood and bowel are toxic.

Coffee Enemas have become a standard in natural healing when liver and blood related cancers are present. Caffeine used in this way stimulates the liver and gallbladder to remove toxins, open bile ducts, encourage increased peristaltic action, and produce necessary enzyme activity for healthy red blood cell formation and oxygen uptake. Use 1 cup of **regular** strong brewed coffee to 1 qt. water.

How to take a therapeutic enema: place the enema solution in a water bag, and hang or hold about 18 inches higher than the body. Attach colon tube, and lubricate with vaseline or K-Y jelly. Lying on the left side, slowly insert the tube about 18 inches into the colon. Rotate tube gently for ease of insertion, removing kinks, so liquid will flow freely. When all solution has entered the colon, slowly remove the tube and remain on the left side for 5 minutes. Then move to a knee-chest position with the weight of the body on the knees and one hand. Use the other hand to massage the lower left side of the abdomen for several minutes. Roll onto the back for another 5 minutes, massaging up the descending colon, over the transverse colon to the right side, and down the ascending colon. Then move onto the right side for 5 minutes, so that each portion of the colon is reached. Get up and quickly expel fluid into the toilet. A sticky grey or brown mucous substance, small dark incrustation chunks, or long, tough ribbon-like pieces will frequently have been loosened and expelled during the enema. These poisonous looking things are usually the obstacles and toxins interfering with normal body functions.The good news is that they are no longer in **you.** You may have to take several enemas before there is no more evidence of these substances.

✤ COMPRESSES: These are used to draw out waste and waste residues such as cysts, growths and abscesses through the skin, or release them into the body's elimination channels. Use alternating hot and cold compresses for best results, applying the herbs to the hot compress, and leaving the ice or cold compress plain. We regularly use Cayenne, Ginger and Lobelia effectively.

❦ Simply add 1 teasp. powdered herbs to a bowl of very hot water. Soak a washcloth and apply til the cloth cools. Then apply a cold cloth dipped in ice water on the area til it reaches body temperature. Repeat several times daily. Green Clay compresses, effective for growths, may be applied to gauze, placed on the area, and left for a day at a time. Simply change as you would any dressing when you bathe.

HEALTHY DRINKS, JUICES & WATERS

Liquids have long been considered an easy way to take absorbable, usable nutrients into the body. Drinks are the least concentrated form of nutrition, but have the great advantage of rapid assimilation. They can break down and flush out toxins quickly, and provide lubrication to the system. The tissues can be flooded with therapeutic, health-giving values in a mild, gentle, and often delicious way. In fact, the body often craves what it needs most, and recognizes natural medicinal drinks as rich in qualities it lacks, such as minerals, proteins, and chlorophyll. Therapeutic liquids can sometimes taste better than anything else.

MEDICINAL DRINKS FOR SPECIFIC AREAS

For both fruits and vegetables, a high quality juicer is the best way to get all the nutrients. However, we have used regular food processor and blender attachments with satisfactory results. Use organic produce whenever possible.

◆ **POTASSIUM BROTH**
The single most effective vegetable juice I know for cleansing, neutralizing acids, strengthening and rebuilding the entire body.

For one 8oz. glass:
3 CARROTS
1/2 BUNCH SPINACH
1/2 BUNCH PARSLEY
3 STALKS CELERY
optional: 2 teasp. BRAGG'S LIQUID AMINOS
Contains approximately 1275Mg. potassium.

◆ **POTASSIUM ESSENCE BROTH**
If you do not have a juicer, use this high potassium drink. While not as concentrated or pure, it is still an excellent source of energy, minerals and electrolytes.

For a 2 day supply: Cover with water in a soup pot:
3-4 CARROTS
2 POTATOES WITH SKINS
1 ONION, OR 4 LARGE GARLIC BULBS
1/2 BUNCH PARSLEY
1/2 HEAD CABBAGE
3 STALKS CELERY WITH LEAVES
1/2 BUNCH BROCCOLI
Simmer covered 30 minutes.
Strain and discard solids.
Add 1 teasp. Vegex yeast paste extract or Bragg's Liquid Aminos if desired for flavor and concentrated B vitamins.
Store in a covered glass container.
Drink broth essence only. Contains approximately 1255Mg. potassium.

GREEN DRINKS & BLOOD TONICS

Green drinks are high in chlorophyllins. The composition of chlorophyll is so close to that of human hemaglobin that these drinks can act as "mini-transfusions" for the blood, and tonics for the brain and immune system. Green drinks also have anti-infective properties, are excellent for mucous cleansing, and alkalize the body.

◆ **EVERGREEN**
A personal favorite for taste, mucous release and improved enzymatic activity.

For 1 drink: Run through a juicer:
1 CORED GREEN APPLE WITH SKIN
1/2 FRESH PINEAPPLE SKINNED AND CORED
1 TUB (4OZ.) ALFALFA SPROUTS
1 t. SPIRULINA OR CHLORELLA GRANULES
3-4 SPRIGS FRESH MINT

◆ **SKIN TONIC**
Deep greens to nourish, cleanse and tone the skin from the inside.

For 2 drinks: Run through a juicer:
1 CUCUMBER WITH SKIN
1 TUB (4oz.) ALFALFA SPROUTS
1/2 BUNCH PARSLEY
3-4 SPRIGS FRESH MINT

◆ **SPROUT COCKTAIL**
A high protein juice particularly good for ending a fast.

For 1 drink: Run through a juicer:
3 TART APPLES WITH SKIN, CORED
1 TUB (4oz.) ALFALFA SPROUTS OR MIXED SALAD SPROUTS
3-4 SPRIGS FRESH MINT

◆ **CARROT JUICE PLUS**
High Beta Carotene enhanced with cleansing properties.

For 2 drinks: Run through a juicer:
4 CARROTS
1/2 CUCUMBER WITH SKIN
2 STALKS CELERY WITH LEAVES
1 T. CHOPPED SEA VEGIES, SUCH AS WAKAME OR DULSE

◆ **KIDNEY FLUSH**
An aid to the water elimination area, with high potassium and blood cleansing properties.

For 3 drinks: Run through a juicer:
4 CARROTS
4 BEETS WITH TOPS
4 CELERY STALKS WITH LEAVES
1 CUCUMBER WITH SKIN
8-10 SPINACH LEAVES, WASHED

CLEANSING PURIFYING FRUIT DRINKS

Fruits are wonderful for a quick system wash and cleanse. Their high water and sugar content speeds up metabolism to release wastes fast. However, because of this rapid metabolic use, pesticides, sprays and chemicals on fruits can enter the body rapidly. **Eat organically grown fruits whenever possible.** Wash fruit well if commercially grown.

Fresh fruit juices have an alkalizing effect on the body, and are high in vitamins and minerals. Fruits and fruit juices have their best nutritional effects when taken alone. Take them before noon for best cleansing benefits and energy conversion.

◆ **BLOOD BUILDER**
A blood purifying drink with natural Iron enrichment.

For 1 1/2 quarts:
2 CUPS GRAPE JUICE, OR LIQUEFY 2 BUNCHES GRAPES IN THE BLENDER
2 CUPS ORANGE JUICE, OR 6 ORANGES PEELED AND JUICED
1 CUP LEMON JUICE, OR 8 LEMONS PEELED AND JUICED
1 CUP WATER
1/4 CUP HONEY

◆ **STOMACH & BREATH REFRESHER**
This drink alkalizes an acid stomach.

FOR 1 quart:
1 1/2 CUPS GRAPE JUICE , OR 1 LARGE BUNCH GRAPES JUICED
1 1/2 CUPS APPLE JUICE, OR 4 APPLES CORED AND JUICED
1-2 BASKETS FRESH STRAWBERRIES, JUICED
4-5 SPRIGS FRESH MINT LEAVES

◆ **ENZYME COOLER**
An intestinal balancer to help lower cholesterol and allow better assimilation.

For 2 drinks:
1/2 CUP APPLE JUICE OR 1 APPLE CORED AND JUICED
1 1/2 CUPS PINEAPPLE JUICE, OR 1 PINEAPPLE SKINNED, CORED AND JUICED
1/4 CUP LEMON JUICE OR 2 LEMONS PEELED AND JUICED

◆ **DIURETIC MELON MIX**
A good morning drink with diuretic properties. Take on an empty stomach.

For 1 quart: Juice in the blender
3 CUPS WATERMELON JUICE
1/2 CUP PERSIAN MELON JUICE
1/2 CUP HONEYDEW MELON JUICE

◆ **PINEAPPLE CARROT COCKTAIL**
Natural source Beta-Carotene, Bromelain and Vitamin A.

Use a juicer for this if possible. Makes about 1 qt.
1 1/2 CUPS PINEAPPLE JUICE, OR 1 PINEAPPLE SKINNED, CORED AND JUICED
4 CARROTS JUICED
1/2 CUP PARSLEY CHOPPED AND JUICED

CLEANSING BROTHS & HOT TONICS

Clear broths are a very satisfying form of nutrition during a cleansing fast. They are simple, easy, inexpensive, can be taken hot or cold, and provide a means of "eating" and being with others at mealtime without going off a liquid program. This is more important than it might appear, since solid food, taken after the body has released all its solid waste, but before the cleanse is over, will drastically reduce the diet's success.

Hot tonics are neither broths nor teas, but unique hot combinations of vegetables, fruits and spices with purifying and energizing properties. The ingredients provide noticeable synergistic action when taken together, with more medicinal benefits than the single ingredients alone. Take them morning and evening for best results.

◆ ONION & MISO BROTH
To alkalize the system.

For 6 servings:
Sauté 1 CHOPPED ONION in 1/2t. SESAME OIL for 5 minutes
Add 1 STALK CHOPPED CELERY WITH LEAVES, and sauté for 5 minutes more
Add 1 QT. WATER or VEGETABLE STOCK
Cover and simmer for 10 minutes.
Add 3-4T. LIGHT MISO
Remove from heat.
Add 2 GREEN ONIONS and whirl in the blender til liquefied.

◆ ONION & GARLIC BROTH
For mucous release. Very powerful.

For 1 drink:
Sauté 1 ONION and 4 CLOVES GARLIC in 1/2t. SESAME OIL til very soft.
Whirl in the blender. Take in small sips.

◆ COLD DEFENSE CLEANSER
For the minute you feel a cold coming on.

Heat for 1 drink:
1 1/2 CUPS WATER
1 t. garlic powder
1 t. GROUND GINGER
1 T. LEMON JUICE
1 T. HONEY
3 T. BRANDY
1 /2 t. CAYENNE PEPPER
Simmer gently for 5 minutes. Drink in small sips for best results.

◆ STOMACH & DIGESTIVE CLEANSER
Whirl in the blender for 1 8oz. glass:

1/2 CUCUMBER WITH SKIN
2 T. APPLE CIDER VINEGAR
2 PINCHES GROUND GINGER
ENOUGH WATER TO MAKE 8 OZ.

◆ **WARMING CIRCULATION TONIC**
Immediate body heat against aches, shakes and chills.

For 4 drinks:
1 CUP CRANBERRY JUICE
1 CUP ORANGE JUICE
2 T. HONEY
4-6 WHOLE CLOVES
4-6 CARDAMOM PODS
1 CINNAMON STICK
4 T. RAISINS
4 T. ALMONDS
1/4 t. VANILLA
Heat all gently 15 minutes. Remove Cloves and Cardamom. Serve hot.

◆ **BLOOD PURIFYING BROTH**
Very high in potassium and other minerals.

For 6 cups:
Sauté in 2 T. OIL til tender crisp
1/2 CUP CHOPPED BROCCOLI
1/4 CUP CHOPPED LEEKS
1/4 CUP DAIKON RADISH
1/4 CUP CHOPPED CELERY WITH LEAVES
1/4 CUP GRATED CARROTS

Add 6 CUPS RICH VEGETABLE STOCK
1/4 CUP SNIPPED PARSLEY
2 t. BRAGG'S LIQUID AMINOS
2 t. FRESH SNIPPED LEMON PEEL
Serve hot. Drink in small sips.

◆ **MUCOUS CLEANSING BROTH**
Grandma was right. Hot chicken broth really does clear out congestion faster.

For 4 drinks.
Make 1 QT. CHICKEN STOCK. (Boil down bones, skin and trimmings from 1 fryer. Skim off fat and solid pieces)

Sauté in a large pot til aromatic for 5 minutes
3 CLOVES MINCED GARLIC
1 t. HORSERADISH
A PINCH CAYENNE PEPPER
Add stock and simmer for 10 minutes.
Top with NUTMEG and SNIPPED PARSLEY

◆ COLDS & FLU TONIC
This drink opens up nasal and sinus passages right away.

For 2 drinks:
Toast in a dry pan til aromatic
4 CLOVES MINCED GARLIC OR 2 t. LEMON/GARLIC SEASONING
1/4 t. CUMIN POWDER
1/4 t. BLACK PEPPER
1/2 t. HOT MUSTARD POWDER
Add 1 T. OIL and stir in. Toast for 1 minute more.
Add 1 CUP HOT WATER
1 t. TURMERIC
1/2 t. SESAME SALT
1/2 t. GROUND CORIANDER (1 T. FRESH)
1 CUP COOKED SPLIT PEAS (OR 1 CUP FRESH FROZEN)
Simmer 5 minutes, and whirl in the blender. Very potent!.

◆ ALKALIZING APPLE BROTH
This drink balances the acid/alkaline system, and helps lower serum cholesterol.

For 4 drinks:
Sauté in 1 t. OIL til soft
1/2 RED ONION CHOPPED
2 CLOVES GARLIC MINCED
While sautéing, whirl in the blender
1 SMALL RED BELL PEPPER
2 TART APPLES, CORED AND QUARTERED
1 LEMON PARTIALLY PEELED
2 T. SNIPPED PARSLEY
2 CUPS KNUDSEN'S VERY VEGIE-SPICY JUICE (or any good tomato juice)
Add ONIONS AND GARLIC. Blend well.
Heat gently again and serve hot.

◆ REVITALIZING TONIC
This is the authentic "hangover" remedy from the movies where smoke comes out of your ears after one sip. Effective hot or cold. Works every time.

For 1 pitcher:
1 32OZ. CAN TOMATO JUICE OR KNUDSEN'S VERY VEGGIE SPICY JUICE
1 CUP CHOPPED MIXED GREEN ,YELLOW AND RED ONIONS
2 STALKS CELERY CHOPPED WITH LEAVES
1/2 BUNCH PARSLEY CHOPPED
1 1/2 t. HOT PEPPER SAUCE
1/2 t. ROSEMARY LEAVES
1/2 t. FENNEL SEEDS
1 T. CHOPPED FRESH BASIL (OR 1 t. DRIED)
1 CUP WATER
1 t. BRAGG'S LIQUID AMINOS OR TAMARI SAUCE
Pour into a large pot. Bring to a boil. Simmer for 30 minutes.

PROTEIN DRINKS & ENERGY TONICS

You must have protein to heal, and the new breed of protein drinks are a wonderful way to get protein without meat or bulk or excess fat. These drinks obtain protein from several sources so that a balance with carbohydrates and minerals is achieved, and a real energy boost felt.

◆ **MORNING MEAL REPLACEMENT**
Effective non-dairy protein. Whirl in the blender til mixed.

For 4 drinks:
1 CUP SLICED STRAWBERRIES
1 BANANA SLICED
1 CUP PAPAYA CHUNKS
8 OZ. SOFT TOFU, OR 1 CUP AMAZAKE RICE DRINK
2 T. SWEET CLOUD SYRUP, OR BARLEY MALT
1 CUP PINEAPPLE/COCONUT JUICE
1 1/2 t. VANILLA
1 T. WHEAT GERM

◆ **HEAVY DUTY PROTEIN DRINK**
For a hard workout or hard work. Blend all in the blender til mixed.

For 2 drinks:
1 CUP WATER
6T. NONFAT DRY MILK
1 BANANA
2T. PEANUT BUTTER
1 CUP YOGURT
2T. BREWER'S YEAST
1T. WHEAT GERM
1T. ROASTED CAROB POWDER

◆ **PERSONAL BEST V-8**
A delicious high vitamin/mineral drink for body balance and energy. A good daily drink for maintenance and disease prevention. Use a juicer for best results.

For 5-6 glasses:
6-8 TOMATOES, OR 4 CUPS TOMATO JUICE
2 STALKS CELERY WITH LEAVES
1/2 GREEN PEPPER
3-4 GREEN ONIONS WITH TOPS
1/2 BUNCH PARSLEY
2 CARROTS
1/2 SMALL BUNCH SPINACH, WASHED, OR 1/2 HEAD ROMAINE LETTUCE
2 LEMONS, PEELED, OR 4T. LEMON JUICE
optional: 2t. BRAGG'S LIQUID AMINOS and 1/2 t. GROUND CELERY SEED

ABOUT NATURAL WINES

Naturally fermented wine is more than an alcoholic beverage. It is a complex biological fluid possessing definite physiological values. **Wine is still a living food,** and can combine with, and aid the body like yogurt or other fermented foods. Many small, family owned wineries make chemical and additive free wines that retain inherent nutrients, imcluding absorbable B vitamins, such minerals and trace minerals as potassium, magnesium, organic sodium, iron, calcium and phosphorus.

Wine is a highly useful drink for digestion, and in moderation, as a sedative for the heart, arteries and blood pressure. (in fact, tests have shown that a glass or two of white wine with dinner can cut heart disease risk by 50%). Its importance should not be overlooked in a weight loss or fitness program, because a little wine relaxes. When you are relaxed, you tend to eat less. Because of its high density lipoproteins, wine can free the circulation, relieve pain and reduce acid production in the body. It is superior to tranquilizers or drugs for relief of nervous stress and tension.

ALWAYS USE IN MODERATION.

Note: Liquor other than wines is not recommended, even for cooking, when you are involved in a healing program. Although most people can stand a little hard spirits without undue effect, and alcohol burns off in cooking, the concentrated sugar residues won't help a recovering body.

ABOUT MILK

We do not recommend drinking or using cow's milk in cooking when on a healing program, because of its clogging and mucous forming properties. Pasteurized milk is a relatively dead food as far as nutrition is concerned, and even raw milk can be difficult to assimilate for someone with allergies, or respiratory problems.

Happily, there are several delicious, healthy substitutes that can be used for cooking and drinking on almost any healing plan, without sacrificing richness or taste.

SOY MILK is nutritious, versatile, smooth and delicious. It is vegetable based, lactose and cholesterol free, with unsaturated or poly-unsaturated fat. Soymilk contains less calcium and calories than milk, but more proteins and iron. Use it cup for cup as milk for cooking; plain flavor for savory dishes, vanilla flavor for sweet dishes.

ALMOND MILK is a rich non-dairy liquid that can be used as a base for cream soups, sauces, gravies and protein drinks. It can be used cup for cup as milk to enrich any baked recipe. Put 1 CUP ALMONDS in the blender with 2-4 CUPS WATER depending on the consistency desired. Add 1 t. honey, and whirl til smooth.

YOGURT is a good intestinal cleanser that helps balance and replace friendly flora in the G.I. tract. Even though yogurt is dairy in origin, the culturing process makes it a living food, and beneficial for health. Mix equal parts of yogurt with water, chicken or vegetable broth, white wine or sparkling water, and use cup for cup instead of milk in cooking.

ABOUT WATER

Water is second only to oxygen in importance for health. It makes up 65-75% of the body, and every cell requires water to perform its essential functions. **Water maintains** system equilibrium, lubricates, flushes wastes and toxins, hydrates the skin, regulates body temperature, acts as a shock absorber for joints, bones and muscles, adds needed minerals, and transports nutrients, minerals, vitamins, proteins and sugars for assimilation. **Water cleanses** the body inside and out. **When the body gets enough water, it works at its peak. Fluid and sodium retention decrease, gland and hormone functions improve, the liver breaks down and releases more fat, and hunger is curtailed.** To maintain this wonderful internal environment, you must drink lots of pure water, **6 - 8 glasses every day** to replace lost electrolytes and metabolic waste fluid.

However, most of our tap water today is chlorinated, fluoridated, and treated to the point where it can be an irritating disagreeable fluid instead of a valuable benefit. Regular city tap water may contain as many as 500 different disease-causing bacteria, viruses and parasites. Many toxic chemicals and heavy metals used by industry and agriculture have found their way into ground water, adding more pollutants. Some tap water is now so bad, that without the enormous effort our bodies use to dispose of these chemicals, we would have ingested enough of them to turn us to stone by the time we were thirty! Concern about this lack of purity is leading more and more people to bottled water.
For a healing program, several types of water are worth consideration.

MINERAL WATER is usually from natural springs with varying mineral content and widely varying taste. The naturally occurring minerals are beneficial to digestion and regularity, and in Europe this form of bottled water has become a fine art. It is not U.S. government regulated for purity except in California and Florida.

DISTILLED WATER can be either from a spring or tap source, but is "de-mineralized" so that only oxygen and hydrogen remain. This is accomplished by reverse osmosis, filtering or boiling, then conversion to steam and recondensing. It is the purest water available, and ideal for a healing program.

SPARKLING WATER comes from natural carbonation in underground springs. Most are also artificially infused with CO_2 to maintain a standard fizz. This water is an aid to digestion, and is excellent in cooking to tenderize and give lightness to a recipe.

ARTESIAN WELL WATER is the cadillac of natural waters. It always comes from a deep pure source, has a slight fizz from bubbling up under rock pressure, and is tapped by a drilled well. The water never comes in contact with ground contaminants.

NOTE: **Beyond buying bottled water, you can also take steps as an individual to diminish water pollution:** ❦ **Use biodegradable soaps and detergents** ❦ **Don't use water fresheners in your toilets** ❦ **Avoid pouring hazardous wastes such as paint, solvents, and petroleum based oils into drains or sewers** ❦ **Use natural fertilizers such as manure and compost in your garden** ❦ **Avoid using non-biodegradable plastics and polystyrene** ❦ **Conserve water.**

LIGHT MACROBIOTIC & 'NEW AGE' EATING

Macro (long) - biotic (life) stems from the Eastern philosophy of life, and considers the seasons, climate, activity level, farming methods, traditions, and an individual's condition, in determining the way to eat. Other aspects of the macrobiotic way of life include daily exercise, avoiding synthetic clothing, aluminum, Teflon cookware and microwave ovens, expressing gratitude and appreciation, living positively, and an "early to bed and early to rise" habit. Proper orientation to all these considerations, according to this philosophy, leads to happiness, health, freedom and appreciation for the bounties and boundaries of life.

In America, Macrobiotics has rightly become popular as a healing diet, encouraging harmony and balance in the body. It is non-mucous forming, low in fat, high in vegetable proteins and fiber, and very alkalizing. Brown rice, other whole grains, and fresh in-season foods are the mainstays.
While Macrobiotics is flexible and not a set pattern, in general this way of eating consists of about 50-60% whole grains and beans for good complex carbohydrates and plant protein, 25-30% vegetables, 10% soy foods such as tofu, tempeh and miso, 5% sea vegetables, nuts and seeds, 5% fruit, and 5% cultured foods, such as Kefir, Kefir cheese and yogurt, with occasional fish and eggs. Condiments and seasonings are an important part of macrobiotic cooking, not only to enhance flavor, but to promote good enzyme and digestive avtivity.
Favorite Macrobiotic seasonings include gomashio (sesame salt), Kuzu starch, sea salt, daikon radish, ginger pickles, umeboshi plums, tamari soy sauce, tekka, brown rice vinegar and wasabi horseradish, with occasional maple syrup, rice syrup or barley malt for sweetening.

A macrobiotic diet is stimulating to the heart and circulatory systems by keeping the body alkaline and high in natural iodine and potassium, through its emphasis on foods such as miso, bancha tea (Kukicha), Shiitake mushrooms, sea vegetables, tofu and soy foods, and umeboshi plums. It is a diet resistant to disease in strict form; a way of eating that is cleansing and balancing at the same time.In modified, light form, it is a way of eating you can live with in health on a lifetime basis.

HOWEVER, as we learn more about "New Age" ways of eating; Macrobiotics, Fruit cleansing diets, Juice fasting, Mono diets, etc., we find that caution must be used if you are not in a controlled clinical environment. **In their <u>strict cleansing/healing form</u>, these diets should be used only as short term programs.**

There must be balance to your diet. It is largely "civilization" foods and a lack of balance that get us into trouble, that lowers immunity and resistance to disease. Vitamin B_{12} from animal or dairy products is necessary for cell growth, immunity and energy. Protein is neeeded for healing and strength. Complex carbohydrates are essential for endurance and stamina. Minerals are necessary for assimilation and building blocks, and soluble food fiber is integral to effective body cleansing, and weight maintenance. For the best route to long term health, find out what foods have the elements you need in their natural state, and include them in your diet, raw, or simply cooked, on a regular basis. For more on this optimum way of eating, see **"<u>COOKING FOR HEALTHY HEALING</u>", by Linda Rector-Page.**

ABOUT SEA VEGETABLES & IODINE THERAPY

Sea vegetables have superior nutritional content. They transmit the energies of the sea as a rich source of proteins, complex carbohydrates, minerals and vitamins. Ounce for ounce, along with herbs, they are higher in vitamins and minerals than any other food group. **Sea vegetables** are one of nature's richest sources of vegetable protein, and they provide full spectrum concentrations of carotene, chlorophyll, enzymes and soluble fiber. The distinctive salty taste is not just "salt", but a balanced, chelated combination of sodium, potassium, calcium, magnesium, phosphorus, iron and trace minerals. They convert inorganic ocean minerals into organic mineral salts that combine with amino acids. Our bodies can use this combination as an ideal way to get usable nutrients for structural building blocks. In fact, sea vegetables contain all the necessary trace elements for life, many of which are depleted in the earth's soil.

Sea vegetables are almost the only non-animal source of Vitamin B_{12} necessary for cell growth and nerve function. Their mineral balance is a natural tranquilizer for building sound nerve structure, and proper metabolism.

Sea vegetables alkalize the body, reduce excess stores of fluid and fat, and work to transform toxic metals in the system (including radiation), into harmless salts that the body can eliminate. They purify the blood from acidic effects of the modern diet, allowing for better absorption of nutrients. They strengthen the body against disease.

In this era of processed foods and iodine-poor soils, **sea vegetables and sea foods** stand almost alone as potent sources of natural Iodine. Iodine is essential to life, since the Thyroid gland cannot regulate metabolism without it. Iodine is an important element of alert, rapid brain activity, and prime deterrent to arterial plaque. Iodine is also a key factor in the control and prevention of many endocrine deficiency conditions that are prevalent today; breast and uterine fibroids, tumors, prostate inflammation, adrenal exhaustion, and toxic liver and kidney states. Pregnant women who are deficient in iodine are more prone to giving birth to cretin babies, a form of retardation.

Specific Iodine Therapy treatment for each of these conditions is discussed on the specific pages in this book, but **preventive measures** may be taken against these problems by just adding 2 tablespoons of sea vegetables a day to the diet.

Sea vegetables are delicious, and convenient to buy, store, and use as needed in their sun-dried form. Store them in a moisture proof container and they will keep indefinitely. A wide variety of sea vegetables is available today, both in Macrobiotic and regular quality. These include: AGAR AGAR, ARAME, BLADDERWRACK, DULSE, HIJIKI, IRISH MOSS, KELP, KOMBU, NORI, SEA PALM, SPIRULINA, **and** WAKAME. They may be crushed, chopped or snipped into soups and sauces, crumbled over pizzas, and used as toppings on casseroles and salads. When you are using sea vegetables, no other salt is needed, an advantage for a low salt diet.

My favorites for recipes and cooking are: HIJIKI for its curly texture and nutty crisp taste, DULSE with a soft, chewy texture, and strong salty flavor, KOMBU **and** NORI as sweet wrappers for hors d'oeuvres, SEA PALM for exotic taste, and WAKAME as a delicate addition to soups and salads and salads and dips.

Here is a delicious salad, soup and topping blend to add sea vegies to your diet. Just *barely whirl in the blender so there are still sizeable chunks.* They will expand in any recipe with liquid, and when heated will return to a beautiful ocean green color.

SEA VEGIES SUPREME
3/4 CUP CHOPPED DRIED DULSE
1/4 CUP CHOPPED DRIED WAKAME
1/4 CUP DRIED NORI OR SEA PALM
1/4 CUP CHOPPED DRIED KOMBU
1/2 CUP TOASTED SESAME SEEDS

THE LOW SALT DIET

In the past generation, Americans have consumed more NaCl than ever before; too much restaurant food, too many processed and refined foods, too many animal foods. Most people are aware that excessive salt causes heart disease, hypertension, and blood pressure problems. Circulation is constricted, kidneys malfunction, fluid is retained, and migraines occur frequently. Too much salt can produce hyperactivity, aggressive behavior, and poor glandular health.
 A salt free diet is obviously desirable for someone who eats too much salt. However, once the body's salinity normalizes, **some** salt should be brought back into the diet quickly. Adequate salinity is needed for good intestinal tone, strong blood, tissue transportation of nutrients, healthy organs and glands.Too little or no salt can lead to lack of vitality, stagnated blood and loss of clear thinking.

Regular table salt is almost totally devoid of any nutritional value, but there are many other ways to get the good salts that the body needs. Tamari, say sauce, shoyu, misos, umeboshi plums, sea vegetables and salt, herb salts and seasonings, sesame salt, and many fermented foods such as pickles, relishes and olives all have the enzymes and alkalizing properties that make salts usable and absorbable.

LOW SALT, NOT NO SALT, is best for a permanent way of eating.

ABOUT FOOD GRADE HYDROGEN PEROXIDE

Much controversy has surrounded the use of H_2O_2 Food Grade Hydrogen Peroxide for therapeutic anti-infective and anti-fungal applications. Our experience with this source of nascent oxygen has been successful in many areas, **but a great deal of that success is predicated on <u>the way this substance is used</u>.**

Food Grade H_2O_2 is available in three refrigerated forms in most health food stores:

35% FOOD GRADE - is the strongest available solution and **must be diluted** before external or internal use. **Mix 1 oz. of 35% solution with 11 oz. distilled water for 12 oz. of 3% H_2O_2.**
This <u>3% dilute solution </u>may be used internally for serious complaints where higher tissue oxygen is needed to control disease growth, as in asthma, emphysema, arthritis, Candida Albicans, Epstein Barr Virus, certain cancerous growths, and other degenerative conditions such as AIDS and ARC. Like many antibiotics, H_2O_2 will also kill friendly bacterial culture in the digestive tract. Take an acidolphilus supplement or eat some plain yogurt after taking H_2O_2. This solution may be used as an oxygen bath in the spa or tub to energize the body. One cup of the 35% solution may be poured directly into a bathtub or spa full of water. An energy increase is usually noticed right away.

3% FOOD GRADE H_2O_2-DILUTE SOLUTION - this form has been pre-diluted to a ready-to-drink potency, and is usually flavored with lemon. It may be used as a mouthwash, skin spray, or on cotton balls to replace the skin's acid mantle that has been removed by soap. Other uses for this form include housecleaning applications for sparkling appliances, dishes and counters. Therapeutic applications where a **3% dilute solution of H_2O_2** has been effective include athlete's foot, and other fungal conditions; as a douche for vaginal infections; and as an enema or colonic solution during cleansing.

FOOD GRADE GEL - (PEROXY GEL) combined with Aloe Vera juice, Glycerine, and Red Seaweed extract, is the most popular form for general application, with beneficial uses for athlete's foot, minor cuts, burns and bruises, and insect bites. It may be applied topically to affected areas on the skin, or massaged into the soles of the feet where the pores are large. It can reach most parts of the body through them. It may also be taken internally for detoxification, using 1/2 teaspoon of the gel and 1/4 teasp. powdered ascorbate Vitamin C to an 8 oz. glass of water. **1 teaspoon of peroxide gel combination provides 15 drops of 35% H_2O_2.**

For pet health, use 1oz. 3% H_2O_2 to 1 qt. water; for larger animals, use 2oz. to 1 gallon of water.

For plant health and growth, use 1oz. 3% solution in 1 qt. water.

In most applications, especially those where anti-infective and anti-fungal properties are needed, we have found it more beneficial to **use H_2O_2 in an alternating series,** (usually 10 days of use, and then 10 days of rest, or 3 weeks of use, and 3 weeks of rest, in more serious cases)

Directions with this therapeutic product are very specific as to dosage and ailment. Read the bottle label carefully before embarking on a program that includes H_2O_2 to insure success.

OPTIMAL HEALING AFTER SURGERY

STRENGTHENING YOUR BODY FOR SURGERY ✦ ACCELERATING HEALING ✦ CLEANING OUT
DRUG RESIDUES ✦ GETTING OVER THE SIDE EFFECTS

Before you go to the hospital:

Strengthen the immune system.
Include daily: Beta-carotene 25,000IU
                Vitamin E 400IU
                Vitamin C 1000Mg. with Bioflavonoids and Rutin
                B Complex 100Mg. w/ Pantothenic acid 500Mg. for adrenal strength
Eat a high vegetable protein diet. You must have protein to heal.
Take a full spectrum pre-digested amino acid compound, capsules or drink.
Eat plenty of brown rice and other whole grains for complex carbohydrates.
Take a Potassium Broth or juice (see page 33) and/or a protein drink every day.
Strengthen body defense measures.
Include daily: Bromelain 500Mg. (with Quercetin if there is inflammation)
                Biotec million unit S.O.D. 6 daily **or** Germanium 30Mg. capsules (or
                    dissolve 1 gm. of powder in 1 qt. water, and take 2-3 Tblsp. daily).
                Sun Chlorella 20 tablets daily, or 1 packet of powder.
                Crystal Star **MEGA-MINERAL, POTASSIUM SOURCE , ADRN EXTRACT**

When you return home:

Eat a very nutritious diet.
Include frequently: Organ meats
                   Seafoods and baked or broiled fish
                   Brown rice and other whole grains with Tofu
                   Fresh fruits and vegetables
                   Yogurt and other cultured foods for friendly intestinal flora
                   A Potassium Broth or Juice, (Pg. 33) or a **green drink** or **hot energy tonic**
                   A high protein drink such as Nature's Plus SPIRUTEIN or ALL 1
Clean the body and vital organs, to counteract infection.
Include daily for one month: MEGADOLPHILUS or LIFE START 2, 3 t. in juice or water with meals.
                   Crystal Star **LIV-ALIVE CAPSULES** and **LIV-FLUSH TEA**
                   Fresh Carrot juice
                   Wild Cherry bark and Burdock Rt. tea for gland balance
                   Enzyme therapy such as Rainbow Light DETOX-ZYME
                   Beta Carotene or Probiologics AQUEUS LIPISOL for Vit. A uptake
Build the body up.
Include daily for one month: Vitamin B12 SL, or ENER-B VIT. B12 INTERNASAL GEL
                   Vitamin E 400IU with Selenium
                   Enzymatic Therapy LIQUID LIVER WITH GINSENG CAPS.
                   Zinc 30-50Mg. **or** Alta Health SIL-X CAPSULES
                   White Birch Mineral water - food source absorbable potassium.
                   Crystal Star **MIN-ZYME-MINOS DRINK MIX, BODY REBUILDER and ADRN-ALIVE CAPSULES, and MEGA MINERAL CAPS ,.**
                   Carnitine 250Mg. <u>with</u> COQ 10 Mg. as an anti-oxidant.
                   Country Life ENERGIX VIALS 1 daily.
                   Aloe Vera gel to heal scars, lesions and wounds.
                   Shark Liver oil for leukocyte formation to fight infection.

NORMALIZING THE BODY AFTER CHEMOTHERAPY & RADIATION

Chemotherapy and radiation treatments are being widely used by the medical community for several types, stages and degrees of cancerous or malignant cellular growth. While some partial successes have been proven, the after effects are often worse than the disease, in terms of healthy cell damage, body imbalance, and lowered immunity. Many doctors and therapists recognize these drawbacks to treatment with chemotherapy, but under current government, and insurance restrictions, neither doctors nor patients have any other choices.
No other treatments except surgery, radiation and chemotherapy have been officially approved by the FDA in the United States for malignant disease. Exorbitantly high costs of major medical treatment have bound medical professionals, hospitals, and insurance companies in a vicious circle where literally no alternative measure can be used for controlling cancerous growth.

Chemotherapy and radiation costs are currently beyond the financial range of most people, who, along with physicians and hospitals must rely on their health insurance to pay these expenses. However, at the present time, insurance will only pay for "officially approved" chemotherapy and radiation. Neither doctors or hospitals are reimbursed if they use other healing treatments, and everyone, including the patient, is caught in a political and bureaucratic web, where it all comes down to money instead of health.

New testing and research is also abnormally expensive, and lags for lack of funding. Moreover, when a valid treatment is substantiated, there is not even the reasonable investment certainty that government (and therefore health insurance) approval can be achieved through the maze of red tape and political lobbies. This is doubly unfortunate, since there is much research, and many alternative therapies, used with success in Europe and other countries to which Americans are denied access.

Nutritional counselors, holistic practitioners, therapists and others involved in natural healing have done a great deal of research and work toward minimizing the damage, and rebuilding the body after chemotherapy and radiation. These efforts have had notable success, and may be used with confidence by those recovering from both cancer and its current medical treatment.

For three months after chemotherapy or radiation, take the following daily:

☞ **One individual packet of Barley Green granules in water.**

☞ **1 Mega CO Q 10 capsule - 30Mg.**

☞ **1 Germanium tablet - 30Mg. (or dissolve 1 gm. Germanium powder in 1 qt. water. Take 3Tblsp. daily)**

☞ **Ener -B vitamin B$_{12}$ INTERNASAL GEL - 1 dose every other day.**

☞ **Hawthorne extract - 1/2 dropperful under the tongue 2 x daily.**

☞ **Crystal Star LIV-ALIVE CAPS AND LIV-FLUSH TEA , or other good herbal liver cleanser.**

☞ **Ascorbate Vitamin C crystals with Bioflavonoids, 1/4 teasp. in water or juice every hour - supplying approx. 5-10,000Mg, daily.**

☞ **Floradix HERBAL IRON 1t. 3 x daily.**

EXERCISE AS A PART OF HEALTH

BODY BUILDING ✦ SHAPING ✦ TONING ✦ MAINTAINING

BODYWORK & NUTRITIONAL COMPONENTS OF THE NEW PHYSICAL FITNESS

Exercise is an integral part of health. It's not just for athletes anymore. We all know that exercise speeds results in weight loss and heart disease recovery, but regular exercise helps any healing program. It strengthens the whole body - muscles, nerves, blood, glands, lungs, heart, brain, mind and mood. It increases metabolic rate, tissue oxygen uptake, respiratory and circulatory vigor. **Even if you didn't reduce your calorie intake, but added exercise, you would still lose weight and increase body tone.** Every exercise helps. Choose those that work for you conveniently and easily. Every series of stretches and exercises you do tones, elasticizes, shapes and contours your skin, connective tissue and muscles.

AEROBIC EXERCISE is the best for whole body tone; the key to long term weight, and stress control, lower cholesterol, a stronger heart. It also stimulates antibody production, enhancing immune response. Aerobic exercise is easy, and as available as your front door. A daily walk, breathing deeply, for even a mile a day (1/2 mile out, 1/2 mile back) makes a big difference in lung capacity and tissue oxygen. Deep exhalations release metabolic waste along with CO_2, and deep inhalations flood the system with fresh oxygen. The circulatory system is cleansed, heart strength and muscle tone are improved. Sunlight on the body adds natural Vitamin D for skin and bone health. You notice the difference from a fitness walk.

DANCING is another great aerobic exercise. Legs and lungs show rapid improvement, not to mention the fun you have. Any kind of dancing is a good workout, and the breathlessness felt afterward is the best sign of aerobic benefit.

SWIMMING works all parts of the body at once, so noticeable toning improvements come quickly with regular swimming. Just fifteen to twenty steady laps, three or four times a week, and a more streamlined body is yours.

AEROBIC EXERCISE CLASSES are easily available. They are held every day, everywhere, at low prices, with good music and spirit-raising group energy. Workout clothes look great on both men and women. They are comfortable, permit deep breathing, and make you feel good about your body even when you are not exercising.

If your schedule is so busy that you hardly have time to breathe, let alone exercise, but still want the benefits of bodywork, there is an **all-in-one aerobic exercise.** It has gotten resounding enthusiasm, and response rates for aerobic activity and muscle tone - **all in one minute.** The exercise sounds very easy, but is actually very difficult, and that is why it works so well. You will be breathless (the sign of an effective aerobic workout) before you know it.

Simply lie flat on your back on a rug or carpet. Rise to a full standing position any way you can, and lie down flat on your back again. That's the whole exercise. Stand and lie down, stand and lie down - **for one minute.** Typical repetitions for most people with average body tone are six to ten in 60 seconds. Record time for an athlete in top competitive condition is about 20-24 times in a minute. Be very easy on yourself. Repeat only as many times as you feel comfortable and work up gradually. It is worth a try because it exercises muscles, lung capacity and circulatory system so well, but don't overdo it.

Exercise is an integral part of nutrition. We have all experienced the fact that exercise eases hunger. You are thirsty after a workout as the body calls for replacement of water and lost electrolytes, but not hungry. One of the reasons rapid results are achieved in a body streamlining program is this phenomenon. Not only do muscles become toned, heart and lungs become stronger, and fats lost, but the body doesn't call for calorie replacement right away. Its own glycogens lift blood sugar levels and provide a feeling of well-being. **Exercise becomes a nutrient in itself.**

✤ Stretch out before and after a workout to keep cramping down and muscles loose. Get some morning sunlight on the body every day possible for optimal absorption of nutrient fuel.

✤ Whatever exercise program you choose for yourself, make **rest** a part of it. Work out harder one day, go easy the next; or exercise for several days and take two days off. This is better for body balance, and will increase energy levels when you exercise the next time. After a regular program is started, exercise **four days a week** will increase fitness level; exercise **three days a week** will maintain fitness level; exercise only **two days a week** will decrease a high fitness level. But any amount of exercise is better than nothing at all.

The body is an amazing entity. It can be streamlined, toned and maintained, no matter what age or shape you are in, with very little effort. The secret is continuity.

EATING FOR ENERGY & PERFORMANCE

Body building is 85% nutrition. A regular long term, very nutritious diet is the basis for high performance; not protein or even carbo-loading before an event. The major body systems involved in energy production are the liver, thyroid, and adrenal glands. Maximum anabolic effect can be achieved in these areas through food and herbal sources. Complex carbohydrates and minerals are the keys to strength and endurance for both the athlete and the casual body builder. They improve performance, promote storage of muscle fuel, and are easily absorbable without excess fats.

65 - 75% of a high performance diet should be unrefined complex carbohydrates. Good sources are whole grains and pastas, vegetables, rice and beans. **20 - 25%** should be in high grade proteins, from whole grains, nuts, beans, raw dairy products, tofu or other soy foods, yogurt, kefir, and eggs, with some occasional poultry, fish and seafoods. About **10 - 15%** of the diet should be in energy-producing fats and oils necessary for glycogen storage. The best are unrefined, mono or unsaturated oils, a little pure butter, nuts, low fat cheses and whole grain snacks. The remaining fuel, should be in liquid nutrients; fruit juices for natural sugars, mineral waters, and electrolyte replacement drinks for lost potassium, magnesium and sodium, and **plenty of pure water.** When the body senses lack of water, it will naturally start to retain fluid. Waste and body impurities will not be filtered out properly, and the liver will not metabolize stored fats for energy. Six to eight glasses of water a day are a must, even if you don't feel thirsty. It often takes the sensory system time to catch up with actual body needs.

Remember that eating junk foods pays the penalty of poor performance. **Athletes cannot excel by just adding anabolic steroid supplements to an inferior diet. The only effective thing is optimum nutrition.**

Remember that vegetable protein is best for mineral absorption and bone density.

For complete TRAINING & OPTIMAL ENERGY DIETS see "COOKING FOR HEALTHY HEALING" by Linda Rector-Page.

SUPPLEMENTS FOR BODYBUILDING & PERFORMANCE

Nutritional supplementation is excellent for both the serious and casual athlete. It can help build muscle tissue, maintain low body fat, and improve over all strength, endurance and power when the body is under the stress of a workout series. Supplements optimize recuperation time between workouts, are a proven adjunct to fitness and muscle growth, and speed healing from sports-related injuries.

How you take training supplements is as important as **what** you take. Your program will be more productive if you balance supplementation between workout days and rest days. Muscle growth occurs on the "off" days, as the body uses the exercise you have been giving it. In general, increased enhancement can be obtained by taking **vitamins, minerals, and glandulars** on "off" days. **Proteins, amino acids, anabolics and herbs** work best taken on "on" days, before the exercise or workout.

The following schedule contains effective products in each supplementation area:

MINERALS: You must have minerals to run - for bone density, speed and endurance.
- ◆ Potassium/Magnesium/Bromelain- relieves muscle fatigue/lactic acid buildup
- ◆ Cal/Mag/Zinc - a basic maintenance complex to prevent cramping
- ◆ Chromium picolinate, 200Mg. - for sugar regulation and glucose energy use
- ◆ Twin Lab Ultra Fuel or Endurance Quick Fix, Knudsen Recharge, Alacer Hi-K Cola - effective electrolyte mineral replacement drinks
- ◆ Mezotrace - ancient sea bottom minerals and trace minerals

VITAMINS: Anti-stress factors for muscles, nerves and heart.
- ◆ B Complex, 100Mg. or more - for nerve health and muscle cramping
- ◆ Vitamin C, 3000Mg. daily w/ Bioflavs and Rutin for connective tissue strength
- ◆ Vitamin B_{12} sublingual or internasal, for cell development, energy, strength
- ◆ Dibencozide - the most absorbable and usable B_{12} for athletes needs.

ANTI-OXIDANTS: To increase oxygen use in blood, tissues and brain.
- ◆ Vitamin E, 400IU with Selenium - for heart and circulatory health
- ◆ CO Q 10 - a catalyst factor to produce and release energy
- ◆ B_{15}- Di-Methylglycine - to boost oxygen delivery
- ◆ Biotec S.O.D. - 1 million units from sprouts - a free-radical scavenger
- ◆ Country Life ENERGIX VIALS.

RAW GLANDULARS: Growth gland and hormone stimulation
- ◆ Pituitary, 200Mg. - the master gland, for upper body development
- ◆ Adrenal, 500Mg. - for adrenal support and cortex production
- ◆ Liver, 400Mg. - for fat metabolism, and detoxification support
- ◆ Orchic, 1200Mg. - for male testosterone support

FREE FORM AMINO ACIDS: Hormone activators to increase body structure and strength.
- ◆ Arginine/Ornithine/Lysine, 750Mg. - to help burn fats for energy, and reduce useless body fat
- ◆ Carnitine, 500Mg. - to strengthen heart, circulatory system, and metabolize fats
- ◆ Inosine, 1000Mg. - to reduce workout stress, and kick in glycogen use for extra edge performance
- ◆ Branched Chain Complex - BCAA - for ATP energy conversion and rebuilding damaged muscles.
- ◆ Full Spectrum Anabolics - for natural steroids and body growth
- ◆ Pre-digested Amino Acids - pro-proteins for better performance

ENZYMES: To process fuel nutrients for most efficient body use.
- ◆ Pancreatin, 1400Mg. - to metabolize fats, oils and carbohydrates correctly
- ◆ Bromelain/Papain, 500Mg. - for muscle and ligament repair and strength

LIPIDS: Liver cleansers to metabolize fats and help form strong red blood cells.
- ◆ Choline/Methionine/Inositol - a basic liver lipid
- ◆ Methionine/Lysine/Ornithine - with extra fat metabolizing agents

PROTEIN DRINKS: Daily mainstays for extra energy and endurance
- ◆ Nature's Plus Spirutein - a maintenance drink with added body cleansers
- ◆ Joe Weider VICTORY protein powder - a training energy drink
- ◆ RichLife PRO MUSCLE RAPID WEIGHT GAIN - effective for bulking up.
- ◆ Champion METABOLOL 2 - a competition level low fat muscle builder
- ◆ Strength Systems EGG AMINOS DRINK - highest quality egg protein

ELECTROLYTE REPLACEMENTS: Excellent after exertion to replace body minerals
- ◆ Richlife HYDROLOAD
- ◆ Knudsens RECHARGE
- ◆ Twin Lab ULTRA FUEL
- ◆ Strength Systems CARBO COOLERS
- ◆ WHITE BIRCH MINERAL WATER for mega doses of potassium

ABOUT STEROIDS

As the standards of excellence rise in sports and competition, the use of steroids is increasing. Steroid enhancement has now spread beyond the professional and Olympic arenas to dedicated weight lifters, body builders and team players at all levels. **The dangers of steroids far outweigh any advantages.** Steroid use leads to wholesale destruction of glandular tissue, stunted growth from bone closure in males, testicle shrinkage, low sperm counts with sterility noticeable after only a few months of use, enlargement and tenderness of the pectorals, weakening of connective tissue, jaundice from liver damage, circulation impairment, and adverse side effects evidenced in hostile personality behavior and facial changes.

Amino acids, and some herbs and vitamins, can act as natural alternatives to help build the body to competitive levels without these consequences. These "natural steroids" help release growth hormone, promote ammonia and acid detoxification, stimulate immunity and encourage liver regeneration. They maximize potential, promote fast recuperation, increase stamina, and support peak performance.

The following products are for the serious athlete, supplying far more than the usual level of supplementation. They are super-nutrients. The doses are not for regular maintenance.

✤ ANABOLICS, MEGABOLICS, ULTRABOLICS, AMINOBOLICS, etc., **4-6, or 1-2 packs daily** - the mainstay of the dedicated athlete's program. They improve power, strength and endurance, build muscle tissue and stimulate growth hormone.

✤ BRANCHED CHAIN AMINOS, **2-4 daily** - take before a workout for good ATP conversion and rebuilding of damaged muscles.

✤ TYROSINE/ ARGININE/ TRYPTOPHANE/ GLYCINE/ ORNITHINE,, **needed in multigram doses for desired effect,** - to stimulate GH release.

✤ GAMMA ORYZONAL (GO), **500-1500Mg. daily** - a hypothalamus and pituitary stimulator to increase testerone secretion; primarily for maximum weight gain and calorie use, with a noticeable gain in muscle mass and reduction of body fat in 3-4 weeks.

✤ BETA SITOSTEROL, **2-4 daily** - to keep blood fats and cholesterol low, and circulation clear.

✤ INOSINE, **500-1500Mg. daily** - to increase endurance, energy and ATP build up, take 30 minutes before working out.

✤ DIBENCOZIDE B $_{12}$ - the most active form of B$_{12}$ as a steroid alternative.

✤ CHROMIUM PICOLINATE, **250Mg. daily** - enhances muscle growth.

✤ COQ 10, **30-60Mg. daily** - for enhanced flow of oxygen to the cells.

HERBS FOR A WINNING BODY

Herbs act as concentrated nutrients for body building, and offer extra strength for energy and endurance. They work best when taken on exercise days; in the morning with a good protein drink, or 30 minutes before exertion.

The following products are effective for both serious training and casual exercise.

✤ SMILAX **1-2 times daily** - an extract of Sarsaparilla bark and root. Coaxes the body to produce greater amounts of the anabolic hormones, testosterone, cortisone, progesterone.

✤ SIBERIAN GINSENG **2-4 caps daily** - clinically proven to increase stamina, endurance, gland activity, and lean muscle mass, with higher tolerance for stress.

✤ SPIRULINA, **1000Mg. tabs daily** - natural source amino acids, proteins and chlorophyll.

✤ BEE POLLEN & ROYAL JELLY, **2 teasp. or capsules daily** - a perfect concentrated food, with essential amino acids, proteins, enzyme stimulants and B Vitamins.

✤ **Country Life** ENERGIX **vials - 1 daily before a work out -** for stamina and endurance

✤ VEGEX YEAST PASTE EXTRACT, **1 teasp. in a cup of hot water** - excellent source of absorbable B vitamins for workout recovery and nerve strength.

CRYSTAL STAR BODY BUILDING COMBINATIONS:

❦ <u>Mineral formulas</u> - for strong body building blocks, better nutrient absorption, bone density, and endurance -HIGHLY ABSORBABLE MINERAL COMPLEX EXTRACT, MEGA-MINERAL CAPSULES, POTASSIUM **and** CALCIUM SOURCE CAPSULES,

❦ <u>Glandular formulas</u> - for gland and hormone stimulation and growth - MASTER BUILDER **and** ADRN-ALIVE CAPSULES.

❦ <u>Energy formulas</u> - high grade concentrated nutrition for extra endurance and acid detoxification in muscles - SUPERMAX **and** HIGH PERFORMANCE CAPSULES, HIGH ENERGY TEA.

❦ <u>Metabolic formulas</u> - to aid fat metabolism and cell production -LIV-ALIVE CAPSULES **and** LIV TONIC EXTRACT.

❦ <u>Drink mixes</u> - building, rejuvenating drinks with natural source amino acids, proteins, chlorophyll, enzymes and vitamins - ENERGY GREEN **and** MIN-ZYME-MINOS

❦ <u>Drawing & Sweating Body Wrap</u> - use it like a steam room to draw toxic wastes out through the skin after a workout.

BODY WORK FOR BODY BUILDING

Besides your major sport or activity, supplement and strengthen it with auxiliary exercise such as dancing, bicycling, jogging, walking, swimming or aerobics. This will balance muscle use and keep heart and lungs strong.

✤ Recuperation time is essential for optimum growth and strength. Muscles do not grow during exercise. They grow during rest periods. Alternate muscle workouts, and your training days with rest days.

✤ <u>Deep</u> breathing is important. Muscles and tissues must have enough oxygen for endurance and stamina. Breathe <u>in</u> during exertion, <u>out</u> as you relax for the next rep.

✤ Don't forget the importance of water. Good hydration is necessary for high performance, blood circulation, cardiovascular activity and overheating. Take a good electrolyte replacement drink after a workout or anytime during the day.

See SPORTS INJURIES page in this book for more information.

HAVING A HEALTHY BABY

PREGNANCY ✦ CHILDBIRTH ✦ LACTATION

A woman's body changes so dramatically during pregnancy and childbearing that her normal daily needs change. The body takes care of some of this need through cravings, and during this one time of life, the body is so sensitive to its needs, the cravings are ususally good for you. We know that every single thing the mother does or takes in affects the child. The nutritional suggestions here will help build a healthy baby with a minimum of discomfort and excess fatty weight gain that can't be lost after birth.

OPTIMAL EATING FOR TWO

Promise yourself that at least during these few months of pregnancy and nursing, your diet and lifestyle will be as healthy as you can make it. A highly nutritious diet will help pregnancy be more of a pleasure, with less discomfort or risk of complications.

🍎 Eat a high vegetable protein diet, with plenty of whole grains, seeds, sprouts, and fish or seafoods at least twice a week. Have a fresh fruit or green salad every day. Eat lots of high soluble fiber foods like whole grain cereals and vegetables for regularity. Eat complex carbohydrate foods like broccoli and brown rice for strength.

🍎 Drink lots of pure water, mineral water and juices throughout the day to keep the system free and flowing. Carrot juice at least twice a week is ideal. Include pineapple and apple juice.

🍎 Eat **folacin rich foods** such as fresh spinach and asparagus for healthy cell growth
Eat **zinc rich foods** such as pumpkin and sesame seeds for good body formation.
Eat **vitamin C foods** such as broccoli and bell peppers and fruits for connective tissue
Eat **alkalizing foods** such as miso soup and brown rice to combat and neutralize toxemia.
Eat **mineral-rich foods** such as sea vegies, leafy greens, whole grains for baby building blocks.

🍎 Take a good protein drink several times a week for optimal growth and energy. The following is a proven example: Mix 1/2 cup raw milk, 1/2cup yogurt, the juice of one orange, 2T. Brewer's yeast, 2T. wheat germ, 2tsp. molasses, 1tsp. vanilla, a pinch cinnamon.

🍎 Eat small frequent meals instead of large meals.

There are several important thing to avoid during pregnancy and nursing, for the greatest health to the baby.

🛑 Don't diet. Lower calories usually mean lower birth weight. Metabolism becomes deranged during dieting, and the baby will receive abnormal nutrition that can impair brain and nerve development. Even if you feel you are gaining too much, a healthy diet is full of nutritious calories, (not empty calories) that you will be able to lose easily after nursing. Until then you are still eating for two.

🛑 Don't restrict your food variety. Eat a wide range of healthy foods to assure the baby access to all nutrients. (Avoid cabbages, onions, and garlic. They upset body balance during pregnancy. Avoid red meats. Most are full of nitrates, and other chemicals the baby can't eliminate.)

🛑 Don't fast - even for short periods where fasting would normally be advisable, such as constipation or to overcome a cold. Food energy and nutrient content will be diminished.

Avoid all processed, refined, preserved and colored foods. Refrain from alcohol, caffeine and tobacco. Avoid X-Rays, chemical solvents, chloro-fluorocarbons such as hair sprays, and even cat litter. Your system may be able to handle these things without undue damage, the baby's can't. Even during nursing, toxic concentrations occur easily.

Don't smoke. The chance of low birth weight and miscarriage is twice as likely if you smoke. Smoker's infants have a mortality rate 30% higher than non-smoker's. Nursing babies take in small amounts of nicotine with breast milk, and become prone to chronic respiratory infections.

OTHER NUTRITIONAL WATCHWORDS:

•**During Labor:** take no solid food. Drink fresh water, have carrot juice, or suck on ice chips.
•**During Lactation:** promote milk quality and richness with almond milk, brewer's yeast, green drinks and plenty of green foods, avocados, carrot juice, soy milk and soy foods, goat's milk and unsulphured molasses.
•**During Weaning:** papaya juice will help slow down milk flow.

HEALTHY PRE-NATAL SUPPLEMENTS

All drugs should be avoided during pregnancy and nursing; including alcohol, tobacco, caffeine, MSG, Saccharin, X-Rays, aspirin, Valium, Librium, Tetracycline, and harsh diuretics.
Especially stay away from recreational drugs; including cocaine, PCP, marijuana, meth-amphetamines, Quaaludes, heroin, LSD and other psychedelics. Even the amino acid L-Phenalalanine can adversely affect the nervous system of the unborn child.

✤ Mega-doses of <u>anything</u> are not good for the baby system.
Remember that the developing child's body is very small and very delicate. Ideal supplementation should be from food-source complexes for best absorbability. Dosage should be about half of normal.

✤ **Take a good <u>pre-natal</u> multi-vitamin and mineral supplement, such as Rainbow Light PRE-NATAL; especially starting six to eight weeks before the expected birth. Clinical testing has shown that mother's who took nutritional supplementation during pregnancy were far less likely to have babies with neural tube and other defects.**

✤ Take a natural mineral supplement such as MEZOTRACE for good body building blocks.

✤ Take extra Folic acid **to prevent neural tube defects;** vitamin B$_{12}$, and vitamin C for good cellular and connecting tissue development.

✤ Take vitamin B$_6$ 50-100Mg. for bloating, leg cramps and nerve strength, and natural vitamin E 200IU, or wheat germ oil for skin and body tone.

OTHER SUPPLEMENTATION WATCHWORDS:

•**During the last tri-mester:** rub vitamin E oil on the stomach and around the vaginal opening every night to make stretching easier and skin more elastic. Begin to take extra minerals as labor approaches for an easier birth.
•**During Labor:** take vitamin E and calcium/magnesium to relieve pain and aid dilation.
•**During Nursing:** calcium lactate is beneficial with calcium ascorbate vitamin C for collagen development. Apply vitamin E oil to alleviate crusting.

HERBS FOR A HEALTHY PREGNANCY

Herbs are perfect for the extra growth requirements of pregnancy, childbirth and nursing. They are concentrated, high mineral foods that are easily absorbed by both mother and child. Herbs are identified and accepted by the body's enzyme activity as whole nutrients, lessening the risk of toxemia or overdose. They have been successfully used for centuries to ease the discomforts of bloating, stretching, and the hormone imbalances of pregnancy, without impairing the development or health of the baby.

Herbs are good and easy for you; good and gentle for the baby.

DURING PREGNANCY:
❦ Take two daily cups of Red Raspberry tea, or Crystal Star MOTHERING TEA, a Red Raspberry blend. Both are safe, high in iron and other minerals, strengthening to the uterus and birth canal, effective against birth defects, long labor and afterbirth pain, and elasticizing for a quicker return to normal.
❦ Take kelp tablets, MIODIN DROPS, or Crystal Star IODINE THERAPY CAPS against birth defects.
❦ **During the last tri-mester,** take Crystal Star PRE-NATAL HERBS for gentle, absorbable minerals and toning agents to elasticize tissue and ease delivery. Other formulas providing herbal minerals include Crystal Star IRON SOURCE, CALCIUM SOURCE, **and** MEGA-MINERAL CAPSULES, SILICA SOURCE **and** HIGHLY ABSORBABLE MINERAL COMPLEX EXTRACTS.
❦ **Five weeks before the expected birth date,** take Crystal Star FIVE WEEK FORMULA capsules to aid in hemorrhage control and correct presentation of the fetus.
DURING LABOR:
❦ Take LABOR tincture drops, or Crystal Star CRAMP CONTROL EXTRACT to ease contraction pain, and PANEX CAPSULES for afterbirth pain.
❦ For false labor, drink 4-6 cups catnip/blue cohosh tea to renormalize. If there is bleeding, take 2 capsules each cayenne and bayberry, and get to a hospital or call your midwife.
DURING NURSING:
❦ Add 2 Tblsp. Brewer's Yeast to your diet, along with Red Raspberry, Marshmallow, or Crystal Star MOTHERING TEA to promote and enrich milk.
❦ Fennel, Alfalfa, Raspberrry Lf., Cumin, or Comfrey Lf. teas help keep the baby colic free.
❦ For infant jaundice, use Hyland's BILIOUSNESS Tabs.
DURING WEANING:
❦ Take Parsley/Sage tea to help dry up milk.

BODYWORK FOR TWO

✚ Be sure to get daily exercise during pregnancy. A good brisk walk for fresh air, oxygen and circulation, and aerobic capacity.
✚ Sunbathe every morning for a half an hour if possible for natural vitamin D, calcium absorption and bone growth.
✚ Consciously set aside a stress-free relaxation time each day. Play your favorite restful music. The baby will know and thrive on it.
✚ If you practice reflexology, do not press the acupressure point just above the ankle on the inside of the leg. It can start contractions.
✚ Rub cocoa butter or wheat germ oil on the stomach and around the vaginal opening every night to make stretching easier and the skin more elastic.
✚ Get plenty of rest and adequate sleep. The body energy turns inward during sleep for repair, restoration and fetal growth.

SPECIAL PROBLEMS DURING PREGNANCY

Illness and body imbalances during pregnancy need to be treated slightly differently than a usual approach. Dosage of any medication, natural or allopathic, should be less than normal to allow for the infant's tiny systemic capacity. The mother's body is very delicately balance and sensitive at this time, and problems can occur easily.

The following schedule contains effective natural products that may be used without harm to the baby.

✤ ANEMIA - Take a non-constipating, absorbable herbal iron, such as Floradix LIQUID IRON, yellow dock tea, or Crystal Star IRON SOURCE CAPSULES. Take a good green drink daily, such as apple/alfalfa sprout/parsley juice, Barley Green Magma, Crystal Star ENERGY GREEN DRINK or Chlorella. Add vitamin C and E to your diet, and eat plenty of dark leafy greens.

✤ BREASTS - **for infected breasts,** 500Mg. Vitamin C every 3 hours, 400IU vitamin E, and Beta Carotene 10,000IU daily. Get plenty of chlorophyll with green salads, green drinks, or green supplements such as Chlorella, Crystal Star ENERGY GREEN DRINK or Green Magma.

- **for caked or crusted breasts,** simmer elder flowers in oil and rub on breasts. Wheat germ oil, almond oil and cocoa butter are also effective.

- **for engorged breasts during nursing,** apply ice bags to the breasts to relieve pain.

✤ CONSTIPATION - use a simple soluble fiber laxative, such as Yerba Prima COLON CLEANSE, or Crystal Star CHO-LO FIBER TONE, or a gentle herbal laxative such as Herbaltone. Add additional fiber fruits such as prunes and apples to your diet.

✤ FALSE LABOR - Catnip tea or red raspberry tea will help.

✤ GAS & HEARTBURN - This is usually caused by an enzyme imbalance. Take papaya or bromelain chewables or papaya juice with a pinch of ginger, or Comfrey/Pepsin tablets.

✤ HEMORRHOIDS - Take cascara sagrada or stone root capsules as needed, or Crystal Star HEMRREZE CAPSULES. (These may also be used effectively mixed with cocoa butter as a suppository.)

✤ INSOMNIA - take a liquid or herbal calcium supplement, such as Crystal Star CALCIUM SOURCE CAPSULES, or HIGHLY ABSORBABLE CALCIUM EXTRACT, with Chamomile tea

✤ MORNING SICKNESS - use homeopathic IPECAC and NAT. MUR, add vitamin B 100Mg. 2x daily, sip mint tea whenever queasy, and see MORNING SICKNESS program in this book.

✤ MISCARRIAGE - **for prevention and hemorrhage control** - drink red raspberry tea every hour with 1/4t. ascorbate C powder added, and take drops of Hawthorne or Lobelia extract every hour. See the MISCARRIAGE PREVENTION program in this book for complete information.

✤ POST-PARTUM SWELLING & DEPRESSION - Homeopathic ARNICA.

✤ STRETCH MARKS - Apply wheat germ, avocado, sesame oil, vitamin E, or A D& E oil. Take vitamin C 500Mg. 3-4 times daily for collagen development. See **Stretch Marks** program in this book for more information.

✤ TOXEMIA - take several green drinks such as apple/alfalfa sprout/parsley or Barley Green Magma for a "chlorophyll cleanout". Add vitamin C 500Mg. every 3-4 hours, and 10,000IU Beta-carotene and B Complex 50Mg. daily. Enzymatic Therapy MUCOPLEX and DGL have also been helpful, as has iodine therapy via daily kelp tablets.

✤ UTERINE HEMORRHAGING - Take bayberry and cayenne capsules, and get to professional help immediately.

✤ VARICOSE VEINS - Take vitamin C 500Mg. with Bioflavonoids and Rutin, 4 daily. Drink and apply Crystal Star VARI-VEIN TEA to swollen veins.

PREVENTING **SIDS** - SUDDEN INFANT DEATH SYNDROME: If the baby has a weak system, or poor tissue or lung development (signs that it is a candidate for this condition) give a weak ascorbate vitamin C with bioflavonoids solution in water daily.

HERBAL REMEDIES FOR CHILDREN

A child's body responds very well to herbal medicines. Unless unusually or chronically ill, a child is born with well-developed, powerful immune system, and this inherent resistance ability is a key factor in understanding children's diseases. They often only require the subtle, body strengthening forces that herbs or homeopathic medicines supply. The more highly focused medications of allopathic medicine can have drastic side effects on a small body. We have found that children will drink herbal teas, take herbal drops and syrups, and dissolve homeopathic medicines in the mouth much more readily than you might think. Kids don't want to be sick, they aren't stupid, and they will instinctively recognize natural things that are good for them. The remedies and methods listed in the following section are building, strengthening and non-traumatic to a child's system. Check suggested dosage amounts according to child's age on page 10. Conditions not listed below have their own specific page in the "AILMENTS" section of this book.

☺ ACUTE BRONCHITIS - Give thyme, mullein or plantain tea every 3-4 hours. Chamomile and honey tea will help curb bronchial inflammation. B & T COUGH & BRONCHIAL SYRUP.

☺ CHEST CONGESTION - Herbal steam inhalations with eucalyptus oil, tea tree oil, or Crystal Star RESPIRATOR TEA will help keep lungs mucous free and improve oxygen uptake. Hydrotherapy baths with calendula flowers or strong comfrey tea will induce cleansing perspiration and neutralize body acids. Peppermint and raspberry tea are effective. Apply a soothing chest rub with Tiger Balm, White Flower or calendula oil to loosen congestion after a bath.

☺ CONSTIPATION - Soak raisins in Senna tea and feed to child for almost instant relief. Give weak licorice or mullein tea, molasses in water, or one teaspoon Psyllium husk in Aloe Vera juice 2 times daily. A gentle catnip enema will effectively clear the colon of impacted waste, and allow the body to rid itself of diseased bacteria.

☺ CRADLE CAP - Use vitamin E or jojoba oil, and massage in gently for 5 minutes. Leave on for 30 minutes, then brush scalp with soft baby brush and shampoo with Tea Tree oil or Aloe Vera shampoo. Repeat twice weekly.

☺ CUTS, BURNS & BRUISES - Apply Tea Tree oil, calendula ointment, B & T CALIFLORA GEL, or aloe vera gel every 2 or 3 hours, then apply vitamin E oil at bedtime. Apply B & T ARNIFLORA GEL for bruises and swelling.

☺ DIAPER & SKIN RASH - Mix comfrey, golden seal and arrowroot powders with aloe vera gel and apply to rash. Or use calendula ointment, liquid lecithin, or slippery elm powder. Dab on mineral water, or rub on vitamin A, D & E oil, or TEA TREE CREAM. Expose the child's bottom to sunlight for 20 minutes every day possible for vitamin D nutrients. Wash diapers in water with a teasp. of tea tree oil. An oatmeal bath will neutralize acids coming out through the skin.

☺ DIARRHEA - Give carob powder in apple juice every three hours, and offer several apples every day. Give slippery elm mixed with a little skim milk, or peppermint tea twice daily. Feed plenty of brown rice and yogurt for B Complex vitamins and friendly intestinal flora. Red raspberry, chamomile, and thyme teas are also helpful.

☺ EARACHE - Use mullein essence or garlic oil ear drops directly in the ear. Or mix vegetable glycerin and witch hazel, dip in cotton balls and insert in ear to draw out infection. Give lobelia extract drops in water or juice for pain. See EAR INFECTION PAGE for more information.

☺ FEVER - Catnip tea and catnip enemas will help a moderate fever. The diet should be liquids only - juices, herb teas, such as peppermint and red raspberry, water and broth for at least 24 hours til the fever breaks. A fever is usually a body cleansing and healing process; **a result of the problem, a part of the cure.** See FEVER page in this book for more information. See a doctor if fever is very high.

☺ **GAS & FLATULANCE** - Soak anise seed, dill seed, carraway seed or chamomile in water or juice and strain off. Give tablespoons of liquid every 3-4 hours until digestion rebalances.

☺ **INDIGESTION** - Give chamomile, fennel or catnip tea, or a little ground ginger and cinnamon in water. Use soy milk or goats milk instead of cows milk for digestability. Give a teaspoon of acidolphilus liquid before meals and eating to build healthy flora.

☺ **INSECT BITES & STINGS** - Apply B & T SSSSTING STOP CREAM for pain and itch. (May also be used as a repellent). Or apply TEA TREE OIL. Give vitamin C 100-500Mg. chewables every 4-5 hours to neutralize poison. Use vit. B_1 as a natural insect repellent, 100Mg. 2x daily.

☺ **JAUNDICE** - Give Hyland's BILIOUSNESS TABS. Prick a 100IU vitamin E oil capsule and squirt in mouth. Give a little lemon water with maple syrup.

☺ **MUMPS -** Give 10 drops mullein/lobelia tincture in water every few hours. Give Crystal Star **ANTI-BIO DROPS** in water every few hours to clear the lymph glands. Offer lots of juices and liquids with a pinch of ginger powder in each for stomach cleansing. Take ginger or vinegar/sea salt baths. Make sure the child gets plenty of rest and sleep. Catnip, fenugreek, and scullcap teas are all effective.

☺ **PARASITES & WORMS** - Give raisins soaked in senna tea to cleanse the intestines. Use a garlic enema, or insert a garlic clove in the rectum at night. Give chlorophyll liquid, wormwood tea or herbal pumpkin tablets.

☺ **SORE THROAT** - Give Crystal Star **COFEX TEA** as a throat coat at night for almost immediate relief. Give pineapple juice 2-3x daily as an anti-viral. Use NF Factors HERBALSEPTIC to numb the throat. Mild zinc lozenges and licorice sticks or tea are also effective.

☺ **TEETHING** - Rub gums with honey, a little peppermint oil, or a few drops of lobelia tincture. Give weak catnip, fennel or peppermint tea to soothe irritation. Add a few daily drops of A, D & E oil to food.

☺ **THRUSH FUNGAL INFECTION** - Give Natren LIFE START daily, chewable vitamin C 100Mg. and vit. A 10,000IU. Thrush is often caused by widespread anti-biotic use. Give garlic extract drops in water, or squirt a pricked garlic oil cap in the mouth..Give acidolphilus liquid by mouth, and use as a suppository in the rectum.

☺ **WHOOPING COUGH** - Give Crystal Star **ANTI-SPAZ and ANTI-BIO CAPSULES,** lobelia tincture or Nature's Way ANTSP EXTRACt to control involuntary coughing. Add 10,000IU vitamin A, and 2 cups of red clover or ephedra tea daily. Apply hot ginger/garlic compresses to the chest, and use a eucalyptus steam at night. Give a liquid diet during acute stage with plenty of juices, broths and pure water.

☺ **WEAK SYSTEM** - Add a mineral supplement in liquid or chewable form, such as Floradix MULTIPLE, or Mezotrace MULTI-MINERAL COMPLEX. Give apple and carrot juices. Include a chewable vitamin C wafer every day as a preventive against disease exposure.

ALWAYS KEEP TEA TREE OIL AND "RESCUE REMEDY" HOMEOPATHIC DROPS ON HAND. THEY CAN HANDLE MOST MINOR CHILDHOOD EMERGENCIES NATURALLY AND EFFECTIVELY.

❦ **TEA TREE OIL** - For infections of all kinds where antiseptic or antifungal activity is needed; mouth, tooth, gum, throat, ringworm, fungus, etc. Effective on stings, bites, burns, sunburns, cuts, wounds and scrapes.

❦ **RESCUE REMEDY** - For respiratory problems, coughing, gas, stomach, constipation and digestive upset. A rebalancing calmative for emotional stress and anxiety.

❦ To help prevent contagious disease after exposure, give 1 cayenne capsule 3x a day, 2 chewable vitamin C 500Mg. wafers 3x a day, and a cup of roasted dandelion root tea daily, for the next 3 or 4 days

HEALTHY PETS

NATURAL HEALING FOR ANIMALS

Cats and dogs usually need more nutrition than is found in most commercial animal foods. Most pet foods are derived from low quality ingredients rejected for human consumption. Pet foods that are advertised as "Complete and balanced" are usually based on uncertain minimum nutrition requirements designed only for <u>adequate</u> health, not optimal health. Many vitamins and minerals are lost or lacking through non-standardized "mixmaster" processing that relies heavily on chemical additives to make the food palatable, and the shelf life long. Veterinarians today are seeing many premature and chronic health problems that seem to stem from substandard, poor quality, processed foods.

In general, animals thrive on the healthy foods and balanced diet that is good for people. Whole grains, a little meat, and lots of fresh water every day are basic. And just like people, animals need fresh greens, to keep immunity strong and their systems clean and regular. Unfortunately, also just like people, busy schedules and fast feeding make it difficult to insure that your animals are getting all the nutrition they need. Herbs, homeopathic medicines and high quality natural supplements can help maintain and restore pet health.

❤ DIET FOR A HEALTHY PET: Most pets should have some fresh vegetables every day. Greens keep their systems clean and healthy. Mix them with a little fish, raw liver and kidney, chicken, low ash canned or dry food. Most animals like cucumbers, green peppers, carrots, green onions, parsley, celery and tomato juice.

♥Add whole grains every day for fiber and complex carbohydrates, either from a high quality kibble, or stale bread, crackers or cereal from the kitchen.

♥Give them some dairy foods several times a week. Most animals like cheese, yogurt, kefir, cottage cheese, goat's milk and sour cream.

♥A little fruit is good occasionally to loosen up a clogged system, but give sparingly. Most animals like raisins, coconut, cantaloupe and apples.

♥Have fresh water available all day long. Most animals need lots of liquids every day.

♥A good sample meal for general health can be made up all at once and divided between feedings. Mix lightly: 1 small can, or about 6-8 oz. meat, 3t. Brewer's yeast, 1 raw egg, 1 cup chopped vegetables, a little broth or water to moisten. THEY'LL LOVE IT.

♥Avoid junk foods and refined foods for your pets. They are even worse for their smaller, simpler systems than they are for you.

❤ SUPPLEMENTS FOR A HEALTHY PET: Food source supplements are wonderful for animals. Wheat germ oil, Spirulina, kelp, brewer's yeast, bran and lecithin are all good for keeping animals as well as people in tip top condition.

Crystal Star has a very successful food and herbal supplement for animals.

HEALTHY LIFE ANIMAL MIX™ is a delicious food sprinkle packed with nutrients for a shiny coat and eyes, for healthy gums and teeth, for good temperament, regularity, immune strength and freedom from fleas and ticks. HEALTHY LIFE gives animals the valuable benefits of concentrated greens to keep the blood strong, the body regular and the breath and stomach sweet. It is rich in Beta Carotene for natural immune strength. HEALTHY LIFE is high in anti-oxidants such as vitamin C and E to help control arthritis and displaysia symptoms, and help prevent damage from rancid fats or poor quality foods. It is full of natural enzymes for easier digestion and regularity. All kinds of animals love it, from hamsters to horses. Some of them (including our own) won't eat without it!

Homeopathic remedies are also wonderful for animals, both in liquid and tablet form. They are effective, gentle, non-toxic, and free of side effects. They heal without harming.

Keep TEA TREE OIL, food grade **1%** H_2O_2, (1oz. 3% solution in 1 qt. water) and RESCUE REMEDY EXTRACT on hand for your pets. These natural medicinals can handle many minor emergencies, and even some major problems. All are effective and non-toxic, and can be used externally as well as internally

❤ BODYWORK FOR A HEALTHY PET: Brush and comb your animals often. It keeps their coats shiny, circulation stimulated, and they like the attention.

♥Avoid commercial, chemical-impregnated flea collars. They often have DDT or a nerve gas in them.

♥Sprinkle cedar shavings around your animal's sleeping place to keep insects away and make the area smell nice.

♥Use Nature's Miracle Liquid for accident clean-up. It is all natural, non-toxic, and it works.

GIVE YOUR PETS LOTS OF LOVE AND AFFECTION. IT IS ALWAYS THE BEST MEDICINE FOR HEALTH AND HAPPINESS. THEY NEED IT AS MUCH AS YOU DO.

ALTERNATIVE NUTRITIONAL HEALING FOR ANIMALS

ARTHRITIS: ☙ Avoid refined and preserved foods, especially white flour and sugar.
☙ Reduce red meat and canned foods. Add green and raw foods.
☙ Make a comfrey/flaxseed or alfalfa tea, and add to animal's drinking water.
☙ Give 2 teasp. cod liver oil 100-200IU vitamin E daily, 6-8 alfalfa tablets and 1/4 teasp. sodium ascorbate, Ester C powder, or vitamin C crystals daily.
☙ H_2O_2 1% solution in water - 1 teasp daily for 1 month.
☙ Give Crystal Star RTH EASE CAPSULES and TEA, (1/2 dose)
☙ Give Crystal Star HEALTHY LIFE ANIMAL MIX 2 teasp. daily.

BAD BREATH:
☙ Feed more fresh raw foods, less canned processed foods. Snip fresh parsley into food at each meal.
☙ Sprinkle a little spirulina powder or liquid chlorophyll on food.
☙ Give Dr. Goodpet GOOD BREATH homeopathic remedy.

BLADDER INFECTION/INCONTINENCE:
☙ Give vitamin C 250Mg. 2-3 times daily, B Complex 10-20Mg. once daily.
☙ Put the animal on a liquid diet for 24 hours with vegetable juices and broths - no solid foods. Offer lots of fresh water.
☙ Give magnesium tablets, 100Mg. daily for a week.

CANCERS/LEUKEMIA/MALIGNANT TUMORS:
☙ Give buffered vitamin C as sodium ascorbate powder, 1/4 teasp. twice daily for larger animals, and cats with Leukemia, or Alacer Emergen-C in water. As tumor starts to shrink, decrease vitamin C to a small daily pinch.
☙ Feed fresh garlic cloves, or Garlic/Parsley tablets daily.
☙ Give vitamin E 200IU daily, and apply vitamin E oil locally if there is a tumor or malignancy.
☙ Give 1 teasp. Cod liver oil, or Beta Carotene 10,000IU daily.
☙ Give dilute **1%** food grade H_2O_2- 2-3 teasp. daily to both dogs and cats.
☙ Dilute a golden seal/echinacea extract to 1/2 strength. Give 1/4 teasp.daily.

COAT & SKIN HEALTH:

- Add lecithin granules or Crystal Star HEALTHY LIFE MIX to food daily.
- Add 2 teasp. cod liver oil to food daily.
- Give vitamin E 100IU daily. Apply E oil or jojoba oil to affected skin areas.
- Add 1 teasp. Spirulina or kelp powder to food daily.
- Give Dr. Goodpet SCRATCH-FREE to curb itching and dry hot spots.

CONSTIPATION:

- Add more greens and vegies to the diet; decrease canned food.
- Add Crystal Star HEALTHY LIFE MIX for soluble food fiber.
- Mix a little garlic powder with 1 Tblsp. olive oil and add to food.
- Exercise the animal more often. Let it outside more often for relief.

CUTS & WOUNDS:

- Apply a golden seal/myrrh solution, or comfrey salve.
- Give vitamin C crystals (as sodium ascorbate if possible) 1/4-1/2 teasp. in a cup of water. Apply directly, and give internally throughout the day.
- Apply vitamin E oil. Give vitamin E 100IU daily.
- Apply calendula ointment.
- Apply Nutrition Resource NUTRIBIOTIC SPRAY as needed.
- Apply Aloe vera gel and give desiccated liver tabs or powder in food daily.

DEHYDRATION:

- This is a major emergency for cats. Check for dehydration by pulling up the scruff of the neck. If skin is slow to return, animal is dehydrated. Take to a vet as soon as possible.
- Make a comfrey tea immediately. Force feed if necessary about 2oz. an hour Mix a little bran, tomato juice, sesame oil. Feed each hour til improvement.
- Try to feed green vegies; especially celery, lettuce and carrots for electrolyte replacement. Once the crisis has passed, add kelp or spirulina to the diet.
- Check for worms, often a cause of dehydration.
- Give the animal lots of love and attention. Dehydration is often caused by depression. The animal simply curls up and will not eat or drink anything. RESCUE REMEDY is excellent in this case.

DIARRHEA:

- Diarrhea is often caused by spoiled food, non-food items, worms or harmful bacteria. Put the animal on a short 24 hour liquid diet with vegetable juices, broths, and lots of water.
- Give yogurt or acidolphilus liquid at every feeding til diarrhea ends.
- Give Brewer's yeast and 1 teasp. carob powder at every feeding.
- Sprinkle crushed activated charcoal tablets on food.
- Use Dr. Goodpet DIAR-RELIEF homeopathic remedy.

DISTEMPER:

- If the problem is acute, put the animal on a short liquid diet with vegetable juices, broths, and plenty of fresh water.
- Give vitamin C crystals (sodium ascorbate if possible), 1/4 teasp. mixed in a cup of water, and divided throughout the day. If there is severe vomiting and loss of fluids, give some of the vitamin C liquid every hour. Or give Dr. Goodpet CALM STRESS homeopathic remedy to calm vomiting.
- Add 1/2 dropperful B Complex liquid and 1 teasp bonemeal to food daily.
- Give dilute (1 drop in 2 teasp. water) golden seal/myrrh, or echinacea tincture. Or give echinacea tea to flush and neutralize toxins.
- Give yogurt or acidolphilus liquid to rebuild friendly flora and immunity.
- Give fresh garlic, or a garlic/honey mixture daily. Add raw liver or desiccated liver tablets several times a week.
- Add brown rice and bran to daily food for B vitamins and system tone.

ECZEMA:
    ↝ Give Zinc 25Mg. internally, and apply zinc ointment to infected areas.
    ↝ Mix cottage cheese, corn oil, vitamin E oil, and Brewer's yeast. Give 1 Tblsp. daily. Or give 1 teasp. cod liver oil mixed with 1 Tblsp. Garlic powder daily.
    ↝ Give 1-2 teasp. wheat germ daily. Apply locally to sores.
    ↝ Reduce meat and canned foods. Add fresh vegies and greens to the diet.

EYE & EAR INFECTION:
    ↝ Add Beta carotene 10,000IU, 1 teasp. cod liver oil, and vitamin E 100IU to the diet. Cod liver oil and E oil may also be applied locally.
    ↝ Give goat's milk daily in food, and apply with cotton balls to the eye.
    ↝ Use Dr. Goodpet EYE-C homeopathic remedy for eyes, EAR RELIEF for ears.
    ↝ Give homeopathic Nat. Mur in early stages, and Silicea in later stages for reversal of cataract development.
    ↝ Apply an eyebright herb tea or Crystal Star EYELIGHT TEA to infected area.

FLEAS/TICKS/MITES:
    ↝ String eucalyptus buds around animal's neck and sleeping area.
    ↝ Put eucalyptus, pennyroyal, and citronella oils on pets collar.
    ↝ Rub rosemary, myrrh, or tea tree oil directly on animal's coat between shampoos to drive off insects and leave a nice scent. Stuff a pillow with rosemary, pennyroyal, eucalyptus and mint leaves, and place on animal's bed.
    ↝ Sprinkle Crystal Star HEALTHY LIFE MIX, Dr. Goodpet FLEA RELIEF homeopathic remedy, or brewer's yeast on food daily.
    ↝ Give 1/2 of a 100Mg. vitamin B_1 tablet daily to ward off insects.
    ↝ Apply Tea Tree oil directly on the insect to kill it. Apply jojoba oil on the bitten place to heal it faster.

GAS & FLATULENCE:
    ↝ Give alfalfa tabs, spirulina, or dilute chlorophyll liquid at each feeding.
    ↝ Sprinkle a pinch of ginger powder on food at each feeding.
    ↝ Give comfrey, chamomile or peppermint tea daily.

GUM & TOOTH PROBLEMS:
    ↝ Apply a dilute golden seal/myrrh or propolis solution to gums.
    ↝ Give and apply dilute chlorophyll liquid solution.
    ↝ Give a natural fresh foods diet, adding crunchy raw vegies and whole grains.
    ↝ Apply vitamin E oil, tea tree oil, or calendula oil to gums.

HIP DISPLAYSIA & LAMENESS (SEE ALSO ARTHRITIS):
    ↝ Mix 1 teasp.sodium ascorbate, or Ester-C crystals in water and give throughout the day, every day.
    ↝ Mix 1 teasp. bonemeal powder with a cup of tomato juice, 1 teasp. bran and 1/2 teasp. sesame oil and give daily.
    ↝ Mix 2 teasp. Cod Liver oil, 1 Teasp. bonemeal, 1 Tblsp. Lecithin. Give daily.

INTESTINAL & STOMACH PROBLEMS:
    ↝ Put the animal on a short liquid diet for 24 hours, with water, broth and green juices, to clear the intestines. Then feed yogurt or liquid acidolphilus and fresh foods for 2-3 days. Give Comfrey tea in the water bowl.
    ↝ Give Crystal Star HEALTHY LIFE MIX with extra garlic powder daily.

MANGE & FUNGAL INFECTION:
    ↝ Put drops of tea tree oil in the animals shampoo and use every 2 or 3 days.
    ↝ Apply Pau de Arco salve, zinc ointment, fresh lemon juice to relieve area.
    ↝ Add bonemeal powder to food to ease tension and curb frantic licking. Or use Dr. Goodpet CALM -STRESS homeopathic remedy.
    ↝ Apply dilute echinacea tincture, or golden seal/echinacea/myrrh water solution to affected areas daily. Also sprinkle on food.

❧ Use Nutrition Resource NUTRIBIOTIC SPRAY on the areas several times daily.

❧ Give 1 teasp. lecithin granules daily. Mix 2 teasp. cod liver oil with 1 Tblsp brewer's yeast and 2 teasp. desiccated liver powder and give daily.

OVERWEIGHT:

❧ Reduce canned foods. Increase fresh foods, whole grains and organ meats.

❧ Give Crystal Star HEALTHY LIFE MIX for fiber without calories.

❧ Add more exercise to the animal's life.

PREGNANCY & BIRTH:

❧ Give red raspberry tea daily during the last half of gestation for easier birth.

❧ Give daily spirulina tabs or powder for extra protein.

❧ Give desiccated liver tabs, extra bonemeal. and cod liver oil daily.

❧ Give extra vitamin C 100Mg. chewable, and vitamin E 100IU daily.

RESPIRATORY INFECTIONS & IMMUNE STRENGTH:

❧ Put animal on a short liquid diet for 24 hours to cleanse the system, with vegetable juices, broths and water. Offer comfrey tea to flush toxins faster.

❧ Add 1 teasp. Bee Pollen, vitamin E 100IU, and 1/4 teasp. vitamin C (as sodium ascorbate if possible) dissolved in a cup of water to diet.

❧ Add dilute **1%** food grade hydrogen peroxide to the diet for oxygen therapy.

❧ Add 2-4 garlic tablets and 6 alfalfa tablets to the daily diet.

❧ Give Crystal Star HEALTHY LIFE MIX for immune strength, and COFEX TEA for dry hacking cough.

WORMS & PARASITES:

❧ Build up immunity for the best long term solution with Crystal Star HEALTHY LIFE MIX on a daily basis.

❧ Put the animal on a short 24 hour liquid fast with **water only** to weaken the parasites. Then give Crystal Star VERMEX CAPS as directed in water or an electuary for 3-7 days. Repeat process in a week to kill hatched eggs.

❧ Give garlic and cloves daily til worms are gone.

❧ Give spirulina for a month after worming to rebuild immune strength.

AILMENTS
IN ALPHABETICAL ORDER

EACH AILMENT PAGE CONSISTS OF A FOUR POINT PROGRAM:
FOOD THERAPY, VITAMIN/ MINERAL THERAPY, HERBAL THERAPY AND **BODYWORK.**

These programs can be used in several ways, according to the individual person's needs. A mixture of remedies may be employed in each area, or just one or two areas may be used. Pick the suggestions that you feel instinctively strong about. They are invariably the best for you, and will be the easiest to incorporate into your lifestyle.

ALL THE REMEDIES HAVE BEEN FOUND EFFECTIVE, BUT EVERY PERSON HAS A DIFFERENT BODY AND IS A DIFFERENT INDIVIDUAL. HEALING AND RESPONSE SEEM TO ACCELERATE WHEN A PERSON PICKS OUT HIS OWN AREAS OF NATURAL THERAPY.

◆ **Bold print entries** indicate the most successful, or most often used therapeutics.

◆ Where a method has also proven effective for children, a small child's face ☺ appears at the end of the recommendation.

◆ Where a method has proven particularly successful for women, a female symbol ♀ appears at the end of the recommendation.

◆ Where a method has proven particularly successful for men, a male symbol ♂ appears at the end of the recommendation.

All recommended doses are daily unless otherwise specified. Dosage listed is for the major time of healing, and is not to be considered as maintenance or long term.

The traditional rule of thumb for natural healing is one month for every year you have had the problem.

❖ Note: At the time of this writing, L-Tryptophane has been recalled by the FDA, and is not available until a safe source is found. It is recommended in this book as an effective sleep aid and relaxant, with every expectation of its safe return to the public.

ABSCESSES

BOILS ◆ SUPPERATING SORES

FOOD THERAPY	VITAMINS/ MINERALS	HERBAL THERAPY	BODYWORK
Go on a short 1-3 day juice diet (pg.27), followed by a fresh foods cleansing diet to remove toxins.	Beta-carotene A , 100,000IU daily for 1 week. **with** Vit. E 400IU 2x daily.	**Echinacea extract 3x daily under the tongue.**	Take a catnip enema to clean out toxins.
Mix grated garlic with lemon juice. Apply.	Vit. C ascorbate powder, 3-5 grams daily.	Propolis tincture - apply directly, take internally, 2x daily.	Apply an epsom salts compress.
Boil flax and fenugreek together. Mash pulp. Apply to abscess.	Zinc 50-100Mg. daily.	Crystal Star ANTI-BIO caps; 6 daily for 3 days, 4 daily for 1 week. **with** Crystal Star CLEANSING & FASTING TEA for 1 week.	**Apply a St. John's wort poultice.**
Eat yogurt, kefir, acidolphilus for friendly intestinal flora.	Liquid chlorophyll - apply locally. Take internally, 3t. daily.	**Black walnut tincture. Take internally. Apply directly.**	Apply Nature's Herbs BLACK OINTMENT.
Drink 6-8 glasses of pure water a day.	**Apply tea tree oil.**	Apply aloe vera gel.	Apply Echinacea salve or cream, or Echinacea tincture drops.
	Apply calendula gel.	Apply a green clay compress 2x daily.	Expose the area to early morning sunlight for 15 min. a day.
	Take MEGA-DOLPHILUS 3x daily. **with** Garlic caps, 2 caps 3x daily.		
	Apply Nutrition Resource NUTRIBIOTIC SPRAY as needed.		

COMMON SYMPTOMS: Inflammation and infection of the skin layers; supperation; weeping pus-filled sores.

COMMON CAUSES: Toxicity of the system; acid condition allowing a staph infection; viral infection.

65

ACIDITY ✧ ACIDOSIS

RESTORING ACID/ ALKALINE BODY BALANCE

FOOD THERAPY

🐾 Go on a short 24 hour (pg. 28) liquid fast to cleanse acid wastes. Then eat alkalizing foods: salads, green vegies, sprouts, apples, figs, potatoes, beets, cucumbers, carrots, goat's milk, vegie juices, etc.

🐾 Drink a daily 8oz. glass mix of tomato juice, wheat germ, brewer's yeast, lecithin. ♂
or
Drink 1-2 glasses of cranberry juice daily ♀

🐾 Crystal Star MIN-ZYME-MINOS DRINK MIX daily in water.

🐾 Eat smaller meals. Chew slowly.

VITAMINS/ MINERALS

✢ **Ascorbate vit. C crystals 3000Mg. daily.**

✢ HCl tabs after meals.
or

✢ High potency digestive enzymes at meals.

✢ B Complex 100Mg. with extra Pantothenic acid 500Mg. 2 daily.

✢ Twin Labs LIQUID K 2t. daily.

✢ Source of Life FOOD SENSITIVITY SYSTEM daily.

HERBAL THERAPY

🐾 Crystal Star FIBER & HERBS COLON CLEANSE CAPS to clean out acid waste.

🐾 Take 2 Ginger caps daily **and** use ginger compresses on the kidneys to increase elimination of toxins.

🐾 Effective teas:
Catnip ☻
Chamomile ♀
Fennel

BODYWORK

❖ Mild exercise every day for body oxygen.

❖ Have a little wine before dinner to relax and reduce body acid.

❖ Avoid yeasted breads, pasteurized dairy, red meats, processed sugars til condition clears.

❖ **Crystal Star ALKALIZING ENZYME BODY WRAP for almost immediate change in body pH.**

❖ REFLEXOLOGY POINT:

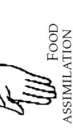

FOOD ASSIMILATION

COMMON SYMPTOMS: Frequent skin eruptions; arthritic symptoms; burning stools, anal itching; acid stomach; bad breath and body odor; chronic poor digestion.

COMMON CAUSES: Mental stress and tension; excess acid-forming foods (caffeine, fried foods, tobacco sweets).

ACIDOSIS is often related to or caused by arthritis, diabetes or borderline diabetes. Refer to those pages in this book.

ACNE ✧ PIMPLES ✧ BLEMISHES

FOOD THERAPY	VITAMINS/ MINERALS	HERBAL THERAPY	BODYWORK
❧ Go on a short 1-3 day liquid cleanse (pg.27) to clear out acid wastes. Use apple, carrot, pineapple and papaya juices. Then eat lots of fresh foods. One salad every day. Add often to the diet: whole grains, green vegies, brown rice, seafood, sea vegetables, sprouts, low fat dairy, apples.	✤ Mix 1/4 teasp. vitamin C crystals with 1 Tblsp. acidolphilus liquid and take 4 x daily.	❦ Relieve infection and inflammation first with Crystal Star ANTI-BIO CAPS OR EXTRACT, 4 x daily for 1 week. then take	❖ Apply H_2O_2 peroxy gel to affected areas for 1-2 months. Do not squeeze. Blemishes and black-heads will come to the surface and be eliminated.
	✤ Beta carotene 100,000IU with vitamin D 1000IU daily	❦ High potency royal jelly 2 teasp. daily ♀ with	❖ Rub face with insides of papaya and cucumber skins to neutralize acid wastes.
	✤ ACT CLEAR pancreatin to digest oils with 1 Tblsp. Omega 3 Flax or fish oil daily. or 1 packet GREEN MAGMA	❦ Crystal Star BEAUTIFUL SKIN TEA. Drink & apply with cotton balls. or ❦ Crystal Star THERADERM CAPS as directed.	❖ Steam face with SWISS KRISS herbs; or eucalyptus and thyme.
❧ NO red meats, white flour or sugar, soft drinks, caffeine, fried foods, candy, pasteurized dairy.	✤ Zinc 50-100Mg daily with B_2 100Mg. daily.	❦ Apply a Golden Seal and Myrrh solution, or ❦ Propolis tincture directly to sores. ♂	❖ Get some early morning sun on the face every day possible. Get fresh air and exercise daily, lots of rest to eliminate toxins.
❧ NO JUNK FOODS.	✤ Enzymatic Therapy DERMA CLEAR cream & soap, with ACNE-ZYME.		
❧ Rub on lemon juice or aloe vera gel at night. Wash in the morning.	✤ Apply tea tree oil to sores 3x daily. Use tea tree soap.	❦ Drink and pat on daily Burdock/Sarsaparilla/ Sassafras tea for pH balance. ♂	
❧ Drink 6-8 glasses of bottled water daily.	✤ Apply 2-3 Nutrition Re-source NUTRIOBIOTIC LIQUID CONC. drops directly and massage in.	❦ Evening primrose oil 4-6 daily, with Kelp 6 tablets daily.	

COMMON SYMPTOMS: Inflamed and infected pustules on the face, chest and back. Often itching and scarring.

COMMON CAUSES: Hormone (particularly Pituitary) imbalance during high growth years; bad diet, especially saturated fats and fried foods and excess sugar; (a rise in blood sugar is multiplied by 5 when it gets to the skin. Sugar saturated skin is very susceptible to the bacterial infection of acne) liver toxicity and malfunction; poor digestion of fats and oils; EFA deficiency; poor elimination and constipation; allergy-causing facial cosmetics; impure blood; overeating and lack of green vegies.

67

ADRENAL GLAND HEALTH

FOOD THERAPY

❧ The importance of good diet is essential to adrenal health. Eat small, instead of large meals, low in sugar and fats. Eat lots of fresh foods, brown rice, and whole grains.

❧ See DIET FOR HYPOGLYCEMIA in this book.

❧ Take 2 T. each daily:
Brewer's yeast
Wheat germ

❧ Make a mix of Flax seed/Bran/Broth/Honey. Take some each day to feed adrenals.

VITAMINS/ MINERALS

❖ **Adrenal complex glandular, such as Country Life ADRENAL WITH TYROSINE. ♂**

❖ Enzymatic Therapy LIQUID LIVER WITH SIBERIAN GINSENG. ♂

❖ **Pantothenic acid 500-2000Mg. daily. with**

❖ Tyrosine 500Mg. daily.

❖ B Complex 100Mg.

❖ Ascorbate vitamin C - 3000Mg, or Ester C 1500Mg. daily.

❖ High potency digestive enzymes, such as Rainbow Light DOUBLE STRENGTH ALL-ZYME, to stimulate adrenal cortex production.

❖ **Vitamin E 400IU daily.**

HERBAL THERAPY

❧ Crystal Star ADRN-ALIVE CAPSULES or ADRN EXTRACT, 2 x daily with BODY REBUILDER CAPS to stimulate hormone rebalance.

❧ **High potency Premier One or YS ROYAL JELLY, 2 t. daily. (highest source of natural pantothenic acid available)**

❧ Miodin 1-2 drops daily ♀

❧ Siberian Ginseng caps 2 daily. ♂

❧ Effective teas:
Licorice Rt.
Hawthorne
Gotu Kola
Ginger

❧ Astragalus/Ginseng capsules, 4 daily. ♂

BODYWORK

❖ Stimulation and nourishment of the adrenals is an aid in the healing of Arthritis, Bronchitis, Hypoglycemia, exhaustion, fatigue, and the hormone imbalances found in P.M.S. and menopause

❖ REFLEXOLOGY POINT:

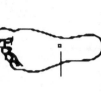

ADRENALS

COMMON SYMPTOMS: Lack of energy and alertness; a sense of being 'driven' and anxious , followed by great fatigue; low blood pressure and poor circulation; moodiness; irritability; low immunity; brittle nails, dry skin.

COMMON CAUSES: Stress; poor diet with too much sugar and refined carbohydrates; over use of alcohol or recreational drugs; too much caffeine; vitamin B and C deficiencies.

AGE SPOTS ✧ LIVER SPOTS

FOOD THERAPY

🌿 Go on a short liquid diet (pg.27) to clear the liver of toxins. **Age spots are often the visible sign that the body is throwing off metabolic wastes through the skin**

🌿 Then drink carrot/beet/cucumber juice once a week for the next month to keep the liver clean.

🌿 Follow the LIVER CLEANSING PROGRAM in this book. Include lots of fresh foods and green salads. Avoid acid forming foods such as red meat, caffeine, etc.

🌿 Avoid rancid nuts and oils.

🌿 Take 2 T. Brewer's yeast daily.

VITAMINS/ MINERALS

❖ **Ascorbate vitamin C crystals 1/4 teasp. in water 4 x daily.**
with
❖ **Beta Carotene A 100,000IU and vitamin D 1000IU daily to clear the liver.**

❖ **Take vitamin E 400IU and apply to spots. ♂**

❖ Rainbow Light DETOX-ZYME 3-4 daily.

❖ **High Omega 3 fish or flax oil 3 x daily.**

❖ B Complex 100Mg.

❖ **Evening Primrose oil 2-4 daily.**

HERBAL THERAPY

🌿 **Biotec AGELESS BEAUTY 4 daily to metabolize rancid fats in the Liver ♀**

🌿 Crystal Star LIV-ALIVE CAPSULES and LIV FLUSH TEA.
with
HERBAL ENZYMES CAPSULES as a liver digestive stimulant.

🌿 Premier One high potency ROYAL JELLY, 2 teasp. daily. ♀

🌿 Apply Dong Quai extract to spots. Take Dong Quai/Ginseng capsules 3-4 daily. ♀

🌿 Effective teas:
**Rose Hips
Chamomile
Dandelion Root
Take both internally and apply to spots.**

🌿 Take a glass of lemon juice and water daily, and apply lemon juice to spots.

BODYWORK

❖ Avoid excess sun exposure.

❖ REFLEXOLOGY: press point on stomach just above the navel. Stroke downward in the area of the liver under the right breast.

❖ FOOT REFLEXOLOGY:

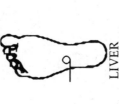

LIVER

❖ **Rub on H$_2$O$_2$ PEROXY GEL every night for 1-3 months til clear.**

COMMON SYMPTOMS: Brown mottled spots on the hands, neck and face.

COMMON CAUSES: Liver malfunction and exhaustion; poor assimilation and digestion.

AGING & LONGEVITY

FOOD THERAPY	VITAMINS/ MINERALS	HERBAL THERAPY	BODYWORK
Include high fiber foods daily, from fruits, vegetables, whole grains, to assure a free flowing system.	Ester C with Bioflavs. 1-3000Mg. daily.	Sun CHLORELLA TABS OR DRINK daily.	Do deep breathing and mild stretching exercises every morning - outdoors if possible for early sunlight and to keep oxygen levels high.
Keep the body alkaline through greens, soy foods, and sea vegies.	CO Q 10 3-4 daily, with vitamin E 400IU with Selenium, and Beta-Carotene 25,000IU.	Crystal Star MIN-ZYME-MINOS DRINK MIX daily.	Take a walk every day, especially after your largest meal, for circulation and enzyme activity. **Exercise is a nutrient in itself.**
Eat fish or seafood every week for Omega 3 oils, and iodine for metabolic balance.	Biotec EXTRA ENERGY ENZYMES 3 daily. with Mezotrace SEA MINERAL COMPLEX 2 daily.	**Ginkgo Biloba 2 daily. with bee pollen daily.** or Premier One or YS ROYAL JELLY 2 t. daily.	
Eat cultured foods to promote friendly intestinal flora; yogurt, kefir, sauerkraut, etc., a glass of wine at dinner.	All 1 VITAMIN/ MINERAL DRINK daily. ♂	Siberian Ginseng tea or caps daily for men. ♂ Dong Quai/Damiana caps or extract for women. ♀	**Take an occasional "oxygen bath" with 1/2 cup 35% food grade H_2O_2 in spa or bath.**
Drink 6-8 glasses of bottled water daily.	Ener-B internasal B_{12}.	Efamol EVENING PRIMROSE OIL caps 2-4 daily. ♀	*No smoking.* Besides all its other well documented hazards, smoking uses up available body and tissue oxygen.
Avoid refined foods, red meats, fried foods, and caffeine.	Solaray CHROMIACIN 2 X daily.	Atomodine drops in water for iodine therapy and metabolic increase. (Add wheat germ oil for oxygen)	Remember that it is normal to eat and sleep less as metabolism slows.
	Enzymatic Therapy LIQUID LIVER W. SIBERIAN GINSENG ♂		
	Twin Labs CHOLINE OR CHOLINE/ INOSITOL.		

COMMON SYMPTOMS: Memory loss and impairment; loss of sex drive; low immunity; a decrease in lean body mass; poor digestion, assimilation and elimination; arthritic and joint stiffness; decreased physical activity; weakened respiratory capacity; poor skin, organ and muscle tone; thyroid decrease.

REMEMBER: THAT AGE IS NOT THE ENEMY; ILLNESS IS. KEEP IMMUNITY STRONG. SYSTEMATICALLY UNDEREAT TO KEEP SLIM AND WEIGHT DOWN. (EXTRA WEIGHT AGES SEXUALLY, PHYSICALLY AND MENTALLY). ENJOY A REGULAR SEX LIFE. (ENDOCRINE ACTIVITY KEEPS YOU YOUNG). OFFER LOTS OF LOVE AND AFFECTION. THERE IS NOTHING LIKE LOVE AND EMOTIONAL INVOLVEMENT TO KEEP LIFE YOUTHFUL, INTERESTING AND WORTHWHILE..

AIDS ✧ ACQUIRED IMMUNE DEFICIENCY ✧ ARC ✧ AIDS RELATED COMPLEX

FOOD THERAPY

🌰 Diet should be the highest possible nutrition A modified macrobiotic diet is ideal for high resistance and immune strength.

🌰 The intestinal pH environment must be changed to optimize disease protection. **See diet for AIDS & ARC on the following pages.**

🌰 Take 3-4 glasses of fresh carrot juice daily or 300,000IU Beta Carotene to stimulate effective T cell activity.

🌰 Take a potassium broth or essence every day for ongoing detoxification.

🌰 NO junk foods; particularly no caffeine, sugar, alcohol or tobacco.

🌰 **Avoid all pleasure drugs.**

VITAMINS/ MINERALS

❖ **Egg yolk lecithin. Active Lipids that render the cell walls resistant to attack.**

❖ Effective anti-oxidants:
  ◆ **Germanium 150Mg. 6 x daily with Astragalus 2 daily.**
  ◆ **COQ 10 30 Mg. 2 x daily for strong T-Cells and T-Cell formation.**
  ◆ **H₂O₂ PEROXY GEL rubbed on the feet, or 3% liquid, 1T in 8oz. water taken internally.**
  ◆ **Ester C powder with Bioflavonoids, 10-30 grams daily by injection or orally.**

❖ Effective enzymes:
  ◆ **Rainbow Light DETOX-ZYME with meals.**
  ◆ **Biotec EXTRA ENERGY ENZYMES S.O.D.**

❖ **Megadolphilus LIFE START #2, 3 teasp. daily for G.I. balance. The HIV virus lives in the intestinal tract.**

❖ Pro-biologic aqueous solution LIPISOL for Beta-carotene uptake.

HERBAL THERAPY

🐾 **Crystal Star DETOX, ANTI-BIO CAPS or EXTRACT, and HERBAL DEFENSE TEAM CAPS or EXTRACT as directed.**
  with

🐾 **LIV-ALIVE CAPS or LIV TONIC EXTRACT. The liver must be working for the immune system to be restored.**
  and

🐾 **ADRN ALIVE CAPS or EXTRACT for exhausted adrenals. ANEMIGIZE CAPS for stronger blood and energy.**

🐾 **Sun CHLORELLA, 2 packets daily with Enzymatic Therapy LIQUID LIVER WITH SIBERIAN GINSENG**

🐾 **Echinacea extract 3 x daily to encourage interferon**

🐾 **St John's Wort extract** proven effective against retro viruses.

🐾 **Aloe Vera juice 3 glasses daily to curb virus spread, with Garlic extract caps 8 daily.**

🐾 **Country Life ENERGIX VIALS 1 daily**

BODYWORK

❖ **IT IS ABSOLUTELY NECESSARY TO CLEAN THE LIVER FOR THERE TO BE ANY HEALING.**

❖ **REFLEXOLOGY POINT:**

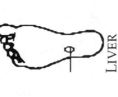
LIVER

❖ Avoid anal intercourse. Avoid needle-injected and all pleasure drugs. Practice safe sex. Make sure any blood transfusion plasma has been tested for HIV virus.

❖ Take a colonic once a week til recovery is well underway to remove infected feces from the intestinal tract.

❖ Get fresh air and sunlight on the body every day. Get mild exercise daily, and lots of rest.

❖ See Overheating therapy on the next page.

THE HOLISTIC APPROACH TO AIDS & ARC

More and more people with this tragic disease are turning to alternative therapies and taking responsibility for their own research and treatment. This kind of direct action enables things to move very fast, and we can get a much clearer understanding of treatment and response. Indeed there are enough success stories just in the last eighteen months from the people themselves, and the holistic practitioners working with them, to sense a small triumph for natural healing therapies. A much more positive picture is emerging. AIDS, ARC, and other immune deficiency diseases are no longer seen to be inevitably fatal as they were before. Holistic programs are frequently causing symptoms to abate and gradually disappear. The advance of the virus itself has been slowed in many instances, and improved longevity and quality of life are observed even in full-blown AIDS cases. As more and more people with these diseases see their own progress, return to work, and pick up their lives, more expertise is coming into the field; holistic physicians, homeopaths, naturopaths, chiropractors, therapists, nutritional counselors and others.

California cities have become the leader in this effort, and a mecca for dedicated people with the latest knowledge and successful therapies. Seek them out if you need help in this area. We are seeing improvement, energy return, and diminishment of symptoms every day.

The following schedule is an updated listing of holistic therapies we are aware of that have achieved measureable success with AIDS and ARC. Doses are generally quite high when beginning these therapies, and may be reduced as improvement is observed. Treatments may be used together or separately as desired by each individual, along with the recommendations of a competent professional with personal case knowldge.

❖ **ASCORBATE VITAMIN C CRYSTALS** - use calcium ascorbate, or a mixed mineral ascorbate with bioflavonoids; to flush and detoxify the tissues. Take ORALLY 10-20 teasp. daily for 2-3 weeks, then reduce to 10 grams twice a week. Mega-doses may be resumed as necessary. INTRAVENOUS dose - 100-150 grams daily for 2-3 weeks, reducing to 30 grams every week for maintenance.

❖ **VITAMIN E** - 1000IU daily, **WITH SELENIUM** as sodium selenite drops or selenomethionine.

❖ **RAW THYMUS EXTRACT** - 1 tablet 3 x daily or 1/2 dropperful 2 x daily to strengthen immunity.

❖ **ECHINACEA EXTRACT OR PAU DE ARCO EXTRACT** - 1/2 dropperful 3 x daily, to stimulate production of interferon, interleukin and lymphocytes, **OR** 4-6 cups daily of the following immune restorative tea: Steep for 30 minutes: Prince Ginseng Roots, dry Shiitake Mushrooms and soaking water, Echinacea Angustifolia and Purpurea Root, Schizandra Berries, Astragalus, Ma Huang, Pau de Arco Bark and St. John's Wort.

❖ **ACIDOLPHILUS CULTURE COMPLEX WITH BIFIDUS** - refrigerated, highest potency, 3 teasp. daily with BIOTIN 1000MG.

❖ **FRESH VEGETABLE JUICES** - a good juicer such as Champion is critical to juice potency. Take Carrot/Beet/Cucumber juice 1-3 x daily with garlic extract and Flax oil added, to detoxify the Liver. Chew 1-3 DGL tablets during the day to neutralize released acids.

❖ **AGED ALOE VERA JUICE** - 2-3 glasses daily; found to block the virus spread from cell to cell.

❖ **EGG YOLK LECITHIN** - highest potency from Jarrow Corp.

72

❖ ANTI-OXIDANTS - such as COQ 10 30Mg., Germanium 100-150Mg. AND Octacosanal 1000Mg. to overcome the side effects and nerve damage from AZT, and to strengthen white blood cell and T-cell activity. Take with Quercitin Plus with Bromelain 500Mg. 3x daily, and high potency digestive enzymes, such as Rainbow Light Detox-Zyme.

❖ CARNITINE - 500Mg. daily for 3 days. Rest for 7 days, then take 1000Mg. for 3 days. Rest for 7 days. Take with high omega 3 fish or flax oils, 3-6 x daily, or Evening Primrose oil 1000Mg. 3 x daily.

❖ VITAMIN B COMPLEX - 100-200Mg. 3 x daily, with extra Pantothenic Acid 250Mg. and Zinc 30-60Mg.

❖ HYDROGEN PEROXIDE, food grade PEROXY GEL OR 3% SOLUTION - by injection with a qualified practitioner or orally 1T. in 8oz. of water, 3-4 x daily, or rubbed on the feet morning and evening. Alternate use, one week on and one week off for best results.

❖ GERMANIUM - highest potency 200Mg. 3x daily. with ASTRAGALUS capsules.

❖ SUN CHLORELLA - 15-20 tablets or 2 packets of granules daily for immune building.

❖ SHARK LIVER OIL - increases leukocytes and white blood cell activity to fight infection.

❖ ST. JOHN'S WORT EXTRACT OR CRYSTAL STAR " ANTI-VI" EXTRACT (50% St. John's Wort/50% Lomatium) 3 x daily.

❖ OVERHEATING THERAPY has been effective against AIDS by speeding up metabolism and inhibiting growth of the invading virus.

COMMON SYMPTOMS: Extreme fatigue; lack of energy; inability to heal even minor ailments; progressive degeneration of the body; fever; night sweats; constant respiratory infections; chronic diarrhea.

COMMON CAUSES: Breakdown of the immune system due to abuse of drugs and infective needles; malnutrition on a wide scale; virulent infection that the body cannot fight; infected blood transfusion; toxic pleasure drugs; anal sex with an HIV positive person; widespread antibiotic and vaccination use.

NOTE: It is easy to transfer HIV virus through anal intercourse, more difficult through vaginal or oral sex. Enzymes in the saliva, friendly flora in the intestinal tract, and HCl in the stomach produce a hostile environment that destroys the virulence of the virus. There is no such protection in the colon. Many people test "HIV positive" with no symptoms of AIDS or ARC.

Depression of the immune system is believed to occur when the HIV virus slips through the intestinal wall and into the bloodstream. The immune system attacks the virus with macrophages that then die and are removed through the lymphatic system. This toxic waste is finally dumped into the colon on its last leg of clearance from the body, but in an unprotected colon without friendly bacteria or a good defensive pH environment, new HIV virus hatch from the dead macrophages, and multiply in the feces all over again to repeat the same cycle. The immune system cannot detect the virus in the colon and does not marshal its forces until it is in the bloodstream; often too late if immune defenses are exhausted.

The following protocol for treating AIDS is based on a fresh foods macrobiotic diet, colon cleansing and the addition of friendly flora to create a hostile environment for the growth of the pathogenic bacteria.

73

DIET DEFENSE AGAINST AIDS & ARC

A high resistance, immune-building diet is primary to success in overcoming this condition. It is a major disease, and treatment must be approached with vigorous commitment. The intestinal environment must be changed to create a hostile environment for the pathogenic bacteria. (This protocol is also effective against Candida Albicans and some types of Cancer) The following liquid and fresh foods diet is for the ill person who needs drastic measures - a great deal of concentrated defense strength in a short time. It represents the first "crash course" stages of the change from cooked to living foods. It has been successful in the reversal of HIV positive to HIV negative, and in great improvement of full-blown AIDS cases. The space in this book only allows for an abbreviated form of this diet. The complete program with supporting recipes, may be found in "COOKING FOR HEALTHY HEALING" by Linda Rector-Page.

This is a modified macrobiotic diet, emphasizing more raw than cooked foods, and **mixing in acidolphilus powder with foods that are cooked** to convert them to living nourishment with friendly flora. As with other immune depressing viral diseases, the pathogenic HIV bacteria live on dead and waste matter. We have found that for several months at least, the diet should be vegetarian, low in dairy, yeasted breads and saturated fats, and eliminating meats, fried foods, and dairy products except yogurt and kefir, Coffee, alcohol, salt, sugars and all refined foods must be avoided, and of course, all drugs should be excluded, (even prescription drugs if possible). The ultra purity of this diet controls the multiple allergies and sensitivities that occur in immune deficiencies, yet still supplies the needs of a body that is suffering primary nutrient privation. For most people, this way of eating is a radical change, with major limitations, but the health improvement for AIDS and ARC is excellent.

THE FOLLOWING IS A SUGGESTED DAILY OUTLINE:

ON RISING: take 2-3 Tblsp. cranberry concentrate in 8 oz. of water with 1/2 teasp. ascorbate vit. C crystals added; **or** cut up 1/2 a lemon (with skin) and blend in the blender with 1 tsp. honey and 1 cup distilled water. Strain. **Add 1/2 teasp. Natren LIFE START 2** lactobacillus complex or **Alta Health CANGEST** to either of these drinks.

Take a brisk walk for exercise and morning sunlight.

BREAKFAST: have a glass of fresh carrot juice with 1 T. Bragg's LIQUID AMINOS, **and** whole grain muffins or rice cakes with kefir cheese;
or a cup of yogurt with sesame seeds, walnuts and fresh fruits added;
or a cup of soy milk mixed in the blender with a cup of fresh fruit, some walnuts, and 1/2 t. Natren LIFE START 2.;
or oatmeal, amaranth or buckwheat pancakes with yogurt and fresh fruit.

MIDMORNING: take a weekly colonic. On non-colonic days, take a potassium broth or essence with 1 Tblsp. Bragg's liquid aminos **and** 1/2 teasp ascorbate vitamin C crystals added;
and have another fresh carrot juice, or pau de arco tea, with 1/2 teasp. Natren LIFE START 2 powder added.

LUNCH: have a fresh green salad with lemon/flax oil dressing, with some tofu, avocado or sprouts;
or an open-faced sandwich on rice cakes or a chapati with fresh vegies and soy or yogurt cheese;
or a cup of miso soup with rice noodles or brown rice;
or some steamed vegies and tofu with millet or brown rice;
Take a cup of pau de arco tea or aloe vera juice with 1/2 teasp. ascorbate vit. C and 1/2 teasp Natren LIFE START 2.

MIDAFTERNOON: have a carrot juice with Bragg's LIQUID AMINOS and 1/2 teasp. Natren LIFE START 2 added;
and a green drink such as Sun CHLORELLA, BARLEY GREEN MAGMA, or Crystal Star ENERGY GREEN, with 1/2 t. ascorbate vitamin C crystals added.

DINNER: have a baked potato with Bragg's LIQUID AMINOS,soy cheese or kefir cheese and a green salad;
and another potassium broth or essence with 1/2 teasp. Natren LIFE START 2 added;
or black bean or lentil soup and a tofu and vegie casserole;
or a fresh spinach or artichoke pasta with steamed vegies and lemon/flax oil dressing;
or a Chinese steam stir-fry with shiitake mushrooms, brown rice and vegetables.
Sprinkle a little Natren LIFE START 2 or Alta Health CANGEST powder over any cooked food at this meal.

BEFORE BED: take a glass of aloe vera juice with 1/2 teasp ascorbate vit. C crystals and 1/2 teasp. Natren LIFE START 2;
and a fresh carrot or papaya juice, or alkalizing drink such as Crystal Star MIN-ZYME-MINOS.

Unsweetened mild herb teas and bottled water are recommended throughout the day for additional toxin cleansing and alkalizing.
1/2 teasp. ascorbate vitamin C powder may be added to any drink throughout the day to bowel tolerance for optimum results.

AIR POLLUTION & SMOG

WAYS TO GUARD AGAINST ITS EFFECTS IN YOUR BODY

FOOD THERAPY	VITAMINS/ MINERALS	HERBAL THERAPY	BODYWORK
Drink only pure water. about 6 glasses daily	Beta-Carotene A 100,000IU daily. with	Crystal Star MIN-ZYME-MINOS DRINK MIX daily. and/or HEAVY METAL CAPS 2 daily. ♂	Get lots of body oxygen. Take a walk every day, breathing deeply of fresh air.
Eat a high fiber, high vegetable protein diet, low in fats and sugars.	Vit. C w/ bioflovonoids 5,000Mg. daily. and	H₂O₂ food grade gel rubbed on the soles of the feet every 2 or 3 days to keep body oxygen high.	Use an air ionizer if possible, where pollutants are worst.
Eat Miso soup and Miso foods often to neutralize environmental toxins.	Vit. E w/ Selenium 400IU 2 x daily.	Garlic 4 tabs daily. Kelp 6-8 tabs daily.♀	Take warm relaxing baths. Use a dry skin brush to remove toxins on the skin.
Take 2 T. daily each: Brewer's yeast Wheat germ	Effective anti-oxidants: DMG B₁₅ 125Mg. daily. COQ 10 30Mg. 2 x daily. Chlorella 15 tabs daily.	Barley Green Magma or Crystal Star ENERGY GREEN DRINK MIX daily.	See ALLERGIES SECTION in this book for more information.
	Glutathione 2 daily.		
Add more green leafy vegetables to the diet.	Zinc 75-100Mg. daily.♂		
	Pantothenic acid 250Mg. 2x daily.		
	Biotec SOD 6 daily for free radical scavenging.		
	Kal PYCNOGENOL for effective defense against free radicals. ♂		

COMMON SYMPTOMS: "Allergy type" reactions of coughing, wheezing, congestion, chronic bronchitis, emphysema, respiratory infections; difficulty in breathing; headaches; skin itching and rashes; eyes itching and burning; asthmatic symptoms.

COMMON CAUSES: Smoking and being around a smoker; auto engine exhaust; industrial/chemical pollutants in the air; heavy metals carried in the air by winds; agriculture and fossil fuel pollutants.

✳ Also see IMMUNITY: BUILDING, STRENGTHENING & MAINTAINING IT IN TODAY'S WORLD in this book.

76

ALCOHOL ABUSE

FOOD THERAPY

🐾 Go on a short juice fast (pg. 26 or 27) to clean out alcohol residues.

🐾 **Then follow the hypoglycemia diet in this book for 3 months. Avoid all refined foods, sugars, caffeine, fried foods, heavily spiced foods. They aggravate the craving for alcohol.**

🐾 **The diet should be high in Magnesium. Most alcoholics have a severe deficiency;** include wheat germ, bran, Brewer's yeast, whole grains and cereals, brown rice, green leafy vegetables, potatoes, miso, low fat dairy, eggs and fish.

🐾 Take a Vegex broth at night to curb craving.

VITAMINS/ MINERALS

❖ Mega-vitamin therapy is effctive here. **To curb alcohol craving, take either of the following combinations daily with meals for a month:**
2 Glutamine 500Mg.
2 Cysteine 500Mg.
2 B Complex 100Mg.
3 Ascorb. Vit. C 1000Mg.
2 Niacinamide 500Mg.
2 Zinc 50Mg.♂
or

❖ **3 Solaray Chromiacin
2 Twin Lab GABA Plus
3 Glutamine 500Mg.**

❖ 2 Tryptophane 500Mg.♀

❖ Enzymatic Therapy LIVATOX 3 daily.

❖ B₂ 300Mg. with Folic acid 800Mg. and Choline 600Mg. daily

❖ **DLPA 750Mg. with Tyrosine 500Mg. and 500Mg. Magnesium.♀**

HERBAL THERAPY

🦂 Spirulina 500Mg. or 1 packet of Sun Chlorella or Crystal Star ENERGY GREEN DRINK MIX daily.

🦂 Rainbow Light DETOX-ZYME 3 daily.♂

🦂 Crystal Star LIV-ALIVE CAPS and LIV-TONIC EXTRACT for detox-ification, ADRN EXTRACT and HIGH ENERGY TEA for energy support.

🦂 Raw Brain glandular **with Taurine 2 daily and Zinc 50Mg.** to calm nerves and withdrawal effects. ♂

🦂 Evening Primrose oil caps 2-4 daily. ♀

🦂 4 Chaparral caps or 2 cups Angelica tea every time craving occurs

BODYWORK

❖ **Acupuncture is successful in curbing addiction to alcohol.**

❖ Keep system oxygen high. Get some fresh air and exercise every day.

❖ Keep the liver clean. No detox program will work without concentrated, continued effort in this area. See Liver Detox program in this book.

❖ Be sure to follow a High Mineral Diet for a solid nutritional foundation. (See COOKING FOR HEALTHY HEALING by Linda Rector-Page)

COMMON SYMPTOMS: Alcohol addiction, and inability to stop drinking; short term memory loss; liver disease; high blood sugar; nervousness and poor coordination; high LDL cholesterol and blood sugar malfunction; malnourishment, especially mineral deficiency.

COMMON CAUSES: Excessive intake of alcohol influenced by Hypoglycemia, poor diet high in refined and sugary foods, deficient in fresh and high mineral foods; excessive daily stress and tension; emotional problems.

ALLERGIES ✧ ENVIRONMENTAL & SEASONAL

FOOD THERAPY	VITAMINS/ MINERALS	HERBAL THERAPY	BODYWORK
✤ Go on a short mucous cleansing diet (pg.25) to release allergens from the body. Then begin a diet with non-mucous-forming foods: fresh vegetables and fruits, whole grains, cultured foods such as yogurt, raw dairy, seafoods.	✤ High Omega 3 fish or Flax oils 3 x daily.	✤ Crystal Star ALRG CAPS or ALRG-HST EXTRACT.	✤ Diet change is the single most beneficial thing you can do to control allergies.
	✤ Ascorbate Vitamin C or Ester C powder with bioflavonoids 1/4-1/2t. every 3 hours to flush and detoxify tissues; then reduce to 5000Mg daily.	✤ Crystal Star RESPIRATOR CAPS and TEA.	✤ Relax. Stress and tension aggravate allergies.
		✤ Evening Primrose oil caps 4 daily. ♀ or	
		✤ High potency Royal Jelly 2 teasp. daily. ♂	✤ Take a daily walk with deep breathing exercise.
✤ Lemon water in the morning, and a green drink during the day will flush excess mucous and support clean body energy.	✤ Quercetin Plus 1000-2000Mg. daily with Bromelain 500Mg. for antigen induced allergies.	✤ Crystal Star ADRN-ALIVE CAPSULES or ADRN EXTRACT and POLLEN-EX TEA. 2 x daily.	✤ Use COCA'S PULSE TEST or muscle testing to identify allergens.
	✤ B Complex 100Mg. with extra Pantothenic acid 1000Mg.	✤ Germanium 30Mg. daily with Suma.	✤ Stop smoking. It magnifies allergies more than almost any other practice.
✤ Avoid all refined and preserved foods, sugars, caffeine, oxalic acid forming foods, dairy products and other mucous-forming foods during healing.	✤ Alta Health CANGEST ENZYMES 3 X DAILY.	✤ Effective extracts: Bilberry Ginkgo Biloba leaf Lobelia 10 drops 3 x daily.	
	✤ Raw Adrenal 2 x daily. ✤ Raw Thymus 3 x daily.		
✤ Drink bottled water.	✤ Manganese 5Mg. 2 daily	✤ Unsprayed Bee Pollen 3 t daily. ♂	

COMMON SYMPTOMS: Runny nose and eyes; chronic lung, bronchial and sinus infections; skin itching and rashes; asthma; migraines; edema; menstrual disorders; hypoglycemia; learning disabilities.

COMMON CAUSES: Excess mucous and waste accumulation in the body due to poor diet; junk foods; adrenal exhaustion; stress; hypoglycemia; candida albicans yeast overgrowth; EFA deficiency; free radical damage; elevated histamine levels.

ALLERGIES ✧ FOOD SENSITIVITY & INTOLERANCE

FOOD THERAPY

🐚 Go on a short **24 hour fast** (pg. 27) to clear the system of allergens. **Then follow a diet emphasizing fresh organically grown produce and grains.**

🐚 **Avoid common allergens: mushrooms, pasturized dairy foods, wheat, eggs, yeast, sugar, corn, nightshades.**

🐚 Include lots of manganese-rich foods: buckwheat, nuts legumes, blueberries.

🐚 **Eat plenty of cultured foods to add friendly flora to the G.I. tract.**

🐚 Take 2 T. apple cider vinegar/honey at each meal to acidify saliva.

VITAMINS/ MINERALS

✤ **Quercetin Plus with Bromelain 3 daily.**

✤ Ester C up to 5000Mg. daily to help the liver produce anti-histimines.

✤ **Alta Health MANGANESE WITH B₁₂ SUBLINGUAL.**

✤ A full spectrum digestive enzyme such as Rainbow Light ULTRA-ZYME or Alta Health CANGEST. ♂ and/or Betaine HCl with meals

✤ Rainbow Light FOOD SENSITIVITY CAPSULES with meals.♀

✤ Liquid Chlorophyll 1t. 3 x daily before meals.

HERBAL THERAPY

🐚 **Y.S. bee pollen/royal jelly/honey combination, 2t. daily.**♂

🐚 Crystal Star ANTI-HST CAPSULES or ALRG-HST EXTRACT to help the liver normalize anti-histimine production.

🐚 Barley Green Magma 1 packet daily, **or** Crystal Star ENERGY GREEN.

🐚 Aloe Vera juice daily. ♂

🐚 Comfrey/Pepsin tabs

🐚 Crystal Star HERBAL ENZYMES after meals to aid food assimilation. ♂

🐚 Natra Bio homeopathic
◆ FOOD ALLERGY - GRAIN
◆ FOOD ALLERGY -DAIRY.

BODYWORK

✤ Many childhood allergies are the result of feeding babies meats and pasteurized dairy foods before 10-12 months. Babies do not have the proper enzymes before this time to digest these. Feed mother's milk, soy milk, or goat's milk for at least 8 months to avoid food allergies.

✤ Use COCA'S PULSE TEST or muscle testing to identify allergens.

✤ Use a garlic/catnip enema to cleanse the digestive tract, and balance colon pH.

✤ REFFLEXOLOGY POINT

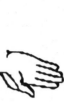

FOOD ASSIMILATION

COMMON SYMPTOMS: The inability to eat normal amounts of a food; cyclical headaches; hypoglycemia;hyperactivity in children; excessively swelled stomach, nausea or tiredness after eating; palpitations, sweating, mental fuzziness after eating.

COMMON CAUSES: Eating chemically altered, sprayed, injected or processed foods that the body cannot handle; overconsumption of too few foods; food additives such as nitrites and sulfites; stress; poor diet; alkalosis with low gastric pH and enzyme deficiency; insufficient sleep; emotional trauma; chronic infections; eating a particular allergen food.

＊ **See COOKING FOR HEALTHY HEALING" BY LINDA RECTOR-PAGE for a full diet to overcome food allergies.**

FOOD THERAPY	VITAMINS/ MINERALS	HERBAL THERAPY	BODYWORK
Follow the HEALTHY HEART DIET in this book Eat vegetable protein brain foods: eggs, soy foods, sea vegetables, whole grains, nuts, seeds, fresh vegetables, etc. Your diet should be low fat, low salt, low meat, and low dairy with plenty of soluble fiber.	Niacin therapy 250-500Mg. 3 x daily. with Omega 3 fish or flax Flax oils 3 x daily.	Crystal Star MENTAL CLARITY CAPSULES. (Do not take if there are blood pressure problems)	Get daily mild exercise and/or use hot and cold hydrotherapy for brain and circulation stimulation.
Take the following mix every morning with juice or cereal: 1T. Lecithin granules 1T. Brewer's Yeast 1T. Wheat Germ oil 1T. Oat or Rice Bran 1T. Blackstrap Molasses 1T. Canola oil ♂	Ester C w/ Bioflavs up to 3000Mg. daily. with PC 55 Phosphatidyl Choline 3 x daily or Choline 1-5 grams daily with pantothenic acid 250Mg. for uptake,	Ginkgo Biloba extract or capsules 2-3 x daily. Premier 1 or YS Royal Jelly 2-3t. daily. ♀	Decrease prescription diuretics if possible. They leach potassium and nutrients needed by the brain.
Drink only bottled water for good blood circulation and brain health.	Twin Lab LIQUID K or WHITE BIRCH MINERAL WATER 2 t. daily. ♂	Ginseng/Gotu Kola capsules 2 daily. or Siberian Ginseng extract drops in water.♂	Avoid aluminum and alum containing products: cookware, deodorants, cannned foods, salt,buffered aspirin, antacids, refined and fast foods, relishes, pickles, tobacco, etc. Read labels!
	Vitamin E 400IU daily, with Beta carotene 25M.	Crystal Star MEGA-MINERAL CAPSULES with CREATIVI-TEA 2 x daily.♀	
	Cal/Mag/Zinc 4 daily to lower blood aluminum.	Garlic 4 capsules daily.	Reflexology pressure points for the brain: ◆ Squeeze all around the hand and fingers. ◆ Pinch the end of each toe. Hold for 5 seconds.
	ENER-B vit. B₁₂ nasal gel every 2-3 days.	Crystal Star POTASSIUM SOURCE CAPS and/or SILICA SOURCE EXTRACT 4 x daily.♀	
	Glutamine and/or Glycine 500Mg. with B₆ 250-500Mg. ♂		

COMMON SYMPTOMS: Loss of ability to think clearly and remember past or present facts, names places, etc; loss of touch with reality; befuddlement.

COMMON CAUSES: Poor or obstructed circulation; arteriosclerosis; anemia from long or excess drug use; decrease in hormone output; lack of exercise and body/brain oxygen; lack of enough pure water; fluid accumulation in the brain; thyroid malfunction; emotional shock, such as the death of a spouse.

FOOD THERAPY	VITAMINS/ MINERALS	HERBAL THERAPY	BODYWORK
❧ Eat iron-rich foods for red blood formation: Liver, organ meats, figs, seafood, beets, brown rice and whole grains, eggs, grapes, raisins, almonds, yams, etc.	✤ ENER-B VIT. B_{12} internasal gel every 3 days. **and** Floradix LIQUID IRON 2 x daily **with** Betaine HCl or Alta Health MANGANESE at meals for best uptake.	❧ Crystal Star ANEMI-GIZE CAPSULES, IRON SOURCE CAPSULES or HIGHLY ABSORBABLE IRON EXTRACT 3 x daily til blood count improves. **or**	✤ Take a good protein drink (pg. 39) or a good green drink (Pg. 34) every morning.
❧ Eat manganese-rich foods for iron uptake.		❧ ENERGY GREEN DRINK MIX 2 x daily.	✤ Get some mild exercise daily to enhance oxygen uptake. Get morning sunlight every day possible for vit. D.
❧ Eat cultured foods for friendly bacteria and B_{12} production: Yogurt, kefir, soyfoods.	✤ Sun CHLORELLA 15-20 tabs daily.	❧ Spirulina 6 tabs daily.	✤ Avoid pesticides, sprays and fluorescent lighting that cause mineral leaching from the body.
	✤ B Complex 100Mg, with extra B_6 and B_2.	❧ Effective teas: Yellow Dock Pau de Arco Dandelion Root	
❧ Eat potassium rich foods, or take a potassium broth (Pg. 33) til blood count improves.	✤ Enzymatic Therapy LIQUID LIVER WITH GINSENG 2 x daily.♂ **or**	❧ Effective capsules: ◆ Beet root ◆ Siberian Ginseng ♂ ◆ Dong Quai ♀ ◆ Kelp ◆ Crystal Star POTASSIUM SOURCE CAPSULES	
❧ Take 2T. each daily: Brewer's yeast, wheat germ, sesame seeds.	✤ Desiccated Liver 6 daily.		
	✤ Kal Folic Acid w / B_{12}.	❧ REMEMBER: Food or herbal iron souces are best for absorbability.	
❧ Avoid acid-forming foods: sodas, caffeine, red meat, etc.	✤ Vitamin. E 400IU with COQ 10 for healthy liver/spleen function.		

COMMON SYMPTOMS: *Weakness, dizziness, headaches, palpitations, lack of sexual energy, gastro-intestinal bleeding; ulcers; slow healing; fatigue; pallor; violent mood swings; irritability; spots before the eyes.*

COMMON CAUSES: Recurring infections and diseases indicating low immunity and mineral deficiency; B 12 and folic acid deficiency; poor diet, poor food assimilation; Candida Albicans, Lupus, or other auto-immune condition; excessive menstruation; lack of green vegetables; alcoholism.

81

ANOREXIA NERVOSA ✧ BULEMIA ✧ MALNUTRITION

FOOD THERAPY

🐚 Emphasis must be on high nutrition for rebuilding and regeneration.
Eat a high vegetable protein, high complex carbohydrate diet. NO junk foods, heavy starches or sugars..

🐚 Breakfast is important, with whole grain cereals, and/or a good protein drink such as Nature's Plus SPIRUTEIN OR All 1.

🐚 Take 2 T. each daily:
Brewer's Yeast
Wheat Germ
Blackstrap Molasses

🐚 Eat slowly; chew well; small meals for better absorption.

🐚 Have a green drink or carrot juice often for blood building energy.

VITAMINS/ MINERALS

❖ ENER B VIT. B$_{12}$ inter-nasal gel or folic acid with B$_{12}$ for cell growth and energy.

❖ Gamma Oryzonal (GO) 60Mg. for better calorie utilization, with BCAAs for muscle growth.♂

❖ A GABA compound for stress relief and nerve rebuilding, such as Natrol SAF OR Country Life RELAXER CAPSULES. with

❖ Ester C WITH BIOFLAVS. 3000MG. daily for tissue collagen growth

❖ Potassium liquid 3 x daily. Much is lost from vomiting and laxatives.

❖ A good food source mutiple, such as Rainbow Light MASTER NUTRIENT SYSTEM.

HERBAL THERAPY

🐚 **Crystal Star BODY REBUILDING CAPSULES WITH ADRN-ALIVE CAPS 2 each daily.**
and

🐚 ANEMI-GIZE CAPSULES for red blood cell rebuilding.

🐚 Crystal Star ENERGY GREEN DRINK for herbal nutrition and minerals.

🐚 Ginseng/ Gotu Kola caps to stimulate a healthy appetite.♂

🐚 **High potency Premier 1 or YS ROYAL JELLY 3-4 t. daily.**

🐚 Alta Health SIL-X caps or Crystal Star SILICA SOURCE EXTRACT for collagen/tissue growth.

🐚 MEGA-DOLPHILUS powder 1/4t. 3x daily for food absorption.

BODYWORK

❖ Get some mild exercise every day for lung and heart rebuilding.

❖ Psychological counseling is often helpful here for an understanding of the problem, and in begin-ning to deal with it.

❖ HAND REFLEX POINT:

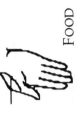

FOOD ASSIMILATION

COMMON SYMPTOMS: Extreme malnutrition from vomiting/laxatives that discharge most nutrients; abnormal desire for thinness at any cost.

COMMON CAUSES: Eating disorders are often caused by emotional problems that end up turning into this form of psychosis.

APPENDICITIS

CHRONIC

FOOD THERAPY

☙ Go on a short vegetable juice diet (Pg.26) to clear and clean the intestines. Take one potassium drink (Pg. 33) daily during this fast.

☙ Then, eat sweet fruits for a day to encourage healing.

☙ Then, resume a mild foods simple diet and include a glass of carrot juice daily for 2 weeks.

☙ Avoid refined and fried foods on a continuing basis.

☙ Make sure the diet is high in soluble fiber for prevention.

☙ Take no solid food or laxatives during an attack.

VITAMINS/ MINERALS

❖ Beta Carotene 25,000IU 4x daily,
with
Liquid Chlorophyll in water 3 x daily.

❖ Natren MEGADOLPHILUS POWDER 1/4t. in water 4 x daily **or New Chapter BIO-FLORA for friendly bacteria and enhanced peristalsis.**

❖ Ester C or ascorbate vit. C crystals 1/4t. in water 4 x daily.

❖ **Vit. E 400IU 2 x daily.**

❖ Living Source STRESS MANAGEMENT COMPLEX multi-vitamin daily.
and
Rainbow Light ULTRA ZYME TABLETS at meals.

❖ **Zinc picolinate 30Mg.**

HERBAL THERAPY

🦂 Crystal Star MIN-ZYME-MINOS DRINK MIX for alkalinity and better food absorption.

🦂 Crystal Star ANTI-BIO CAPSULES OR EXTRACT every 2 hours to lower infection and inflammation.

🦂 Effective Teas:
Alfalfa
Slippery Elm

🦂 Solaray REFRESH CAPSULES or Yerba Prima COLON CARE SYSTEM after an attack for 6 days to clean the colon of infection.

🦂 Echinacea extract 4 x daily under the tongue.

BODYWORK

❖ **If there is danger of appendix rupture, you need surgery. DON'T DELAY!**

❖ **Do not take high colonics or enemas during an attack.**

❖ Keep the colon clean. Constipation is usually the cause of an attack. Use a mild catnip enema. ☺

❖ Use alternating hot and cold cayenne/ginger compresses on affected area & along spine.

❖ REFLEXOLOGY POINT:

APPENDIX

COMMON SYMPTOMS: Intense sharp pain on the right side at the waist.

COMMON CAUSES: Poor diet, lacking in fiber and roughage; too many antibiotics; too many laxatives resulting in lack of peristalsis and friendly bowel flora.

ARTERIOSCLEROSIS ✧ ATHEROSCLEROSIS

FOOD THERAPY	VITAMINS/ MINERALS	HERBAL THERAPY	BODYWORK
Follow the HEALTHY HEART DIET in this book. As a rule, vegetarians have healthier hearts and arteries.	Vital Health FORMULA 1 chelation therapy with EDTA.♂ and CO Q 10 10Mg. 2x daily.	Crystal Star CARDI-STRENGTH CAPSULES or HAWTHORNE EXTRACT 2 x daily. and/or HEMA-CLEANSE TEA. ♀	Arteriosclerosis is not only preventable, but reversible.
Avoid saturated fatty foods such as red meats, full-fat dairy products, fried foods and refined low fiber foods.	Lecithin 1900Mg. daily with Chromium picolinate 2 daily.	Ginkgo Biloba extract under the tongue 2-3x daily and	Stop smoking. Keep your weight down. Relax. The stress and tension from these life styles can cause big artery problems.
Eat plenty of high fiber whole grains and lots of fresh greens.	High omega 3 fish or flax oils 3 x daily.	Sun Chlorella tabs 15-20 tabs or 1 packet daily.	A little wine at dinner can relax stress and raise HDLs.
Take one cup daily of the following mix: 2t. wheat germ 2t. honey 1T. lecithin in 1 cup fenugreek tea.	High potency Pancreatin as a fat and oil digestant. ♂	Apple Pectin 4 x daily.♂	Take a brisk walk daily. Then use a dry skin brush over the body to stimulate circulation. or
	Country Life B₁₅ DMG SUBLINGUAL as a prime anti-oxidant.	Lecithin 1900Mg. daily with Garlic caps and vitamin E 400IU with selenium daily.	Take an alternating hot and cold shower to increase blood flow.
Eat smaller meals, esp. at night. Have a little wine at dinner for digestion/relaxation.	Ester C 3000Mg. daily with bioflavonoids.	Evening Primrose oil caps, 4-6 daily for 1 month, then 3-4 daily.	Love and affection, both given and taken, really reduces heart and arterial problems.
	Niacin 500Mg. 2 x daily with Zinc 50Mg. daily to raise HDL levels.	Ginseng/Cayenne capsules 4 daily.♂	
	Beta Carotene 25,000IU 2 x daily.	Butcher's Broom for a limited time to increase circulation and thin sluggish blood.	

COMMON SYMPTOMS: Poor circulation with cold hands and feet; mild heart attacks; difficulty in thinking and breathing; blurred vision; high blood pressure.

COMMON CAUSES: Too much saturated fat and refined food in the diet; smoking; obesity; stress; lack of aerobic exercise; too much caffeine and alcohol; excess salt.

ARTHRITIS

OSTEOARTHRITIS ✦ RHEUMATOID ARTHRITIS

FOOD THERAPY

☙ Diet change is the single most beneficial thing you can do to control the causes and symptoms of arthritis. See the following pages for a brief control diet. See "COOKING FOR HEALTHY HEALING" by Linda Rector-Page for a complete diet with corresponding recipes.

☙ A proper diet can prevent or neutralize arthritis even in long-standing cases. A modified macrobiotic diet can be particularly helpful. (See page 42).

☙ Start a healing program with a short juice fast to clear out toxic wastes. (Pgs. 26)

☙ Foods to avoid: refined, fatty and salty foods pasteurized dairy, pastries, sugars, caffeine, red meats, and highly spiced foods.

VITAMINS/ MINERALS

❖ Quercetin Plus w/Bromelain 2 daily.
   or
❖ Biotec EXTRA ENERGY S.O.D. w/ CATALASE and Betaine HCl at meals.

❖ DLPA 750Mg. or GABA as needed for pain.♀

❖ Source Naturals GERMANUM 100Mg. with COQ 10 30Mg. 2x daily

❖ Ester C 500Mg. with Bioflavonoids 10 daily for collagen synthesis.

❖ Solaray CAL / MAG WITH BORON AND D for uptake. and

❖ Omega 3 Flax oil 3 x daily.

❖ Oral Chelation 2 packets daily. ♂

❖ Niacin therapy 1000Mg. 3 x daily

❖ Country Life LIGATEND as needed for flexibility and B Complex 100Mg. daily.

HERBAL THERAPY

❧ Crystal Star R^TH EASE CAPS AND/ OR TEA as directed, with 4 each LIV-ALIVE AND ADRN-ALIVE CAPSULES daily.

❧ Ginkgo Biloba extract capsules 250Mg. daily. with

❧ Alta Health SIL-X silica extract caps. 3 daily.

❧ Effective capsules:
   Yucca 4 daily
   Devil's Claw Rt. 4 daily
   Turmeric 4 daily
   Alfalfa 10 daily
   Kelp 8 daily

❧ Pantothenic acid therapy sources:
   ◆Premier 1 or YS Royal Jelly 2 t. daily.
   ◆Enzymatic Therapy ADRENAL COMPLEX

❧ Evening Primrose oil 4 daily. ♀

❧ Aloe Vera juice 1 glass daily.♂

❧ Sun CHLORELLA 2 packets or 20 tabs daily

BODYWORK

❖ Use hot and cold Hydrotherapy showers
   or
   hot epsom salts baths.

❖ Crystal Star ALKALIZING ENZYME HERBAL WRAP.

❖ Apply H_2O_2 PEROXY GEL to soles of feet every 24 hours for tissue oxygen and flexibility.

❖ Massage painful joints with TIGER BALM, WHITE FLOWER OIL, B & T TRI-FLORA GEL, or ALOE VERA GEL.

❖ Have a good chiropractic adjustment.

❖ Apply for pain relief: CAMO CARE CREAM TRIFLORA ANAGESIC GEL OR herbal compresses cayenne/ginger cajeput/wintergreen

❖ NO SMOKING. Tobacco is a nightshade plant. N.B. Motrin is also a nightshade derivative. It is anti-inflammatory but should not be used by nightshade sensitive people.

85

There are two major categories of arthritis: ◆ **Osteoarthritis**, the most common type, is a "wear and tear" disease primarily affecting the bones with a breakdown in the cartilege that normally protect the ends of the bones. This buffer cartilege prevents bone ends from rubbing together, wearing each other away, and causing a great deal of pain. The joints are also painfully affected, as osteoarthritis often forms calcified deposits in them.

◆ **Rheumatoid arthritis** is a systemic disease, a chronic inflammation of the joints, muscles, ligaments and tendons. Crippling and deformities of the affected areas are the end result.

COMMON SYMPTOMS: ◆ OSTEOARTHRITIS: Stiffness, pain, immobility of the joints; bone deterioration; inorganic sediment in the joints; pain and swelling in the joints and spine during damp weather.

◆ RHEUMATOID ARTHRITIS: Inflammation and swelling of the joints; pain affecting the whole body; destruction of cartilege tissue due to poor calcium assimilation; digestive problems; great fatigue; anemia; ulcerative colitis; chronic lung and bronchial congestion; neurological depression; liver malfunction.

COMMON CAUSES OF BOTH OSTEOARTHRITIS & RHEUMATOID ARTHRITIS: Calcium depletion; osteoporosis; gland and hormone imbalance; prolonged use of anti-arthritic drugs, like cortisones, that eventually impair the body's own healing powers; poor diet, lacking in fresh vegetables and high in acid and mucous-forming foods; auto-toxemia from poor bowel movements and constipation; inability to relax resentments and a negative attitude toward life that lock up the body's healing ability.

Overheating therapy is effective in controlling and improving Arthritis symptoms. See Airola, "HOW TO GET WELL" for this technique.

CLEANSING DIET FOR ARTHRITIS

The following brief **beginning diet** program for Arthritis may be used for several weeks to help detoxify the body and flush out inorganic mineral deposits. Small and subtle dietary changes are not successful in reversing arthritic conditions. Vigorous diet therapy is necessary. For permanent results, the diet <u>must</u> be changed to non-mucous-forming.

ON RISING: take a glass of lemon juice and water, **or** a glass of fresh grapefruit juice, to flush out inorganic mineral wastes released during the night.

BREAKFAST: have a glass of cranberry, grape or papaya juice, with some fresh fruits and yogurt. Sprinkle on the following mixture: 2T. **each:** toasted wheat germ, toasted sunflower seeds,lecithin granules, and brewer's yeast.

MIDMORNING: take a potassium broth or juice, **or** a green drink such as BARLEY GREEN or Crystal Star ENERGY GREEN.

LUNCH: have a salad with lots of leafy greens, marinated tofu, and lemon/oil dressing,**and/or** a glass of carrot juice.

MIDAFTERNOON: have some miso soup with sea vegies, **or** a cup of Alfalfa/Mint, or Crystal Star LICORICE MINTS tea.

DINNER: have a cup of black bean or vegetable soup and a large dinner salad with sesame or poppy seed dressing. Add a salmon or sea food dish, or a whole grain and vegetable casserole.

BEFORE BED: take a glass of cranberry juice, **or** a glass of celery juice (to put inorganic mineral deposits into solution), **or** a cup of VEGEX YEAST PASTE broth.

FOOD THERAPY

- Go on a short mucous cleansing liquid diet (Pg.25) for a week. **Then follow a NON-MUCOUS-FORMING, LOW SALT DIET for the next 3 months.** (See next page for a brief version), or "COOKING FOR HEALTH HEALING" by Linda Rector-Page for a complete version, of this diet.)

- **Eat only fresh raw foods during an attack. Include fresh apple or carrot juice daily. Make a syrup of pressed garlic juice, cayenne, and honey. Take 1t. daily.**

- Avoid all foods with sulfites and MSG. Avoid sugars, refined and preserved foods, caffeine, red meats, and white flour foods.

- Reduce salt, starches, fried foods and dairy.

- Maintain a vegetarian diet if possible.

VITAMINS/MINERALS

- ✤ Ester C or ascorbate vit. C powder w/ Bioflavs. & rutin 5000Mg. daily. with
- ✤ BetaCarotene100,000IU or **Quercetin Plus 1000-2000Mg. daily, with Bromelain 500Mg. and vitamin C 3000Mg.**
- ✤ Pantothenic acid therapy sources:
  - ◆ High potency Royal Jelly or Bee Pollen 2 t. daily
  - ◆ Pantothenic acid caps 1000Mg. daily with PABA
  - ◆ B Complex 150Mg. daily.♂
- ✤ Raw Adrenal complex and/or Raw Thymus glandular 2 x daily.
- ✤ Bioforce ASTHMASAN DROPS as directed.♂
- ✤ Alta Health MANGANESE WITH B_{12} 2 x daily.
- ✤ **Use food grade H_2O_2 at 3% dilute solution in 8oz. water in a vaporizer at night for relief and nascent tissue oxygen.**

HERBAL THERAPY

- ❧ Crystal Star **RESPIRCAPS** and **RESPIRTEA, or ALRG-HST EXTRACT** with **ADRN-ALIVE CAPSULES or ADRN SUPPORT EXTRACT**

- ❧ Crystal Star **ANTI-SPAZ CAPSULES** ☺ as needed every hour to control spasmodic wheezing. with DEEP BREATHING or OPEN UP TEA to release mucous congestion.

- ❧ Lobelia tincture under the tongue as needed in emergencies. ☺

- ❧ **Mix fresh grated horseradish and lemon juice. Take a spoonful and hang over a sink to expel mucous in large quantity.**

- ❧ Therapeutic teas: Comfrey/Fenugreek Slippery Elm Elecampane

- ❧ Ginkgo Biloba extract under the tongue.

BODYWORK

- ✤ **Use eucalyptus oil in a vaporizer at night.** ☺

- ✤ **NO smoking. Avoid tobacco smoke.**

- ✤ Massage and gently scratch the lung meridian from top of the shoulder to end of the thumb to clear chest of mucous. Massage between the shoulder blades.

- ✤ Get deep breathing outdoors oxygen every day possible. Take a walk or other aerobic exercise. Exhale strongly to expel toxins.

- ✤ REFLEXOLOGY POINT:

ADRENALS

COMMON SYMPTOMS: Difficult breathing; choking; wheezing; coughing; difficulty in exhaling.

COMMON CAUSES: Poor diet with too much sugar, pasteurized dairy products, and fried foods; allergies to wheat, milk, or preservatives; adrenal exhaustion and imbalance; hypoglycemia; poor circulation.

Asthma is generally a chronic and severe condition requiring much supplementation from vitamins and herbs, and strict adherence to an allergen-free, vegetarian diet. As with most chronic diseases, the term of natural healing is one month for every year of the problem.

Overcoming chronic respiratory problems is always more successful when the program is begun with a short elimination cleanse. This allows the body to rid itself of toxic wastes and mucous accumulations before beginning a change in eating habits. Improved diet and eating habits will eliminate the dairy products, starches and refined foods inherently causing the congestion. Even though respiratory diseases stem from different conditions, all will benefit from this initial cleanse. Symptomatic relief is often felt in 24-48 hours.

MUCOUS CLEANSING DIET FOR ASTHMA & RESPIRATORY DISEASE

Follow for one week at a time as needed for mucous release.

ON RISING: take a glass of cranberry, apple or grapefruit juice. **or** a glass of hot water, lemon juice and honey, **or** a glass of hot water, cider vinegar and honey.

BREAKFAST: take a potassium broth (Pg. 33) with liquid chlorophyll, Sun CHLORELLA or Bragg's LIQUID AMINOS added. Take 2-3 garlic capsules and 1/2 teasp. ESTER C or ascorbate vitamin C crystals in water.

MID-MORNING: have a glass of fresh carrot juice, **and/or** a cup of comfrey/fenugreek or Crystal Star RESPIRTEA.

LUNCH: have a hot vegetable broth, onion soup, or miso soup, **or** Crystal Star MIN-ZYME-MINOS DRINK. Take 2-3 more garlic capsules and 1/2 teasp. ESTER C or vitamin C crystals.

MIDAFTERNOON: have a cup of cleansing herb tea, such as alfalfa/mint or Crystal Star OPEN UP TEA; **OR** another green drink such as Sun CHLORELLA or BARLEY GREEN MAGMA.

DINNER: have a hot vegetable/onion broth or miso soup, **or** another glass of carrot juice. Take 2-3 more garlic capsules, and 1/2 teasp. ESTER C or ascorbate vitamin C crystals.

BEFORE BED: take another hot water, lemon and honey drink, **or** hot apple or cranberry juice.
N.B. Salts should be kept low during this diet, but a little Bragg's LIQUID AMINOS can be added to any broth or juice for flavor.
◆ Try to stay away from cortisone compounds that eventually weaken the immune system, and from over-the-counter drugs that often simply drive the congestion deeper into the lungs and tissues.

See "COOKING FOR HEALTHY HEALING" by Linda Rector Page for the complete diet.

ATHLETE'S FOOT ✧ FUNGAL SKIN INFECTIONS

FOOD THERAPY

❧ Avoid acid-forming foods such as red meats, caffeine and fried foods.

❧ Eat plenty of cultured foods such as yogurt, tofu and kefir to keep the body alkaline and nutrients absorbed.

❧ Drink 6-8 glasses of water daily.

❧ Add lots of fresh fruits and vegetables to the diet during healing.

❧ Apply a honey/garlic poultice to the area to impede bacterial growth.

❧ Daub cider vinegar between the toes 3 or 4 x daily. Wipe inside of shoes with vinegar.

VITAMINS/MINERALS

✤ Zinc 50Mg. 2 x daily with Alta Health MANGANESE & B₁₂ daily.

✤ Vit. E 400IU 2 x daily. Also apply to sore area.

✤ Acidolphilus powder 1/2t. 3 x daily. Also dissolve in water and apply to area directly.

✤ Apply tea tree oil 2-3x daily to area.

✤ Lysine 1000Mg. daily.

✤ Crush or open the following. B₂ 500Mg., Niacin 1000Mg., Pantothenic acid 500Mg. Mix with 2 t. sesame oil and 2 t. Brewer's yeast. Apply to area at night. Put on an old sock to cover and leave on overnight.

✤ Apply a few drops of Nutrition Resource NUTRIBIOTIC LIQUID SPRAY and massage in.

HERBAL THERAPY

❧ Apply Echinacea cream.

❧ Apply Black Walnut tincture. ♀

❧ Apply Tea Tree oil as needed.

❧ Evening primrose oil caps 4 daily for 2 weeks for fungal peeling.

❧ Mix whey and Slippery Elm with water. Apply.

❧ Dust feet with Myrrh/Golden Seal powder.

❧ Apply Aloe Vera gel.

❧ Apply Witch Hazel.

❧ Open a Crystal Star WHITES OUT # 2 CAPSULE Apply directly to toes.

❧ Apply Lomatium extract to area, or Crystal Star ANTI-VI EXTRACT.

BODYWORK

✤ Keep feet well aired. Go barefoot as much as possible. Expose feet to natural sunlight every day to inhibit fungal growth.

✤ Use castile or tea tree oil soap.

✤ Apply N.F. HERBAL-SEPTIC LIQUID daily to affected area. ☺

✤ Apply food grade H₂O₂ 3% PEROXY GEL to area.

COMMON SYMPTOMS: Skin infection between the toes; dry, itchy, scaly, cracked, bleeding and tender. Weeping bacterial odor.

COMMON CAUSES: Tight or non-porous shoes, so that perspiration cannot evaporate; yeast overgrowth; low immunity allowing unfriendly bacteria to thrive and take hold.

BACK ACHE ◇ LOWER BACK PAIN

LUMBAGO ◆ HERNIATED DISC ◆ SCOLIOSIS

FOOD THERAPY

❧ Uric acid aggravates back pain. Avoid red meats, pasteurized dairy and caffeine.

❧ The diet should be high in minerals and vegetable proteins. **Vegetarians have stronger bone density.** Take a high mineral drink daily , such as Crystal Star **MIN-ZYME-MINOS or ENERGY GREEN**
or
A protein drink such as Nature's Plus SPIRU-TEIN.

❧ Drink 6 glasses of pure water daily to keep kidneys flushed and functioning well.

❧ A potassium broth once a week (Pg.33) for strength and kidney cleansing.

VITAMINS/ MINERALS

❖ **Mezotrace MINERAL COMPLEX 3 x daily.**

❖ Stress B Complex with extra B$_6$ 100Mg. daily.

❖ Alta Health Manganese with B$_{12}$ for spine cell development .

❖ DLPA as needed for chronic pain. ♀
or
Country Life LIGATEND as needed.

❖ Apply DMSO or MINERAL ICE for local pain. ♂

❖ **Vit. C 3-5000Mg. with bioflavs. and Emulsified A & D daily for connective tissue.**

❖ Bromelain 500Mg 2 x daily, with a high magnesium CAL/ MAG FORMULA.

HERBAL THERAPY

❧ Crystal Star SILICA SOURCE or HIGHLY ABSORBABLE MINERAL COMPLEX EXTRACTS for good collagen growth. and/or

❧ BONZ CAPSULES OR TEA for strengthening.

❧ Crystal Star RELAX CAPS or ANTI-SPAZ CAPSULES or PANEX CAPSULES as an anti-inflammatory.

❧ Effective compresses:
Hops/Lobelia
Comfrey/Lobelia
Horsetail

❧ **Alta Health SIL-X 3 x daily for building.**

❧ Nature's Way ANTSP tincture as needed.

❧ Crystal Star BLDR FLUSH TEA if kidneys are inflamed.

BODYWORK

❖ **Exercise is the single most important factor in treating and preventing back pain. Mild but regular exercise will build back strength gradually.**

❖ Apply wet heat packs to spine and lower back.

❖ Massage into back:
B&T TRIFLORA GEL
WHITE FLOWER OIL
CAJEPUT/ WINTERGREEN

❖ Get plenty of bed rest with head and legs propped up.

❖ REFLEXOLOGY POINTS:

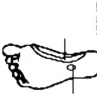

SPINE & KIDNEY

COMMON SYMPTOMS: Spinal stress and pain; inability to do even small bending or pushing actions.

COMMON CAUSES: Poor posture; improper lifting, sitting or standing; kidney malfunction; high heels; overweight; protein, calcium and other mineral deficiency; green vegetable deficiency; osteoporosis or osteoarthritis; congenitally poor alignment.

BAD BREATH

FOOD THERAPY

- Start with a short 24 hour liquid diet (Pg.26) with apple juice and psyllium husks to cleanse the bowel.

- Then follow a diet with lots of crunchy fresh fruits and green vegetables. Eat high chlorophyll foods like parsley and sprouts.

- Eat plenty of cultured foods such as yogurt, tofu and kefir for better digestive activity.

- Have a glass of lemon juice and water every morning, and drink 6 glasses of water daily to keep the kidneys clear.

- Eat lighter less concentrated foods.

- Avoid red meats, fried foods, and heavy sweets.

VITAMINS/ MINERALS

❖ **Acidolphilus 4-6 x daily**

❖ **Betaine HCl before each meal.**

❖ **Liquid chlorophyll in water after meals or take a green drink such as BARLEY GREEN MAGMA or Crystal Star ENERGY GREEN DRINK once a day.**

❖ Vitamin C 1000Mg. with 500Mg. bioflavs. daily.

❖ **Zinc 50Mg. 2 x daily.**

❖ B Complex 100Mg.daily.

HERBAL THERAPY

❧ **Chew propolis lozenges.**

❧ Crystal Star HERBAL ENZYMES at meals. and/or

MEAL'S END TEA for good digestion and fresh breath after eating.

❧ Effective teas:
Comfrey/Peppermint
Fenugreek
Rosemary
Alfalfa/Mint

❧ Clean teeth and mouth with Myrrh gum powder, or use Toms TOOTHPASTE with MYRRH

❧ Use tea tree oil mouthwash.

❧ **Put pinches of cloves, ginger, cinnamon, nutmeg or anise in a cup of water and drink as a natural antacid.**

BODYWORK

❖ Eat smaller, more frequent meals, and chew well for best enzyme activity.

❖ Keep colon and bowel clean with a gentle herbal laxative such as HERBALTONE, or a fiber drink such as Crystal Star CHO-LO FIBER TONE.

❖ Exercise to cleanse metabolic wastes being improperly expelled through breath and lungs.

❖ REFLEXOLOGY POINT.

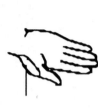

FOOD ASSIMILATION

COMMON SYMPTOMS: Bad taste in the mouth; mouth odor.

COMMON CAUSES: Improper diet; enzyme deficiency; constipation; stress and anxiety; gum disease; food intolerances; HCl deficiency; low grade chronic throat infection; smoking; poor digestion; liver malfunction; post-nasal drip.

BEDWETTING

FOOD THERAPY

❧ Avoid oxalic acid-forming foods, such as cooked spinach, sodas, rhubarb, caffeine, cocoa, chocolate, etc.

❧ **No junk foods. Avoid refined sugars, excess salts and spicy foods as irritants.**

❧ Avoid food colorings, preservatives and pasteurized cow's milk as possible allergens.

❧ Take a small glass of cranberry juice each morning to clean the kidneys.

❧ No liquids before bed. Eat a little celery instead to balance organic salts.

❧ Take a spoonful of honey before bed. ☺

VITAMINS/MINERALS

✤ **Hylands BEDWETTING TABLETS before bed.** ☺

✤ Magnesium 100Mg.

✤ Richlife CHILDRENS CALCIUM CHEWABLES before bed. ☺

✤ New Chapter food source ONLY ONE multiple vitamin for more balanced strength.

HERBAL THERAPY

❧ Crystal Star BLDR-K TEA at dinner. Half strength for children. ☺

❧ **Crystal Star RELAX CAPSULES or STRESS RELIEF EXTRACT in water for stress-related bedwetting.**

❧ Effective teas:
   Cinnamon Bark ☺
   Horsetail at dinner
   Cornsilk
   Oatstraw/Juniper
   Plantain

❧ **Ginkgo Biloba extract drops in water, mixed with a little honey before bed.** ☺

❧ Crystal Star CALCIUM SOURCE CAPSULES or HIGHLY ABSORBABLE CALCIUM EXTRACT drops in water.

BODYWORK

✤ See a good chiropractor if a **compressed nerve** or an **obstruction** is the suspected cause.

✤ Muscle testing **(applied kinesiology) is effective here in determining what allergies may be the cause.**

✤ Good circulation is a key. Good daily exercise is an answer; **especially bicycle riding.** ☺

✤ Leave a night light on so the child will feel free to get up at night.

✤ Give a relaxing massage before bed to ease muscles and fears. ☺

COMMON SYMPTOMS: Involuntary urination during the night beyond toilet training age.

COMMON CAUSES: Excess sugar, salt, spices or dairy in the diet; stress, emotional anxiety; bad dreams; allergies; hypoglycemia or diabetes; compressed nerve or congenital obstruction in the bladder area.

BLADDER INFECTION ✧ BACTERIAL CYSTITIS ✧ INCONTINENCE

FOOD THERAPY	VITAMINS/ MINERALS	HERBAL THERAPY	BODYWORK
❦ Avoid acid and sediment-forming foods, such as caffeine, black teas, tomatoes, cooked spinach, etc. Avoid concentrated starches, fried and fatty foods, sugar, salts, pasturized dairy and refined foods **A yeast-free diet is best, with no baked breads.**	✢ **DDS Milk Free Acidolphilus caps 3 x daily.** with **Garlic caps 6 daily.**	❧ **Crystal Star BLDR-K CAPSULES, or BLDR-K** FLUSH TEA ♀ or PROSCAPS ♂ with **ANTI-BIO CAPSULES if problem is severe.**	❖ **Apply wet heat, or hot comfrey compresses across the lower back and kidneys to relieve pain/ease urination.**
	✢ **Chlorophyll liquid 3 t. daily or Barley Green Magma 15 tabs daily.**	❧ Effective teas: **Cornsilk ♀** Couch Grass Uva Ursi/Nettles Pau de Arco **Dandelion/Juniper Catnip ☺**	❖ **If there is hemorrhage, take 1oz. Marshmallow rt., steep in 1 pt. hot milk. Take every 1/2 hr. to staunch bleeding.**
❦ **Cider vinegar and honey in the morning,** cottage cheese at noon, and a glass of wine at night are beneficial.	✢ **Ascorbate or Ester C 3-5000Mg daily.** with **Beta Carotene 25,000Mg. 4x daily.**		❖ Take a mild catnip or chlorophyll enema to clear acid wastes.
	✢ Enzymatic Therapy ACID-A-CAL 3 X daily to dissolve sediment.	❧ **Ginkgo Biloba Extract 3 x daily, with Crystal Star BLDR-K EXTRACT OR** Plantain/Oatstraw tea 3 cups daily.	❖ **Take hot and cold sitz baths to release fluids and flush out acids.**
❦ Drink 6-8 glasses of water daily to keep acid wastes flushed.	✢ **Take together: Ascorbate or Ester C 1000Mg. 6 tabs daily.** **Bromelain 500Mg. 6x daily.** Lysine 1000Mg.	❧ **High Omega 3 Flax oil with B 250Mg 2x daily.**	❖ REFLEXOLOGY POINT: 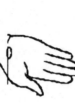 BLADDER
❦ **During acute period:** take a morning cranberry juice, and Carrot/Beet/Cucumber juice every other day to clean kidney infection.		❧ Bioforce BLADDER IRRITATION TINCTURE.	

COMMON SYMPTOMS: **Frequent, urgent, painful urination; pain in lower back and abdomen; often a fever as the body tries to throw off infection; strong odor urine; cloudy urine.**

COMMON CAUSES: Overuse of anti-biotics; venereal disease; stress; spermacide and contraceptives; kidney malfunction; excess acid-forming foods; lack of adequate fluids to keep the body flushed; poor elimination. tampons and diaphragms pinching the neck of the bladder, hampering waste.

93

BODY ODOR

FOOD THERAPY	VITAMINS/ MINERALS	HERBAL THERAPY	BODYWORK
❧ Dab underarms and feet with cider vinegar; or dust with a mix of 2 parts baking soda and 1 part arrowroot.	❖ Zinc 50Mg. 2 x daily.	❧ Fenugreek/comfrey tea	❖ Use a dry skin brush all over the body daily to remove toxins coming out through the skin. Then shower with an oatmeal and honey "scrub" soap.
❧ Go on a short colon cleansing diet (Pg. 26) to eliminate heavy body toxins and detoxify the colon. **Then,** stay with a mainly vegetarian diet, adding occasional chicken and fish. Make sure there is plenty of soluble fiber to keep the colon clear. Avoid red meats, heavy starches and high fat dairy foods.	❖ **Liquid Chlorophyll 1 teasp. before meals.**	❧ Crystal Star HERBAL ENZYMES after meals, **or** Comfrey/Pepsin tabs.	❖ Take a mineral salts bath such as Abracadabra at least once a week. ♀
	❖ **High Omega 3 fish or flax oils to improve circulation and release of serum blood fats.**	❧ Take a green drink such as Sun CHLORELLA GRANULES, **or** Crystal Star ENERGY GREEN DRINK 3-4x a week.	❖ Crystal Star ALKALIZING ENZYME BODY WRAP to alkalize acid wastes coming out through the skin.
❧ **Have a fresh salad with green leafy vegies every day.**	❖ Lecithin 3 caps daily. ♀	❧ Use a good soluble fiber colon cleanser 2-3 x a week, such as Yerba Prima COLON CARE FORMULA, OR Crystal Star CHO-LO FIBER TONE	❖ Wear natural fiber clothing so the skin can breathe. Wear sandals when possible.
❧ Eat small frequent meals. Chew well.	❖ **Odorless garlic caps to control low-grade infection.**	❧ APPLY ALOE VERA GEL under arms. ♀	
	❖ Schiff ENZYMALL TABS with ox bile for better digestion. ♀		

COMMON SYMPTOMS: Foul smelling perspiration.

COMMON CAUSES: Poor digestion; poor diet with green vegetable deficiency; too heavy and too large meals; poor hygiene; chronic low grade infection.

BONES

BREAKS ✦ BRITTLE BONES ✦ CARTILEGE REGROWTH

FOOD THERAPY

🐍 **Vegetarians have denser, better formed bones, and stronger immune systems.** Maintain a mineral-rich vegetable protein diet with whole grain complex carbohydrates.

🐍 Avoid red meats, refined foods, caffeine, & acid-forming foods.

🐍 The liver is vital to bone marrow formation. Keep it clean and healthy.

🐍 **Sugar and citrus inhibit calcium absorption.** Get vitamin C from papayas, bell peppers, broccoli, cantaloupe.

🐍 Good foods for bones: dried fruits, nuts and seeds, honey, a little wine for Boron.

VITAMINS/ MINERALS

❖ Alta Health SIL-X SILICA CAPSULES 2 daily.
　　with
❖ Calcium ascorbate C 3000Mg. daily.
　　and
　　Vit. B₆ 250Mg. daily.

❖ A & D 25M/1M daily
　　with
　　MEZOTRACE 2 daily
　　and vit. E 400IU ♂

❖ **Solaray CALCIUM CITRATE or Enzymatic OSTEOPRIME with Boron for better calcium assimilation.**

❖ **Ener B INTERNASAL B₁₂** every 3 days.

❖ High potency digestive enzymes or Betaine HCl for mineral absorption.

❖ Twin Lab PROPOLIS EXTRACT 2 x daily. ♂

❖ Collagen tablets 6 daily.

HERBAL THERAPY

🐍 **Absorbable minerals are key factors in bone building. Herbs are one of the best ways to get them.**

🐍 Crystal Star BONZ CAPSULES OR TEA daily.
　　and/or
　　ENERGY GREEN OR MIN-ZYME-MINOS DRINK MIX
　　or

🐍 CALCIUM SOURCE CAPS for highly absorbable minerals. ♀

🐍 Crystal Star SILICA SOURCE EXTRACT for collagen formation.

🐍 Effective estrogen balancing herbs for marrow formation:
　　Dong Quai ♀
　　Licorice ♀
　　Black Cohosh
　　Comfrey Root.

🐍 **Solaray ALFAJUICE for active Vit. K and chlorophyll.**

BODYWORK

❖ **Exercise is one of the best ways to build and elasticize bones, and prevent bone loss.**

❖ Get some sunlight on the body every day possible for natural vitamin D.

❖ NO SMOKING. It increases bone brittleness and inhibits bone growth.

❖ Swim or walk in the ocean when possible; or take daily Kelp or Dulse tablets.

❖ Avoid aluminum pots and pans, and fluorescent lighting. Both leach calcium.

COMMON SYMPTOMS: Easy bone breaks; poor bone healing.

COMMON CAUSES: Mineral deficiency or poor assimilation; poor diet with too many refined foods, and too much red meat protein causing excess phosphorus; enzyme deficiency; heavy metal or drug toxicity; steroids; stress; tobacco; too much alcohol.

95

BRAINS ✦ LESS MENTAL EXHAUSTION

MORE MENTAL ACTIVITY

FOOD THERAPY	VITAMINS/ MINERALS	HERBAL THERAPY	BODYWORK
🐍 The brain is a primary health maintenance organ. Good, consistent brain nourishment can straighten out even grave mental, emotional and coordination problems.	✥ Keep brain oxygen high with anti-oxidants: ◆ COQ 10 30Mg. daily ◆ Ener B B_{12} nasal gel ◆ B_{15} DMG sublingual ◆ Carnitine 500Mg. daily	🐍 Crystal Star MENTAL CLARITY CAPSULES, CREATIVI-TEA, and MEDITATION TEA.	✣ Get some mild <u>aerobic exercise</u> daily for brain oxygen. Practice **deep brain breathing.**
🐍 Brain foods are mineral rich, especially in potassium, zinc. magnesium, and iodine Include frequently: **Sea vegetables, fish, sea foods, sprouts, fertile eggs, wheat germ, mono-unsaturated oils, brown rice, tofu, lecithin and brewer's yeast.**	✥ Glutamine pwdr. 1/4 t. <u>with</u> Glycine pwr. 1/4 teasp. ✥ **Organic Germanium 50-100Mg. w/ Suma** and **Choline 600Mg. daily**	🐍 Crystal Star ROYAL MU TEA with Ginseng.♂ 🐍 Effective capsules: ◆ Ginseng/Gotu Kola ◆ Ginseng/Damiana ♂ ◆ Kelp tabs 6 daily.	✣ Cheerfulness, optimism and relaxation assure better brain function. ✣ Tobacco, alcohol, marijuana all inhibit brain release of vassopressin, impairing memory, attention and concentration.
🐍 Take a high protein drink every morning, such as Nature's Plus SPIRUTEIN, or Crystal Star MIN-ZYME-MINOS.	✥ B Complex 150Mg. w/ extra Niacin 500Mg. ✥ Other good nutrients: ◆ Vit. E w/ Selenium ♂ ◆ Phosphatidyl Choline ◆ White Birch min. water ◆ Omega 3 fish/flax oil ◆ Magnesium 800Mg.	🐍 Effective teas: Rosemary Parsley/Sage Gotu Kola 🐍 **Ginkgo Biloba extract 2-3x daily.** 🐍 Evening Primrose oil 2-4 daily for good brain/ electrical connection.♀	✣ REFLEXOLOGY POINT: 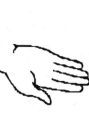 SQUEEZE ALL AROUND HAND FOR BRAIN STIMULATION.

COMMON SYMPTOMS: Lack of concentration and spaciness; inability to remember well or for a reasonable length of time.

COMMON CAUSES: Lack of protein or potassium or other minerals; mental burnout; overwork; lack of a vacation; stress; poor diet.

THE BRAIN is an incredibly sensitive organ. It rsponds quickly but only temporarily to drugs and short term stimulants. The best way to get good long term brain performance is to feed it. Brain nutrients have a far more synergistic effect with the brain than they do on other areas of the body.

BRONCHITIS

FOOD THERAPY

♥ Go on a short **mucous cleansing liquid diet** (Pg. 25) **to clear the body of mucous.** Then follow a basically vegetarian cleansing diet for several weeks, keeping fats, dairy and clogging heavy foods low. **See "COOKING FOR HEALTHY HEALING"** by Linda Rector-Page for a complete non-mucous forming diet.

♥ Take plenty of soups broths, hot tonics, high vitamin C juices and green drinks. Keep salts very low.

♥ Avoid all dairy foods, heavy starches and fatty foods during healing to reduce congestion. Keep the bowels clean so that the system can eliminate mucous well.

VITAMINS/ MINERALS

✤ **Ester C or ascorbate vitamin C crystals in water, 5-10,000Mg. or to bowel tolerance at first, then reducing to 3-5000Mg. daily.** **with**
Bioflavanoids 1000Mg. daily.

✤ **Zinc lozenges as needed with Cysteine 500Mg. for chest congestion.**

✤ Beta Carotene 100,000IU with
Garlic caps 6 daily.

✤ Enzymatic Therapy ADRENAL COMPLEX or THYMUS COMPLEX ♀

✤ **Food Grade H$_2$O$_2$ 3% solution internally 1T. in 8oz. water** to oxygenate lungs and overcome infection. ♂

✤ Standard homeopathic HYLAVIR TABLETS. ☺

HERBAL THERAPY

🐦 Crystal Star ANTI-BIO CAPSULES or EXTRACT **with** RESPIRCAPS **and** OPEN UP TEA.

🐦 Crystal Star CRISIS CAPS 4 as needed to relieve acute conditions quickly.

🐦 Lobelia tincture 3-4 times daily as needed.

🐦 Effective teas:
Ephedra
Elecampane
Coltsfoot
Wild Cherry
Hyssop/Horehound
Ginkgo Biloba Lf.

🐦 **Cayenne/Ginger capsules 4-6 daily. Apply Cayenne/Ginger compresses to the chest.**

🐦 Use Olbas inhaler or lozenges.

BODYWORK

✤ Avoid smoking and secondary smoke. Get fresh air and sunshine, away from environmental pollutants that cause chronic bronchial congestion.

✤ **Take a hot sauna or steam bath and follow with a brisk rubdown.**

✤ **Use eucalyptus, winter-green, or mullein oils in an inhaler at night.**

✤ Rub tea tree oil on the chest.

✤ Apply alternating hot and cold witch hazel compresses to the chest to stimulate circulation.

✤ **Do deep breathing exercises daily in the morning and before bed to clear lungs.**

COMMON SYMPTOMS: <u>ACUTE BRONCHITIS:</u> Slight fever; inflammation; headache, nausea, and body aches; cough. <u>CHRONIC BRONCHITIS:</u> Difficult breathing; coughing and wheezing; fatigue; low grade lung infection.

COMMON CAUSES: High mucous and acid-forming diet; suppressive "cold preparations"; lack of exercise and poor circulation; low immunity and fatigue.

97

FOOD THERAPY

❧ The diet should be light, low fat, and high in minerals and trace minerals to lay a solid foundation for strong capillaries and skin.

❧ Eat vitamin K rich foods, such as alfalfa sprouts, green peppers, citrus fruits and green vegetables.

❧ Avoid pasteurized dairy foods during healing.

❧ Take a green drink once a week for prevention. (Pg. 34), or Crystal Star ENERGY GREEN DRINK MIX.

VITAMINS/ MINERALS

❖ Apply DMSO 2 x daily for a week.

❖ Apply Enzymatic Therapy CELL-U-VAR CREAM daily.

❖ Ascorbate vitamin C with bioflavs and rutin 100Mg. every 2 hours during healing.

❖ Omega 3 Flax oil 3 daily for 1-3 months.

❖ Bromelain 500Mg. 2 x daily.♂

or

Quercetin Plus with Bromelain 4-6 daily. Take for 36-48 hours til discoloration subsides.♀

❖ Vitamin K, 4 daily.

❖ Apply Twin Lab POTASSIUM CHLORIDE LIQUID directly.

❖ COLLAGEN tabs or powder daily.

HERBAL THERAPY

❧ Crystal Star SILICA SOURCE or BILBERRY EXTRACT for capillary strength and collagen formation.

❧ Effective applications:
◆ Arnica extract
◆ Aloe Vera gel
◆ White Flower oil
◆ Wheat germ oil
◆ Witch Hazel
◆ Tea Tree oil ☺
◆ Eucalyptus oil.

❧ Solaray Turmeric capsules 4 daily.

❧ Make Rosemary/Thyme tea. Strain and add to a hot bath. Soak 25 min.♀

❧ Crystal Star MIN-ZYME-MINOS DRINK MIX for foundation food minerals and potassium.

❧ Alfalfa or kelp tabs 6-8 daily, or Solaray ALFAJUICE CAPS, as a vitamin K source.

BODYWORK

❖ Apply ice frequently and squeeze bruise to release blood congestion. Rub vigorously.

❖ Apply H₂O₂ PEROXY GEL to bruise 3-4x daily.

❖ Apply B & T ARNIFLORA GEL 3-4 x daily. ☺

❖ Effective compresses:
◆ Comfrey Rt.
◆ Onion
◆ Aloe Vera
◆ Golden Seal

❖ Do not take aspirin if bruising is frequent.

COMMON SYMPTOMS: Black and blue skin discolorations.

COMMON CAUSES: Vit. K deficiency; thin capillary and vein walls; poor collagen formation; mineral-poor diet.

BURNS

FOOD THERAPY	VITAMINS/ MINERALS	HERBAL THERAPY	BODYWORK
🍃 Apply ice water immediately, then vinegar soaked compresses.	✤ Apply vitamin E oil every 3-4 hours. Take vitamin E 1200IU daily for a week.	🍃 Califlora Calendula gel.	✤ Get medical help fast for anything other than a first degree or small second degree burn.
🍃 Drink plenty of fluids. Eat vegetable proteins and mineral-rich foods for fast tissue repair.	✤ Take Ascorbate vit. C 3-5000Mg daily. Make a solution of ascorbate crystals in water and apply.	🍃 Effective compresses: Comfrey/Wheat Germ oil Tea Tree oil. ☺	✤ Flush with cold water; then apply ice packs til pain is relieved.
🍃 Effective compresses: ◆ Honey ◆ Cold black tea ◆ Egg whites or raw potato for scalds	✤ Enzymatic Therapy DEMAZYME CREAM.	🍃 Make a strong tea; Elder blossoms, Red Clover, Yarrow and Golden Seal. Strain and apply. or	✤ Apply Aloe Vera gel and/or ALOE ICE frequently.
🍃 Use baking soda or cider vinegar in warm water for acid/chemical burns.	✤ Apply PABA ointment.	🍃 Comfrey, Nettles, Marshmallow, Scullcap, Red Clover and apply.	✤ If the burn is 3rd degree, treat for shock until help arrives.
	✤ B Complex 100Mg. with extra Niacin 250Mg for fluid loss.	🍃 For immediate relief with no blistering or irritation, dip cotton balls in strong fresh ginger juice or strong black tea and apply.	◆ Cayenne: 1/4t. tincture or 2 opened capsules in 1 tsp. warm water. ◆Cut away loose clothing that has not adhered to the skin.
	✤ Beta Carotene 25,000IU 4 x daily with Zinc 50Mg. 3 x daily.		◆Apply ice water if skin is not charred. If charred, apply cloths dipped in Aloe Vera gel or juice, or a fresh comfrey leaf poultice.
	✤ Enzymatic Therapy ADRENAL COMPLEX for cortex formation.		

COMMON SYMPTOMS: 1st DEGREE - sunburn, minor blistering and pain.
2nd DEGREE - blistering; scarring; gland structure damage; hair follicles burned off.
3rd DEGREE - extensive tissue damage; oozing, charring; severe loss of body fluids; electrolyte loss and shock.

COMMON CAUSES: Chemical and radiation burns; ultraviolet sunlamps , excessive UV sun rays; fire; electrical devices.

BURSITIS

FOOD THERAPY

- Avoid acid-forming foods, such as caffeine, salts, refined foods, red meats, etc.

- Keep the body alkaline with foods like celery, avocados, potatoes, wheat germ, sweet fruits, sprouts, greens, brewer's yeast, oats and sea vegetables.

- Keep the kidneys flushed with a green drink or carrot/beet/cucumber juice.

- Add to the diet for organic calcium uptake: Salmon & sea foods; Dark green leafies; Cultured foods; Broccoli & potatoes.

- See ARTHRITIS DIET in this book for more information.

VITAMINS/ MINERALS

- Quercetin Plus 3 daily with Bromelain 500Mg.

- Country Life LIGA-TEND as needed or 4 daily.

- DLPA as needed for pain. Apply DMSO with aloe vera roll on as needed for pain.

- Biotec SOD EXTRA ENERGY ENZYMES 6-10 daily.

- Enzymatic Therapy ACID-A-CAL CAPSULES to dissolve sediment. with

- Ascorbate vit. C or Ester C with Bioflavs. and Rutin 3000Mg daily for collagen formation.

- Ener-B VIT. B₁₂ NASAL GEL for energy and cell development.

- Solaray BIOZINC or Zinc picolinate daily.

HERBAL THERAPY

- Alta Health SIL-X SILICA for connective tissue growth and health, with Source Naturals ORGANIC GERMANIUM 100Mg. daily.

- Apply B&T TRI-FLORA ANALGESIC GEL.
  or
  Hot comfrey/Olive oil compresses.

- Crystal Star R^{TH} EASE CAPSULES or TEA with ADRN-ALIVE CAPSULES for better essential cortex formation. and RELAX CAPSULES for stress relief.

- Alta Health CANGEST CAPSULES for better acid/alkaline balance.

- High Omega 3 Flax oil 1 teasp 3 x daily.

BODYWORK

- Take a mineral or Epsom salts bath once a week.

- Use Crystal Star ALKALIZING/ ENZYME SPA WRAP to change body pH almost immediately.

- Apply <u>ice packs</u> to inflamed area during acute stages. Apply <u>wet warm compresses</u> during later stages for faster healing.

- Use affected area gently. Intense sports action is inadvisable til trauma is relieved.

- Regular mild aerobic exercise is recommended to keep joint system free.

- Avoid smoking and tobacco as acid-producing habits.

- REFLEXOLOGY POINT:

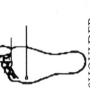

SHOULDER

COMMON SYMPTOMS: Pain, inflammation and tenderness where tendons are near the bones; swelling and redness, especially in damp weather.

COMMON CAUSES: Poor diet causing metabolic imbalance; stress; toxemia; a direct blow to the affected area.

FOOD THERAPY	VITAMINS/ MINERALS	HERBAL THERAPY	BODYWORK
❧ Go on a 24 hour (Pg.27) vegetable juice liquid diet to clear out acid wastes. Then eat lots of fresh raw foods for a month. Have a green salad every day. Take a green drink or carrot/beet/cucumber juice every 3 days to flush the kidneys and rebalance the acid/alkalinity.	✤ **Enzymatic Therapy ACID-A-CAL 3x daily.♀** ✤ Betaine HCl, or Alta Health CANGEST with meals for better mineral assimilation.	❧ **Apply Tea Tree oil 2-3x daily.** ❧ Effective poultices: ◆Green clay mixed w/ liquid chlorophyll. ♂ ◆Flax seed/Garlic	❧ Make a footbath with 2 handfuls of comfrey root to 1 gallon warm water. Soak feet 15 minutes daily. ❧ **Massage affected area with castor oil.**
❧ **Avoid fats, fried foods, sugars and alcohol. Avoid red meats, caffeine, chocolate, sodas, and oxalic acid-forming foods. Eat a low salt diet.** Eat 2-3 apples a day.	✤ Apply DMSO for pain ♂ ✤ **Apply SWEDISH BITTERS and take 1 t. daily.** ✤ Cal/Mag/Zinc 4 daily with B 100Mg. 4 daily. and with Ascorbate vitamin C w/ bioflavs.1000Mg.	❧ **Mix and apply: witch hazel, wintergreen oil, & black walnut tincture.** ❧ Liquid Chlorophyll 3 x daily **with** Crystal Star Echinacea extract.	❧ Apply hot epsom salts compresses. ❧ Avoid antacids. They aggravate and upset. acid/alkaline imbalance. The body needs adequate HCl for proper mineral assimilation.
❧ Rub papaya skins on callouses daily.♀ ❧ Apply olive oil compresses to corns, ❧ Apply raw garlic poultices to bunions.	✤ Vitamin E 400IU daily. Apply E oil daily. ✤ Beta Carotene 50,000IU 2 x daily. ✤ Lecithin 3 daily for smooth skin and improving body flow.	❧ Crystal Star ANTI-BIO CAPSULES or EXTRACT to control staph infection. BLDR-K CAPSULES OR TEA for kidney malfunction. ❧ **Apply H$_2$O$_2$ peroxy gel or 3% solution several times daily for a month.**	

COMMON SYMPTOMS: Staph or strep type infection; pain and inflammation of nodules and growths on the feet.

COMMON CAUSES: Toxemia; sometimes alkalosis; kidney malfunction causing acid/alkaline imbalance; too many sweets, caffeine and saturated fats; excess sebaceous gland output causing poor skin elimination of wastes; poor calcium elimination.

It is vitally important to follow a very concentrated program incorporating several aspects of natural healing. Diet, exercise, enemas, vitamin therapy and herbs all need to be coordinated for there to be remission. A concerted effort is needed for at least 6 months.

FOOD THERAPY

🍃 Follow a strict macro-biotic diet (Pg. 42) during healing. Pay particular attention to vegetable protein foods such as brown rice, whole grains, soy foods, nuts, seeds, and sprouts Have some miso soup, sea vegetables and 2T. brewer's yeast every day.

🍃 Take only fresh juices for 2 days each week. Fruit juices such as cranberry or grape the first day. Vegetable juices such as potassium broth, a green drink, or carrot juice the second.

🍃 Take a carrot/beet/cucumber juice once a week to clean the liver and kidneys.

🍃 Add onions, garlic and cruciferous vegetables and shiitake mushrooms to the diet regularly.

VITAMINS/ MINERALS

❖ The following are effective to combat the effects of chemotherapy and radiation, oxygenate the tissues and deter cancer growth:
◆ Biotec EXTRA ENERGY SOD
◆ Germanium 100Mg.
◆ Green Magma 2 packs
◆ Sun CHLORELLA 20 daily
◆ Biotec GLUTATHIONE

❖ Effective anti-oxidants:
◆ COQ 10 30 Mg.
◆ Beta carotene 100,000IU
◆ Probiologics LIPISOL
◆ Ester C w/ Bioflavonoids
◆ Vit. E w/ Selenium
◆ Vit B_{12} w/ Folic acid (esp. for lung cancer0

❖ Rainbow Light DETOX-ZYME with meals.

❖ Food grade PEROXY GEL rubbed on the feet, or taken at 3% dilution 1t. in 8z. water daily to increase body oxygen uptake.

❖ Twin Lab LIQUID K PLUS

❖ Alta Health CANGEST

HERBAL THERAPY

🍃 Enzymatic Therapy SIBERIAN GINSENG EXTRACT capsules daily with Pau de Arco or Calendula tea 4 cups daily.

🍃 Effective unsaturated fatty acids therapy (esp. for breast and uterine cancers).
◆ Evening Primrose oil
◆ Omega 3 Fish or Flax oil

🍃 Effective Iodine therapy:
◆ ATOMODINE or MIODIN
◆ Crystal Star MIN-ZYME-MINᴐS DRINK
◆ Kelp tabs 8-10 daily

🍃 Crystal Star DETOX CAPSULES as directed. with HIGHLY ABSORBABLE MINERAL COMPLEX EXTRACT 3 x daily.

🍃 Natren LIFE START 2 1/2t. 3 x daily.

🍃 Herbs to reduce the effects of chemotherapy:
◆ Licorice
◆ Astragalus.
◆ Barley Green Magma

BODYWORK

❖ Avoid tobacco, synthetic estrogens, X-Rays, caffeine, junk foods and preserved foods.

❖ Take a coffee enema once a week for a month (1 cup strong brewed in a qt. of water.) or chlorella implants.

❖ Get some sunlight on the body every day possible (esp. for organ cancers).

❖ Effective poultices for external growths:
◆ Garlic/onion
◆ Comfrey lf.
◆ Green Clay

❖ Get aerobic exercise regularly. It is a nutrient in itself. No healing program will make it without some exercise.

102

DIET DEFENSE AGAINST CANCER

The natural healing world has concentrated on cancer problems intensely in the past few years, and has learned and realized much about how to deal with this often unnecessary killer. Even though today's statistics show that 30% of all Americans will contract some kind of cancer in their lives, new evidence is indicating that 90% *of all cancer* is environmentally caused and therefore preventable. Diet and nutrition are by far the most important of the environmental factors. It is definitely felt that America's enormous incidence of breast and colon cancer, 500% compared to the rest of the world, is due to poor nutrition.

❦ **Cancers are opportunistic, attacking when immune defenses and bloodstream health are low.**

❦ Most cancers are caused or aggravated by poor diet and nutrition. Many cancers respond well to diet improvement.

❦ Accumulated deficiencies come over a long period of time - too much refined food, fats and red meats; too little fiber, fresh foods and food source vitamins and minerals. These deficiencies eventually change body chemistry. The immune system cannot defend properly when biochemistry is altered. It can't tell its own cells from invading toxic cells, and sometimes attacks everything or nothing in confusion.

❦ Cancerous cells seem to crave dead de-mineralized foods, and starving them out feels like any drug withdrawal. The fight against this isn't easy, but as healthy cells rebuild, the craving subsides.

❦ Cancers also seem to live and grow in the unreleased waste and mucous deposits in the body. Avoid red meats, pork, fried foods, refined carbohydrates, sugars, caffeine, and preserved or colored foods of any kind, and heavy pesticides and sprays. These substances clog the system so that the vital organs cannot clean out enough of the waste to maintain health. They deprive the body of oxygen use, and provide little or no usable nutrition for building healthy cells and tissue. Avoid antacids. They interfere with enzyme production, and the body's ability to carry off heavy metal toxins.

❦ LOVE YOUR LIVER! It is the main organ to keep clean and working well. It is a powerful chemical plant in the body that can keep the immune system going, healthy red blood cells forming, and oxygen in the bloodstream and tissues.

❦ The answer to cancer seems to lie in promoting an environment where cancer and degenerative disease can't live; where inherent immunity can remain effective. These diseases do not seem to grow or take hold where oxygen and minerals (particularly potassium) are high in the vital fluids. Vegetable proteins and amino acids in the body allow the maximum use and assimilation of these two elements.

❦ A Macrobiotic Diet is effective against cancer, both as a preventive and as a part of the healing program. Foods that are effective against cancer include green, orange and cruciferous vegetables, garlic, yogurt, fish, sea vegetables and seafood, apples, carrots and tomatoes.

❦ Overheating therapy has been effective against cancer. See Paavo Airola's book HOW TO GET WELL.

❦ Regular exercise is almost a "cancer defense" in itself, as it enhances oxygen use and accelerates passage of material in the colon.

❦ Don't become discouraged, no matter how many times you have to return to a juice and raw foods diet. We have seen many prople overcome this "incurable" disease.

See *"COOKING FOR HEALTHY HEALING"* by Linda Rector-Page for a complete diet program for cancer control.

COMMON SYMPTOMS: Chronic constipation or diarrhea; sudden appearance or enlargement of growths; enlarged or swollen organs; internal bleeding and non-healing wounds; blood passing in the stool; unexplained chronic pain in a specific area.

COMMON CAUSES: Poor diet with too many refined foods, junk foods, caffeine, alcohol, tobacco, etc., all of which deprive the body of oxygen use; low nutrition and protein, preventing healthy cell and tissue formation on a continuing basis; over-use of drugs; stress; an acid, mucous-filled system where the vital organs cannot cleanse enough of the waste to maintain health.

103

CANDIDA ALBICANS ✧ CANDIDIASIS

FOOD THERAPY

🍂 The food and diet recommendations are extremely inportant. Absolutely necessary to control yeast overgrowth.

🍂 For the first several weeks of healing, avoid: ALL ALCOHOL, CAFFEINE SWEETENERS, REFINED AND PROCESSED FOODS. Avoid gluten breads and baked goods, dairy products, except plain kefir and kefir cheese or plain yogurt and yogurt cheese. No smoked, dried, pickled, or cured foods. No mushrooms, nuts or nut butters, except almond and almond butter. No fruits, fruit juices, dried or canned fruit. No black tea, or foods containing alcohol or vinegar.

🍂 Diet foods for the first several weeks: Lots of fresh and steamed vegetables, sea vegetables, poultry, sea-foods, fish, unprocessed oils, eggs, tofu, mayonnaise, miso, brown rice, millet, amaranth, buckwheat, soy or vegetable pastas, herb teas, citrus, rice cakes and crackers.
◆ Try to have a green drink and miso soup every day.

VITAMINS/ MINERALS

❖ For best results, rotate anti-yeast and anti-fungal products, so that yeast strains do not build up resistance to any one formula.

❖ Maintaining bowel flora is critical to overcoming yeast growth.
◆ DDS acidophilus
◆ Yerba Prima Fiberdolph
◆ Nat. Way KYODOLPHILUS
◆ W.H. RELEAF

❖ To kill the yeasts:
◆ CAPRICIN 3 X daily
◆ Rainbow Lt . DETOXZYME
◆ Solaray CAPRYL
◆ Nutrapathic Lab D-YEAST
◆ Nutrition Resource NUTRI-BIOTIC LIQUID CONC.

❖ For allergic reactions:
◆ Rainbow Light ALLZYME
◆ Bromelain 500Mg. with
◆ Ascorbate C 3000Mg. and
◆ Lysine 1000Mg.

❖ For Immune support:
◆ Biotin 1000Mcg. daily
◆ Zinc picolinate
◆ Ascorbate C or Ester C
◆ Beta carotene 100,000IU
◆ B Complex with taurine

❖ For protein/nutrition:
◆ ALL-1 protein drink
◆ Full spectrum pre-digested amino acid cmpd.

HERBAL THERAPY

🐚 Herbs are prime agents for restoring body homeostasis.

🐚 To kill the yeasts:
◆ Pau de Arco tea 4 cups
◆ Crystal Star CANDID-EX CAPS & CRANDIDA TEA
◆ Black Walnut tincture
◆ Garlic 6-10 daily

🐚 For gland balance:
◆ Atomodine
◆ Crystal Star ADRN-ALIVE
◆ Evening Primrose oil caps

🐚 For bowel regulation:
◆ Sonne #7 Bentonite
◆ Barberry tea 2 cups daily
◆ Crystal Star CHO-LO FIBER TONE drink

🐚 To build immunity:
◆ Sun CHLORELLA 20 tabs
◆ Nutrapathic NUTRAMUNE
◆ Echinacea extract
◆ Astragalus & Hawthorne
◆ Raw Thymus
◆ C.S. HERBAL DEFENSE CAPS

🐚 For tissue oxygen:
◆ Germanium 30-100Mg.
◆ Rub H_2O_2PEROXY GEL on abdomen. Take with
◆ Ascorbate C 2000Mg.

🐚 To clean the Liver:
◆ Natren LIFE START 2
◆ Alta Heath CANGEST

BODYWORK

❖ Candida is a state of inner imbalance, not a germ, bug or disease.

❖ A positive mind and outlook are essential to overcome this body stress. Relax and have a good laugh every day. Get enough sleep. Regular exercise is a key for body oxygen use.

❖ Avoid tobacco, alcohol and sugars, Avoid chemical foods and drugs such as Cortisco-steroids, anti-biotics, etc.

❖ Use applied kinesiology to test for sensitivities.

❖ REFLEXOLOGY POINT:

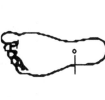

ADRENALS

❖ Soak fungal area in Tea Tree Oil solution. (May also be used as a vag-inal douche in water.)

104

CANDIDA ALBICANS ✧ DAILY DIET FOR THE FIRST MONTH OF HEALING

DIET CHANGE IS THE MOST IMPORTANT AND EFFECTIVE WAY TO REBUILD STRENGTH AND IMMUNITY FROM CANDIDA.

Candida yeasts grow on carbohydrates, preserved, processed and refined foods, molds and gluten breads.

ON RISING: take 2t. cranberry concentrate or 2 T. lemon juice in a glass of water to clean toxins from the kidneys. or a glass of cider vinegar, Sonne # 7 and water if there is flatulence.

BREAKFAST: take **All 1 vitamin/mineral drink** in water or citrus juice;
__then__ have 1 or 2 poached or hard boiled eggs on rice cakes with a little butter;
or almond butter on rice cakes or wheat-free bread;
or oatmeal with butter or Bragg's LIQUID AMINOS;
or amaranth or buckwheat pancakes with a little butter and vanilla.

MID-MORNING: have a green drink (See pg. 34) or Crystal Star ENERGY GREEN DRINK, or Sun CHLORELLA granules;
or a cup of Pau de Arco tea, or Barberry tea, or echinacea extract drops in a glass of water;

LUNCH: have a fresh green salad with lemon/olive oil dressing;
or open face rice cake or wheat and yeast free bread sandwiches, with a little safflower mayonnaise or butter, some greens, seafood, turkey or chicken;
or a vegetable or miso soup with cornbread and butter;
or steamed vegies with sea vegetables, Bragg's LIQUID AMINOS, brown rice and tofu;
or a chicken, tuna or vegetable pasta salad with mayonnaise or lemon/oil dressing.

MID-AFTERNOON: have some rice crackers or baked corn chips with kefir or soy cheese, yogurt cheese, or butter;
or some raw vegies dipped in lemon/oil dressing or spiced mayonnaise; with a small bottle of mineral water and a hard boiled egg with sesame salt or sea vegetable seasoning.

DINNER: have baked, broiled or poached fish with steamed rice or millet, and vegetables;
or a baked potato with Bragg's LIQUID AMINOS, a little kefir or soy cheese, or lemon/oil dressing;
or an oriental stir fry with brown rice and a light miso soup with sea vegies;
or a small omelet with vegetable or seafood filling, and a hot or cold vegetable pasta salad;
or a vegetarian pizza on a chapati or pita crust;
or a tofu and vegetables casserole with Essene bread or corn bread and a leafy green salad.

BEFORE BED: have a cup of herb tea such as chamomile, scullcap, or Crystal Star LICORICE MINTS OR GOODNIGHT TEA.

◆ As you start to see improvement and symptoms decrease, (usually from 1 month to 6 weeks), start to add back some whole grains, fruits, juices, a little white wine, some fresh cheeses, nuts and legumes. Test for food sensitivity all along the way. This next stage usually lasts from 2-6 months.. Go slowly. Add gradually.

Eating sugars and refined foods will allow Candida to grow again!

105

DIAGNOSIS INFORMATION FOR CANDIDA ALBICANS OVERGROWTH

Because much of the traditional medical community has chosen not to recognize, diagnose or treat Candidasis, the alternative professions of Naturopathy, Homeopathy, Chiropractic and Holistic medicine have seen and dealt with most of these cases over the past 8 years. Their energy and dedication have advanced the knowledge and understanding of the symptoms and treatment of Candidiasis to a great degree; better pin-pointing of symptoms and treatment, shortening of healing time, lessening of overkill, and more understanding of the large, overriding psychological aspect of the disease.

Candida Albicans is a strain of yeasts commonly found in the gastro-intestinal and genito-urinary areas of the body. It is generally harmless, but when resistance and immunity are low, this yeast is able to multiply rapidly, feeding on the sugar and carbohydrates in these tracts, releasing many toxins into the bloodstream, and causing far-reaching problems for the body. It is a stress-related disease, brought about because the body is severely out of balance, usually either from repeated rounds of anti-biotics, birth control pills, or cortisones, or a nutritionally poor diet, high in refined sugars, carbohydrates and alcohol, and a life-style short on rest.

The common symptoms for Candida Albicans overgrowth occur in fairly defined stages:

1st symptoms: Bowel problems; heartburn and chronic indigestion with flatulence and bloating; re-occuring cystitis and vaginitis; chronic fungal infections of the skin and nails; athletes foot.

2nd symptoms: Allergy/immune reactions such as Asthma, hives, eczema, hayfever, skin rashes, acne; frequent and chronic headaches and muscle aches; earaches; chronic bronchitis; sensitivity to odors.

3rd symptoms: Central nervous system reactions, such as extreme irritability; confusion, and a "spacey" feeling; memory lapses, and the inability to concentrate; chronic fatigue and lethargy, often followed by acute depression.

4th symptoms: Gland and organ dysfunctions such as hypothyroidism, adrenal failure, and hypoglycemia; ovarian problems, including frigidity and infertility; male impotence and lack of sex drive.

Ask yourself the following questions as a measure of self-diagnosis. "Yes" answers should alert you to Candida.

◆ Have you recently taken repeated rounds of anti-biotic or cortisone drugs?
◆ Have you been troubled by PMS, vaginitis, abdominal pains, prostatitis, or loss of sexual interest?
◆ Are you bothered by unexplained frequent headaches, muscle aches and joint pain?
◆ Do you crave sugar, bread, or alcoholic beverages?
◆ Are you bothered by hives, psoriasis, eczema or chronic dermatitis?
◆ Are you over-sensitive to tobacco, perfume, or other chemical odors?
◆ Do you have recurrent digestive problems, gas or bloating?
◆ Are you now taking, or have you previously taken birth control pills?
◆ Are you bothered by chronic fatigue, depression, poor memory or continuing nervous tension?
◆ Do you feel sick all over, yet the cause cannot be found?

CONTROLLING CANDIDA ALBICANS

Candida Albicans is a modern-day opportunistic strain that takes advantage of a lowered immune system to overrun the body. Keep the liver and immune system strong and active as the primary preventive to recurrence.

A strong immune system is the key to lasting success against Candida overgrowth.

A comprehensive and successful program for overcoming this disease includes the following stages:

◆ Stage 1: Kill the yeasts by changing the diet. Avoid anti-biotcs, steroids, immune suppressing cortisones, and birth control pills unless there is absolute **medical need.**

◆ Stage 2: Cleanse the dead yeast and waste cells from the body with a good soluble fiber cleanser.

◆ Stage 3: Strengthen the digestive system by enhancing its ability to assimilate nutrients. Strengthen the afflicted organs and glands, especially the liver. Restore normal metabolism, and promote friendly flora in the gastro-intestinal tract.

◆ Stage 4: Rebuild the immune system. Stimulating immune well-being all through the healing process supports faster results.

The whole healing/rebuilding process usually takes from 3-6 months or more, and is not easy. Some people feel better right away, others go through a rough "healing crisis". These yeasts are part of the body and killing them off is traumatic. But most people with Candida are feeling so bad anyway, that the treatment and the knowledge that they are getting better, pulls them through the hard times.

Be as gentle with your body as you can. These changes in diet, habits and lifestyle are often radical. Give yourself all the time you need. Go gently, improve at you own pace. Of course you want to get better fast, but doing it all at once can be self-defeating, psychologically upsetting, and very traumatic on the system.

◆ **Remember that Candida can mimic the symptoms of over 140 different disorders. Epstein Barr Virus (Chronic Fatigue Syndrome), Salmonella, internal parasites and Mononucleosis all have similar symptoms to Candida Albicans, but are treated very differently. Have yourself tested for Candida before starting your program to save time and expense, and to get better faster.**

While Candida symptoms seem to appear mostly in women, men and children are also subject to yeast infections. See *"THRUSH"* **in the Children's Ailments section, and** *"FUNGAL INFECTIONS"* **and** *"ATHLETE'S FOOT"* **for more specific information concerning yeast overgrowth in men and children.**

See *"COOKING FOR HEALTHY HEALING"* by Linda Rector-Page for a complete diet program for Candida Albicans.

CARPAL TUNNEL SYNDROME

FOOD THERAPY

🍂 Avoid caffeine, hard liquor and soft drinks. They bind magnesium. Avoid oxalic acid-forming foods.

🍂 Take a glass of lemon juice and water each morning and 2 T. each: Lecithin granules Brewer's yeast

🍂 Go on a short liquid diet for 3 days (Pg. 26) to clean out acids and restore nerve health. Then, eat lots of fresh fruits and vegetables with a green salad every day. Add celery for good cell salt activity, and sea vegetables or miso soup to alkalize.

🍂 Have a green drink (Pg. 34) often, or Crystal Star ENERGY GREEN DRINK, or fresh carrot juice for calcium and magnesium.

VITAMINS/ MINERALS

❖ Vit. B₆ 500Mg daily, with Niacin 500Mg. T.R. 2 x daily. and Ascorbate vitamin C w/ bioflavonoids 3-5000Mg. daily for connective tissue formation.

❖ Quercetin Plus 2 daily, with Bromelain 500Mg. and Ester C with bioflavs. 550Mg. 6 daily.

❖ Country Life LIGATEND as needed. ♂ and/or GABA with Taurine. ♀

❖ DLPA 500Mg. as needed for chronic pain.

❖ Lecithin 19 grain 2 daily.

HERBAL THERAPY

🌿 Crystal Star RELAX CAPS for nerve restoration. with SILICA SOURCE for rebuilding collagen and connective tissue.

🌿 Evening Primrose oil caps 4 daily for prostaglandin formation. ♀

🌿 Ginkgo Biloba extract as needed 2-3x daily.

🌿 Effective extracts: Scullcap Passion Flower Lobelia

🌿 Alta Health SIL-X SILICA 2-3x daily.

🌿 Hylands NERVE TONIC as needed. ♀

BODYWORK

❖ REFLEXOLOGY POINT:

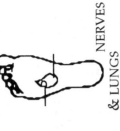

NERVES & LUNGS

❖ Massage affected areas frequently. Apply cajeput oil or WHITE FLOWER OIL.

COMMON SYMPTOMS: Intense numbness, tingling and swelling in the wrist and hand, often also involving shoulder nerves as well; chronic muscular weakness and atrophy; nerve inflammation.

COMMON CAUSES: Vit B₆ deficiency; Magnesium and other cell minerals deficiency; birth control pills creating a B₆ deficiency; leading to the disorder; glandular imbalance during pregnancy; electrical "shorts" in the system from prostaglandin deficiency.

108

CATARACTS ✧ CONJUNCTIVITIS

FOOD THERAPY

❧ The diet should be low in fats, cholesterol, salt, high in magnesium.

❧ FOR CATARACTS:
Blood sugar stability is a key factor. Include green leafy vegies, sea vegetables, seafood, celery, citrus fruits, Brewer's yeast, sprouts, apples and apple juice in the diet.

❧ FOR CONJUNCTIVITIS:
Apply yogurt or grated apple to inflammation.

❧ Avoid all refined carbohydrates and sugars, red meats, caffeine, and tobacco.

❧ Take a potassium broth(Pg. 33) often to feed optical tissue. **and**

❧ A glass of carrot juice daily for three months.

VITAMINS/ MINERALS

❖ Vital Health FORMULA 1 ORAL CHELATION/EDTA.

❖ Enzymatic Therapy ACID-A-CAL CAPS daily.

❖ Effective anti-oxidants:
Vit. E w/ Selenium ♂
Ascorbate Vitamin C
Beta carotene 150,000IU
Glutathione 50Mg. daily.

❖ Vitamin D 1000IU

❖ For cataracts: Histidine 2 daily <u>and</u> QUERCITIN PLUS with BROMELAIN 4-6 daily.

❖ Kal PYCNOGENOL CAPS.♂

❖ For Conjunctivitis: 1 drop castor in the eyes 3 x daily.

❖ B Complex <u>with extra</u> B₂ 100Mg. 3 x daily and B₆ 100Mg. 3 x daily.

❖ Zinc 50Mg. 2 x daily.

❖ GTF Chromium 200Mcg.

HERBAL THERAPY

❧ Crystal Star EYELIGHT TEA as an eyewash. **and**
BILBERRY EXTRACT and/or INSULFORM CAPSULES for sugar regulation.

❧ Aloe Vera juice (without ascorbic acid) drops in the eye 2 x daily.

❧ High potency Royal Jelly 2 t. daily.

❧ Effective teas & eye-washes for cataracts:
Eyebright
Rosehips
Chaparral

❧ Effective teas & washes for conjunctivitis:
Sassafras
Chickweed

❧ Ginkgo Biloba extract or capsules 4x daily.

BODYWORK

❖ A preventive diet and life style are the key to eye health.
Do long slow neck rolls and other good eye exercises (see Bates Method Book).

❖ Avoid long exposure to the sun. Get your exercise early in the day.

❖ **Avoid aspirin and cortisone as detrimental to eye health.**

❖ Palm eyes to release infection and stimulate circulation.

❖ REFLOXOLOGY POINT:

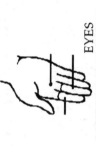

EYES
SQUEEZE AND PRESS

COMMON SYMPTOMS: <u>Conjunctivitis:</u> Inflammation of the eye and eyelid.
<u>Cataracts:</u> Continuing opacity and loss of vision.

COMMON CAUSES: Too much fat, sugar, salt and cholesterol in the diet; Diabetes (See Diabetes Diet in this book); poor circulation and constipation; heavy metal and environmental pollutants; liver malfunction; protein deficiency.

CELLULITE

FOOD THERAPY

🐛 Eat only fruits and fruit juices until noon.
Eat plenty of fresh un-refined foods.
Use only poly-or mono-unsaturated oils.
Avoid all fried and fatty foods.

🐛 Take an olive oil flush and/or a glass of carrot/beet/cucumber juice twice a week to clean the liver so it can metabolize fats well.

🐛 Avoid caffeine carbon-ated drinks, oxalic acid forming foods that cause liver malfunction.

🐛 Eat smaller, more frequent meals, instead of 2 to 3 large ones.

🐛 See "COOKING FOR HEALTHY HEALING" by Linda Rector-Page for a complete cellulite diet.

VITAMINS/ MINERALS

❖ Solaray CENTELLA OR CENTELLA VEIN CAPS. ♀

❖ Enzymatic Therapy CELL-U-VAR TABLETS AND CREAM. ♀

❖ Carnitine 500Mg. daily.
or

❖ Bio-tec AGELESS BEAUTY CAPS for dissolving and flushing rancid and brown fats.

❖ Effective liver aids to help metabolize fats:
◆High potency lipotropics
◆High Omega 3 Flax or fish oils
◆Rainbow Light TRIM-ZYME
◆Source Naturals SUPER AMINO NIGHT CAPS

❖ Esteem Plus 1 daily at lunch as directed.

HERBAL THERAPY

🐛 **Bilberry caps or extract.**

🐛 Crystal Star CEL-U-LITE CAPSULES, 3 daily.
with
THY-METABS CAPSULES if there is a lazy thyroid.

🐛 Apply Yerba Prima VIVALO CREAM.

🐛 Apply H_2O_2 PEROXY GEL to fatty areas. In some cases the fat globules will release coming out through the skin in little white bumps.

🐛 Evening Primrose oil caps 4 daily.
with
Kelp tabs 6 daily or MIODIN DROPS to stimulate metabolism.

BODYWORK

❖ Massage. Massage. From periphery towards the heart. Use a dry skin brush to stimulate lymph glands.

❖ Crystal Star TIGHTENING & TONING BODY WRAP.
and/or
CEL-U-LITE LOTION & DRINK.

❖ Take an hour's walk every day; **especially** _after a heavy meal._ **Exercise 5 minutes before eating to decrease appetite.**

❖ REFLEXOLOGY POINT:

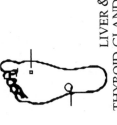

LIVER & THYROID GLAND

COMMON SYMPTOMS: Lumps, bumps and "cottage cheese" around thighs, hips and love handles; fat and other material trapped in pockets beneath the skin; tightness, heaviness in the legs; soreness and tenderness when tissue is massaged.

COMMON CAUSES: Liver exhaustion that results in poor metabolism of fats. Fats are then often thrown off as brown or "chicken fat".

CLEAN THE LIVER FIRST TO CONTROL CELLULITE. THEN FOLLOW THE DIET PLAN IN THIS BOOK FOR EATING LIGHT AND RIGHT.

CEREBRAL PALSY

FOOD THERAPY

❧ Eat organically grown foods as much as possible.
Include plenty of leafy greens in the diet with a fresh salad every day.

❧ Have a potassium broth every other day for 3 months. (Pg. 33)

❧ No refined foods, saturated fats, red meats, fried or fatty foods, caffeine or canned foods.

❧ Take 2 T. each daily:
Brewer's yeast
Lecithin
Wheat germ

❧ A modified macrobiotic diet is effective. (see pg. 42 in this book and "COOKING FOR HEALTHY HEALING" by Linda Rector-Page for a complete daily diet.

VITAMINS/ MINERALS

✤ B Complex 150Mg.daily and Lexon SUPREME B BLEND inositol cocktail powder for muscle atrophy.♂
or

✤ Twin Lab CHOLINE/INOSITOL CAPS.♀

✤ Phosphatidyl Choline or Egg Yolk Lecithin 6 daily. ♂

✤ Effective Anti-oxidants:
Octacosanol 4 daily
Vit. E 400IU 3 x daily
COQ 10 30Mg. daily

✤ Country Life RELAXER (GABA with TAURINE) ♀

✤ Tyrosine 500Mg. daily for L-Dopa formation.

✤ Magnesium 800Mg. for better muscle/nerve coordination.

HERBAL THERAPY

☙ Crystal Star RELAX CAPSULES 2-4 daily as needed for tension. and/or ANTI-SPAZ CAPSULES or CRAMP CONTROL EXTRACT.

☙ Crystal Star MIN-ZYME-MINOS DRINK for stability and alkalinity.

☙ Effective anti-oxidants:
◆ Rosemary
◆ Chaparral
◆ H2O2 GEL applied to affected muscle areas

☙ Ginkgo Biloba extract 3-4 x daily.

☙ Evening Primrose oil caps 6 daily.

☙ An effective tea:
1 part each of Centella, Bilberry, Butcher's Broom, Ginger and Lady Slipper.

BODYWORK

✤ Stay away from all pesticides.

✤ Use hot and cold hydrotherapy to stimulate circulation.

✤ Continuing massage of the muscles is a key deterrent to atrophy.

✤ REFLEXOLOGY POINT:

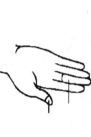

NERVES & MUSCLES

COMMON SYMPTOMS: A muscle-nerve disorder with spastic and uncontrollable muscle movement; often atrophy of the muscles.

COMMON CAUSES: Hereditary through drug abuse or over-use in the mother; malnutrition as an infant; heavy metal poisoning; nerve malfunction through deficient prostaglandin formation.

CHICKEN POX

FOOD THERAPY

☙ Take 2 lemons in water with a little honey every 4 hours to flush the system of toxins and clean the kidneys.

☙ Stay on a **liquid diet for 3 days** with plenty of fruit and vegetable juices Then have some apples, bananas, yogurt, avocados and a fresh salad daily for the rest of the week. **No dairy products except a little yogurt or kefir cheese.**

☙ Dab a little honey or wheat germ oil on scabs to heal and prevent infection.☺

VITAMINS/ MINERALS

❖ Beta carotene 25,000IU.

❖ **Ascorbate vitamin C or Ester C crystals, 1/4 t. every 2-3 hours to bowel tolerance to flush the tissues, relieve the itching, and neutralize the virus.** ☺

❖ Take vitamin E internally 400IU daily. Apply oil to scabs.

❖ Home Health SCAR-GO
or
Enzymatic Therapy DERMA-ZYME OINTMENT to heal scars. ☺

❖ **Zinc 50Mg. 2 x daily for a month after disease has run its course.**

❖ Raw thymus glandular.

HERBAL THERAPY

❧ Crystal Star THERADERM TEA & WASH. Take internally, and apply with cotton balls to lesions.

❧ **B&T CALIFLORA GEL as needed.** ☺

❧ Cayenne/Lobelia caps every 3-4 hours.

❧ **Apply a Golden Seal/ Myrrh solution, or** Yarrow tea to sores.
or
Apply a strong tea of Yellow Dock/Burdock/ Golden Seal every 4 hrs.

❧ **Effective topicals:**
Royal Jelly
Comfrey salve
Aloe Vera gel
St. John's Wort salve

BODYWORK

❖ Use a catnip enema twice during acute stages to clean out toxins.☺

❖ Effective baths for skin itching and healing;
◆ Peppermint/Ginger
◆ Cider vinegar/Sea Salt
◆ Oatmeal

❖ No aspirin. It tends to aggravate sores.

❖ Apply fresh comfrey compresses to sores.

COMMON SYMPTOMS: Mild fever with lots of small lesions all over the body that erupt, crust and leave a small scar.

COMMON CAUSES: Low immunity from a poor diet with too many sugars, sweets, carbohydrates, and mucous-forming foods; lack of green vegetables.

◆ See CHILDHOOD DISEASES AND NATURAL REMEDIES (Pg.57) in this book for more information.

HIGH SERUM CHOLESTEROL ✧ LOW DENSITY LIPOPROTEINS ✧ HIGH TRIGLYGERIDES

FOOD THERAPY

- **Lowering saturated fats in the diet is the key to lowering cholesterol; lowering sugar is the key to lowering triglycerides. Reduce animal fats, red meats, fried foods, high fat dairy foods, salt, sugar, refined foods.**

- Cholesterol in foods (such as eggs) is not the culprit. Excess total (esp. fat) calories are the prime contributor.

- Vegetarians who eat occasional eggs and low fat dairy are at the lowest risk for arterial or heart disease.

- Foods that lower cholesterol: olive and unsaturated oils, whole grains and soluble fiber foods, fresh fruits and vegetables, yogurt and cultured foods, wheat germ, brewer's yeast.

VITAMINS/ MINERALS

- Niacin Therapy:
  - ◆ 1500Mg. daily ♂
  - ◆ 1000Mg. daily ♀
  - ◆ 500Mg TR 2-3x daily with Glycine 500Mg, if sugar sensitive.

- Effective Lipotropics to enhance Liver function:
  - ◆ Choline/Inositol
  - ◆ Carnitine 250Mg. daily
  - ◆ Omega 3 Flax seed oil
  - ◆ Vitamin E 400IU

- Solaray CHROMIACIN for sugar regulation. with Stress B Complex, extra vit. B6 100Mg. and Lecithin 1900 Grains.

- Ester C with bioflavs. 550Mg. 4-6 daily. and vitamin E 800IU.♀

- Apple pectin or activated charcoal tabs 3 daily with meals.

- Health Plus ORAL CHELATION 2 packs daily.

HERBAL THERAPY

- Crystal Star CHO-LO FIBER TONE DRINK morning and evening. and/or CHOL-EX CAPSULES 3 daily for 2 months.

- Crystal Star HEMA-CLEANSE TEA. and/or Hawthorne extract 2-3 x daily.

- Guar gum to form a protective net around blood fat globules and flatten sugar curve. ♀

- Garlic 6 tabs daily for triglycerides.♂

- Sun CHLORELLA TABS 10-20 daily.

- Evening Primrose oil caps 4 daily.

BODYWORK

- No smoking. Nicotine raises cholesterol levels.

- Lose weight. Most overweight people have abnormal biochemistry. A low fat, high fiber diet is the key.

- Eat smaller meals, especially at night. A little wine with dinner reduces stress and raises HDLs.

- Take a brisk daily walk to enhance circulation.

- Ideal cholesterol levels 140-165 mg/dl. (LDL 30-50;HDL 80-90) Ideal triglyceride levels 200-240 mg/dl.

- See HEALTHY HEART DIET in this book; or see "COOKING FOR HEALTHY HEALING" by Linda Rector Page for a complete daily diet.

COMMON SYMPTOMS: Plaque formation on the artery walls; poor circulation; leg cramps and pain; high blood pressure; difficult breathing; cold hands and feet; dry skin and hair; palpitations; lethargy; dizziness; allergies and kidney trouble.

COMMON CAUSES: Stress; diet high in saturated fats, low in soluble fiber; EFA deficiency.

THERE IS A DIRECT RELATIONSHIP BETWEEN HIGH CHOLESTEROL AND HEART AND CIRCULATORY DISEASES.

CHRONIC FATIGUE SYNDROME ✧ EPSTEIN BARR VIRUS

FOOD THERAPY

❧ A highly nutritious diet must be maintained, and foods that build immunity must be emphasized to overcome this virus. Include often: ◆ defense foods, such as cruciferous vegetables; ◆ antibody forming foods, such as onions and garlic; ◆ oxygenating foods such as wheat germ; ◆ high mineral foods such as sea vegetables and whole grains; ◆ soluble fiber foods such as prunes and bran; ◆ cultured foods such as yogurt and miso; ◆ protein foods such as seafood, fish and whole grains.

❧ Take a protein drink every morning such as Nature's Plus SPIRUTEIN, and an alkalizing enzyme therapy drink such as Crystal Star MIN-ZYME-MINOS DRINK each day for a month.

❧ Avoid acid-forming and body stressing foods like junk and fast foods. Omit caffeine, refined sugars and processed foods.

❧ Keep the diet at least 50% fresh foods during intensive healing time.

VITAMINS/ MINERALS

✤ Effective anti-oxidants:
◆ Organic Germanium 30Mg.
◆ CO q 10 30Mg.
◆ Vit. E with Selenium
◆ Chlorella 20 tabs daily
◆ Solaray TRI-O$_2$ CAPS

✤ Vitamin C or Ester C crystals with bio-flavonoids, 1/4t. every 1/2 hour to bowel tolerance to flush the tissues and act as an anti-viral agent.
with

✤ Marine carotene A 100,000IU daily.
and/or
Probiologics LIPISOL for carotene uptake.

✤ Effective energizers:
◆ Country Life ENERGIX VIALS
◆ Country Life B 15 DMG
◆ Ener B$_{12}$ INTERNASAL GEL
◆ Biotec EXTRA ENERGY SOD

✤ Raw Adrenal complex, Raw Thymus and Biotin 1000Mcg. for immune stimulation.

✤ Enzymatic Therapy LIQUID LIVER CAPSULES W/ SIBERIAN GINSENG.

✤ Bromelain 500Mg. daily with Twin Lab LIQUID K.

HERBAL THERAPY

❧ H$_2$O$_2$ food grade PEROXY GEL rubbed onto soles of the feet for nascent oxygen. Use alternating one week on and one week off. Too much reactivates symptoms. A little is great; a lot is not.

❧ Ginkgo Biloba extract 3-4x daily.

❧ Natren LIFE START 2 or MILK THISTLE EXTRACT as effective Liver cleansers.

❧ Crystal Star ADRN-ALIVE CAPS OR ADRN EXTRACT with BODY REBUILDER CAPS. for strength ANTI-VI EXTRACT for anti-viral activity. LIV-ALIVE CAPS AND LIV-FLUSH TEA for the first 3 months.

❧ Effective extracts:
Echinacea
Hawthorne Lf. and flwr.
Siberian Ginseng

❧ Immune building teas:
Pau de Arco
Astragalus
Golden Seal/Myrrh
Dandelion/Red Clover

BODYWORK

❖ Take a daily deep breathing walk for tissue oxygen uptake.

❖ Get some early morning sunlight on the body every day possible for Vitamin D.

❖ Relax. Be optimistic. Mental attitude and frame of mind play a major role in releasing the body from stress, a big factor in lowered immunity.

❖ Immune defense cells are created in bone marrow. Keep new cell development strong with vegetable proteins, B vitamins (esp. B$_{12}$ and Folic acid) and oxygen.

❖ **Avoid tobacco in any form. Nicotine destroys immunity. It takes 3 months to rebuild immune response even after you quit.**

❖ Use hot and cold alternating hydro-therapy to stimulate circulation.

DIAGNOSIS INFORMATION FOR CONTROLLING CHRONIC FATIGUE & E.B.V.

We have now been working with Chronic Fatigue Syndrome and EBV for several years. A number of important things should be recognized to achieve successful and effective control over this condition:

1) These problems represent a degenerative imbalance in the endocrine system and metabolism of the entire body. It is *only* *one* of several viruses causing chronic fatigue symptoms (headaches, muscle aches, pain, etc.)

2) No drugs on the market today help this condition, and most hinder immune response and recovery.

3) Chronic Fatigue and EBV take longer to overcome than Candida or Herpes Virus. It takes *two to four weeks* to notice consistent improvement, and *three to six months or even longer* to feel energetic and normal.

4) Symptoms are controlled immensely by aerobic exercise. Even light stretching, shiatzu exercises, or short walks are noticeably effective when they are done regularly every day.

5) Overheating therapy <u>is</u> effective in controlling and overcoming Epstein-Barr Virus. See Airola "HOW TO GET WELL" for this technique.

5) A good diet is of prime importance in keeping the body clear of toxic wastes and balancing the lymphatic system.

6) Like Candida, these conditions are serious, but be gentle with yourself. Don't get so wound up in the strictness of your program that it further depresses you and takes over your life.

7) The outward symptoms for chronic fatigue conditons are so similar to Mononucleosis, AIDS, ARC, Candida, Lupus and other opportunistic diseases, that it is always best to be tested so that your treatment will be correct.

COMMON SYMPTOMS: <u>First symptoms:</u> Sore throat; high fever; headache and aching joints; fatigue which rest does not help (classic flu or mononucleosis symptoms).
    <u>Second symptoms:</u> Ringing in the ears; exhaustion; chronic depression and irritability; fogginess, spaciness and muddled thinking; low grade infection and fever; moodiness; diarrhea; sharper muscle aches.
    <u>Third symptoms:</u> Extreme fatigue; herpes; aching ears and eyes; weak immune system; paranoia; chronic exhaustion; weight loss and loss of appetite.

COMMON CAUSES: An opportunistic organism that attacks a weakened immune system, particularly if there is a history of Mononucleosis; emotional stress; environmental pollutants; smoking and tobacco; wide spread antibiotics, hydrocortisone or vaccinnations that lower immunity.

POOR CIRCULATION

FOOD THERAPY

- Keep the colon clear with a high fiber diet; at least 60% fresh foods.

- Make the following drink; take some daily: 1/2 cup tomato juice, 1/2 cup lemon juice, 6T. wheat germ oil 1T. brewer's yeast.

- Avoid red meats, fried and fatty foods, caffeine, refined foods, salts and sugar.

- Citrus fruits, juices and dried fruits have good bioflavonoids to strengthen vein and tissue walls.

- See HEALTHY HEART DIET in this book, or "COOKING FOR HEALTHY HEALING" by Linda Rector-Page for a complete diet.

VITAMINS/ MINERALS

- ❖ Niacin Therapy: 250Mg. 3-4x daily, with PABA 500Mg. 2 x daily.

- ❖ Oral Chelation 2 packs daily. ♂ with Ener-B B_{12} every 3 days.

- ❖ High Omega 3 Flax or Fish oils 3x daily.♀

- ❖ Solaray CHROMIACIN CAPSULES 2 x daily. ♂

- ❖ Vit. E w/ Selenium 400IU daily. with Ester C with Bioflavonoids 500Mg. daily.

- ❖ B Complex 100Mg. with extra B_6 250mg. 2x daily.

- ❖ COQ 10 30Mg. daily, or Solaray TRI O_2

- ❖ Twin Lab LIQUID K POTASSIUM 3t. daily.

HERBAL THERAPY

- ❧ Ginkgo Biloba extract 2-3x daily.

- ❧ Bilberry extract daily.♂

- ❧ Crystal Star CARDI-STRENGTH CAPSULES and HAWTHORNE EXTRACT ♀ and/or HEMA-CLEANSE TEA daily as needed.

- ❧ Cayenne/Ginger capsules 2-4 daily.

- ❧ Sun SIBERIAN GINSENG capsules or tea daily.♂

- ❧ Butcher's Broom caps or tea as a naural blood thinner. (Use on a temporary basis)

- ❧ Effective teas: Crystal Star MEDITATION Crystal Star ROYAL MU Kukicha Twig Pau de Arco

BODYWORK

- ❖ Apply alternating hot and cold Cayenne/ Ginger compresses to areas in need of stimulation. Or wrap feet in towels soaked in Cayenne/Ginger solution.

- ❖ Use a dry skin brush over the body before the daily shower.

- ❖ See a chiropractor for a spinal manipulation to clear any obstructions.

- ❖ Take a brisk aerobic walk every day.

- ❖ AROMATHERAPY: Juniper essential oil Cajeput oil

- ❖ Eat smaller meals more often. Avoid large or heavy meals.

COMMON SYMPTOMS: Cold hands and feet; poor memory; numbness; ringing in the ears and hearing loss; dizziness when standing quickly; shortness of breath; high triglyceride and cholesterol levels; varicose veins.

COMMON CAUSES: Cholesterol plaque on artery walls; constipation; lack of exercise; toxic or obstructed system.

116

CIRRHOSIS OF THE LIVER

FOOD THERAPY

🍇 Take a Carrot/Beet/ Cucumber juice daily for 1 week, then every other day for a week, the every 2 days, then every 3 days, and etc. for a month to detoxify the liver.
Then take a glass of lemon juice and water each morning and follow a diet for hypoglycemia. (see appropriate pages in this book, or "COOKING FOR HEALTHY HEALING" by Linda Rector-Page.)

🍇 Drink 2 glasses of carrot juice daily. Eat plenty of fresh fruits and vegetables. Particularly eat vegetable protein, such as sprouts, whole grains, tofu, wheat germ, & brewer's yeast.

🍇 Avoid alcohol, fried or fatty foods, caffeine, salt, sugar and tobacco.

VITAMINS/ MINERALS

✤ Choline 600Mg. daily to prevent fat accumulation in the liver.

✤ Enzymatic Therapy LIVA-TOX 3 daily,or N.F. Factors ALL LIVER.♀

✤ Natren LIFE START 2, 3 x daily to clean and restore liver tissue. with
Beta Carotene 100,000IU daily and

✤ Ascorbate vit. C crystals 5000Mg. daily or to bowel tolerance.

✤ Vit. E 400IU 2 x daily Methionine 2 x daily Folic acid 800Mcg.

✤ B₁₅ sub lingual 1 daily as an anti-oxidant.

✤ Chlorophyll liquid 1t. 3x daily.

HERBAL THERAPY

🍃 Crystal Star LIV-ALIVE CAPS, LIV TONIC EXTRACT, and/or LIV FLUSH TEA (3 cups daily for 3 weeks, then 1 cup daily for a month.)

🍃 Effective teas:
Oregon Grape
Dandelion Root
Hyssop

🍃 Milk Thistle capsules or extract 3 x daily.

🍃 Sun CHLORELLA or BARLEY GREEN MAGMA granules 1 packet daily.

🍃 Make the following tea mix. Take 1 cup daily. Bilberry, Ginkgo Biloba, Ginger.

BODYWORK

✤ Take a coffee enema once a week for a month to flush out and stimulate liver activity.(1 cup strong brewed in a qt. of water), or chlorella implants.

✤ Drink 6-8 glasses of pure water daily. Take an early morning sunbath whenever possible.

✤ REFLEXOLOGY POINT:

LIVER

COMMON SYMPTOMS: Sluggish, reduced energy; exhausted liver, often jaundice; skin itching/ irritation; rings under the eyes.

COMMON CAUSES: Liver toxicity from excess alcohol and/or drugs; excess refined foods and sugars.

CLUSTER HEADACHES

FOOD THERAPY

- Avoid the following foods: pickled fish, smoked meats, aged cheeses, red wines, avocados, caffeine, and chocolate.

- Eat high magnesium foods to reduce throbbing and contractions: dark leafy greens, sea foods and sea vegetables, nuts, whole grains, and molasses.

- Eat vitamin C rich foods: broccoli, green peppers, sprouts, cherries, citrus, etc.

- The food sensitivities accompanying this headache form are often a favorite food that one craves. Watch out for these "trigger foods" and avoid them.

VITAMINS/ MINERALS

- ❖ DLPA 750Mg. for natural endorphin formation.
  and/or
  Twin Lab GABA PLUS, OR Country Life RELAXER CAPSULES for brain stress control.

- ❖ Nature's Plus GERMANIUM 25Mg. WITH SUMA,
  and
  Extra strength Ginkgo Biloba extract capsules.

- ❖ Glutamine 500Mg. 2 or more times daily. ♂

- ❖ Natrol ESTER C WITH BIOFLAVONOIDS 2000Mg. activity daily.

- ❖ Omega 3 fish or flax oils.

- ❖ Nature's Life CAL/MAG PRE-ACIDIFIED LIQUID 3 t. daily. ♂

HERBAL THERAPY

- ❧ Crystal Star MIGR-AID CAPSULES and/or STRESS RELEASE EXTRACT as needed.

- ❧ Feverfew extract as needed for pain, and as a preventive when used on a regular basis. ♀

- ❧ Evening Primrose oil, 4 daily for prostaglandin formation.

- ❧ Crystal Star VALERIAN/ WILD LETTUCE EXTRACT
  or
  Medicine Wheel SERENE EXTRACT as needed. ♀

BODYWORK

- ❖ Biofeedback and relaxation techniques such as meditation, help; especially in conjunction with deep breathing exercises.

- ❖ Get a chiropractic adjustment, or see a massage therapist.

- ❖ **Apply an ice pack on the back of the neck and upper back to reduce swelling and pain.**

- ❖ REFLEXOLOGY POINT:

PRESS AND/OR APPLY ICE.

COMMON SYMPTOMS: Two or more sudden and extremely painful headaches a day, localized over the eyes or a spot on the forehead, usually coming in cycles with long periods of remission; dilated blood vessels with irritated adjacent nerve endings;; localized histimine reaction.

COMMON CAUSES: Vascular changes in the brain; eating allergen foods; prostaglandin deficiency; magnesium deficiency.

COLDS ✧ COUGHS ✧ SORE THROAT

SEE FOLLOWING PAGES FOR WHAT TO DO FOR FLU

FOOD THERAPY

- Go on a liquid diet during acute stages, with green drinks or potassium broth (Pg. 33-34) to clean out toxins and mucous. Then eat lightly when fever and acute stage has passed: fresh and steamed vegetables, fresh fruits and juices, fermented foods for friendly flora.

- Take 2T. cider vinegar, and 2t. honey in water each morning; and 2 T.each lemon juice and honey with 1 t. fresh grated ginger at night.

- Drink plenty of liquids (6-8 glasses daily) to flush the kidneys.

- To release quantities of mucous all at once, take fresh grated horseradish in a spoon with lemon juice, and hang over the sink.

VITAMINS/ MINERALS

- ❖ Ester C or ascorbic acid crystals: 1/4 t every half hour to bowel tolerance to flush the body and neutralize toxins.

- ❖ Low dose Zinc lozenges dissolved under the tongue to kill harmful throat bacteria.
    with
    COQ 10 10Mg. 3 x daily, or Solaray TRI O$_2$

- ❖ Beta carotene 25,000IU 4 x daily.
    with
    Quercetin Plus 3 x daily for inflammation.

- ❖ N.F. HERBALSEPTIC ☺

- ❖ Hylands Homeopathic remedies specific to individual symptoms.

- ❖ Garlic oil caps 6 daily
    with
    Acidolphilus liquid 3t. daily. ☺

HERBAL THERAPY

- ℘ Zand INSURE HERBAL EXTRACT and capsules.

- ℘ Crystal Star ANTI-BIO CAPSULES AND EXTRACT as directed for 4 days
    with
    COLD SEASON DEFENSE CAPSULES and/or
    CHILL CARE TEA ☺ to warm, or OPEN UP TEA as an expectorant.

- ℘ Other effective teas:
    Elecampane
    Horehound
    Coltsfoot

- ℘ Crystal Star CRISIS CAPS every hour during acute stages to promote sweating and eliminate toxins. (Use as a preventive in initial stage)

- ℘ Crystal Star COFEX TEA as a throat coat.

- ℘ Effective capsules:
    Cayenne / Ginger
    Comfrey / Fenugreek

BODYWORK

- ❖ Open all channels of elimination with hot baths, hot broths and tonics, brandy and lemon, and catnip enemas.

- ❖ Apply hot ginger compresses to the chest.

- ❖ Use eucalyptus steams to open sinus passages.

- ❖ See a massage therapist or acupressurist to open up blocked body meridians.

- ❖ Avoid drug store cold remedies. They halt the body cleansing and balancing processes, and generally make the cold last longer.

- ❖ Suck on Zand HERBAL INSURE or propolis lozenges as needed.

A WORD ABOUT THE CHRONIC COLD

There seem to be almost as many cold remedies as there are colds. A **"cold"** is usually an attempt by the body to cleanse itself of wastes, toxins and bacteria overgrowth that have built up to the point where natural immunity cannot handle or overcome them. The glands are always affected, and as the endocrine system is on a 6 day cycle, a normal "cold" usually runs for about a week as the body works through all its detoxification processes. **Sometimes it is just better to let this happen so your body can start fresh, with a stronger immune system.** But it is hard to work, sleep, and be around other people with your misery and cold symptoms.

With this in mind, we have developed a QUICK COLD CHECK that has been successful at minimizing misery while your body gets on with its job of cleaning house.

1) Take a brisk daily walk to rev up the immune system, and get you out of the house into fresh air. A walk puts cleansing oxygen into the lungs, and stops you from feeling sorry for yourself. It works wonders!

2) Take plenty of ascorbate vitamin C or Ester C, preferably in powder form with juice, spread throughout the day. Take Zinc lozenges as needed, and other supplements of your choice.

3) No smoking or alcohol (other than a little brandy and lemon). They suppress immunity. Avoid refined flours, sugar, and pasteurized dairy foods. They increase production of thick mucous.

4) Eat lightly but with good nutrition. During an infection, nutrient absorption is less efficient. A vegetarian diet is the best at this time so the body won't have to work so hard at digestion.

5) Drink plenty of liquids; 6-8 glasses daily of fresh fruit and vegetable juices, herb teas, and water. These will help flush toxins through and out of the system.

6) Keep warm. Don't worry about a fever unless it is prolonged or very high. (See FEVERS AS CLEANSERS AND HEALERS) Take a long hot bath, spa or sauna. Lots of toxins can pass out though the skin. Increase room humidity so the mucous membranes will remain active against the virus or bacteria.

7) Stay relaxed. Let the body concentrate its energy on overcoming the cold. Go to bed early, and get plenty of sleep. Most regeneration of virus-damaged cells occurs between midnight and 4 a.m.

8) Think positively. Optimism is often a self-fulfilling prophecy.

DO YOU HAVE A COLD OR THE FLU? HERE ARE THE DIFFERENCES.

Colds and flu are distinct and separate upper respiratory infections, triggered by different viruses. (Outdoor environment - drafts, wetness, temperature changes, etc. do not cause either of these illnesses.) The flu is more serious, because it can spread to the lungs, and cause severe bronchitis or pneumonia. In the beginning stages the symptoms can be very similar. Both colds and flu begin when viruses - (that unlike bacteria, cannot reproduce outside the cells) - penetrate the body's protective barriers. Nose, eyes and mouth are usually the sites of invasion from cold viruses. The most likely target for the flu virus is the respiratory tract. Colds and flu respond to different treatments. The following symptomatic chart can help identify your particular condition and allow you to deal with it better.

A COLD PROFILE LOOKS LIKE THIS:

✚ Slow onset.
✚ No prostration.
✚ Rarely accompanied by fever and headache.
✚ Localized symptoms such as runny nose and sneezing.
✚ Mild fatigue and weakness as a result of body cleansing.
✚ Mild to moderate chest discomfort, usually with a hacking cough.
✚ Sore throat common.

A FLU PROFILE LOOKS LIKE THIS:

✚ Swift and severe onset.
✚ Early and prominent prostration with flushed, hot, moist skin.
✚ Usually accompanied by high (102°-104°) fever, headache and sore eyes.
✚ General symptoms like chills, depression and body aches.
✚ Extreme fatigue, sometimes lasting 2-3 weeks.
✚ Acute chest discomfort, with severe hacking cough.
✚ Sore throat occasionally.

FLU ✧ VIRAL INFECTION

FOOD THERAPY

❦ **Take only liquids for the first, acute stages of flu. Plenty of hot, steamy chicken soup, hot tonics and broths to stimulate mucous release. Plenty of vegetable juices and green drinks to alkalize the blood and rebuild the blood and immune system.**

❦ When acute stage has passed, stay with a vegetarian, light "green" diet til flu has been overcome. Have a salad every day, fermented foods like yogurt and kefir for friendly flora replacement, and steamed vegetables with brown rice for strength.

❦ Avoid all refined foods, sugar, and pasteurized dairy foods. These increase mucous clogging.

❦ Avoid alcohol/tobacco as immune suppressors.

VITAMINS/ MINERALS

❖ **Homeopathic remedies are excellent against the flu, because they can be so specific as to symptom.**
◆ Boiron Oscillococcinum
◆ B&T Alpha C&F
◆ Hylands remedies specific to throat, cough, aches and fever of the flu.

❖ **Ester C or ascorbic acid crystals: 1/4t. every half hour to bowel tolerance to flush the body and neutralize toxins.**

❖ Zinc Lozenges dissolved under the tongue, to deactivate virus activity in the throat.

or

❖ **N.F. HERBALSEPTIC** ☺

❖ Effective anti-oxidants: CO Q 10, 10Mg. 3 x daily Vitamin E 800IU daily

❖ Raw Thymus tincture to build cell immunity.

❖ **Germanium 100Mg. and Beta carotene 100,000IU as anti-infectives.**

HERBAL THERAPY

❧ **BioForce INFLUAFORCE DROPS AND TABLETS.**

❧ **Crystal Star ANTI-VI EXTRACT as needed several times daily during acute stages til improvement is noticed.**

❧ Effective extracts:
◆ Echinacea angustifolia
◆ St John's Wort
◆ Lomatium

❧ **Crystal Star ENERGY GREEN DRINK MIX** to return body vitality and rebuild healthy blood.
or
MIN-ZYME-MINOS DRINK to alkalize the body and add concentrated food source minerals. ♂

❧ Sun CHLORELLA TABS or GRANULES, KYOGREEN, or BARLEY GREEN MAGMA.

❧ Food grade 3% H_2O_2 (1T. in 8oz. water) as a source of body oxygen and an anti-infective.

❧ Calendula tea 4 cups daily.

BODYWORK

❖ Gargle with a few drops of tea tree oil in water for sore throat.

❖ Get plenty of bed rest, so the body can concentrate on overcoming the virus.

❖ Crystal Star DRAWING & SWEATING HERBAL WRAP to quickly release toxins through the skin.

❖ Use overheating therapy. Take a hot sauna, spa, or bath to help raise body temperature and circulation, to throw off virus quicker. **Heat deactivates viruses.**
◆ **Crystal Star** CRISIS CAPS to raise body temperature and reduce virus multiplication.

FOOD THERAPY

🍃 Add more cultured foods to the diet: yogurt, kefir, sauerkraut, etc. for prevention.

🍃 Avoid high arginine foods, such as coffee, peanut butter, nuts, seeds, corn, etc.

🍃 Keep the diet alkaline: avoid red meats, caffeine, refined and fried foods, sugars, sweet fruits, etc.

🍃 Eat a mineral-rich diet: plenty of salads, lots of raw and cooked vegetables, whole grains. Baked potatoes and steamed broccoli are especially good.

🍃 Take 2T. brewer's yeast every day. Drink a fresh carrot juice once a week.

VITAMINS/ MINERALS

✤ Ascorbate vitamin C crystals. Take 1/4t. every 2-3 hours in juice. Make a strong solution in water and apply directly to sores every half hour til they subside.

✤ Liquid chlorophyll 3t. daily before meals.

✤ Take Lysine 1000Mg daily. Apply SUPER LYSINE PLUS CREAM at first sign.

✤ Natren MEGA-DOL-PHILUS 1/2t. 3 x daily, or LIFE START 2. 😊

✤ Beta carotene 25,000IU 2x daily.

✤ B Complex 100Mg. daily w/ extra B₆ 250Mg.

✤ Hylands HYLAVIR for fever blisters and cold sores. 😊

HERBAL THERAPY

🍃 Aloe Vera juice internally and as a rinse. Apply aloe vera gel frequently.

🍃 Crystal Star HERPEACE CAPSULES 4-6 daily. and/or THERADERM TEA. Apply to sores. Drink 2 cups daily.

🍃 Crystal Star RELAX CAPS as needed to calm the tension often causing sores. ♀

🍃 Apply tea tree oil.

🍃 Apply St. John's Wort Salve. Take St. John's wort capsules or Crystal Star ANTI-VI EXTRACT as anti-virals.

🍃 Burdock tea 2 cups daily to balance hormones.

🍃 White Oak extract as an astringent. ♂

BODYWORK

✤ Effective rinses to alter body and mouth pH:
◆ Golden seal leaf tea
◆ Aloe vera juice
◆ Echinacea solution

✤ Crystal Star MIN-ZYME-MINOS DRINK to alkalize the body for prevention.

✤ Effective topicals: Apply
◆ H₂O₂ peroxy gel
◆ Black walnut tincture
◆ Comfrey/Aloe salve
◆ Red Raspberry tincture
◆ Golden Seal/Myrrh solution. Swish in mouth every 1/2 hour.
◆ B & T SSSTING STOP

✤ Apply ice packs frequently. Follow with vitamin E oil.

✤ Relax more. Get plenty of sleep and rest.

✤ Apply Nutrition Resource NUTRIBIOTIC SPRAY to sore as needed.

COMMON SYMPTOMS: Herpes simplex virus of the face and mouth.

COMMON CAUSES: B Complex deficiency; pre-menstrual tension; over-acid diet; recurring virus infection; emotional stress.

⊛ COLIC ✧ UPSET STOMACH ✧ HICCUPS ☺

FOOD THERAPY	VITAMINS/ MINERALS	HERBAL THERAPY	BODYWORK
Avoid giving cow's milk. (Goats milk or soy milk are both better alternatives.)	Natren LIFE START 1/4t. in water or juice 2-3x daily.	Apply warm ginger compresses to the stomach and abdomen.	Give a catnip enema once a week, or as needed for instant gas release.
If you are nursing, watch your diet very carefully. The baby's digestion is still dependent on yours. Avoid cabbage, brussels sprouts, onions, garlic, yeast breads, fried foods and fast foods. Refrain from red meat, alcohol, refined sugar and caffeine til the child's digestion improves.	Solaray BABY LIFE for mineral and B Complex deficiency.	Turmeric powder 1/4t. in juice or water.	REFLEXOLOGY POINT:
	Solaray BIFIDO-BACTERIA POWDER FOR INFANTS.	Fennel tea or catnip tea, 1t. in water with a little honey.	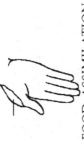
	Small doses of papaya enzymes.	Hyland's COLIC TABS or BILIOUSNESS TABS.	FOOD ASSIMILATION
Make sure baby's food combinations are good if giving any solid food.	B Complex liquid dilute doses in water about once a week.	Peppermint or spearmint tea with a pinch of ginger.	
Give papaya juice or apple juice.		Catnip/peppermint tea.	
Give lemon and honey in water.			

COMMON SYMPTOMS: Excess gas and abdominal discomfort.; burping; hiccups.

COMMON CAUSES: Poor diet with too many acid-forming foods, or poor food combining; introduction of protein foods too soon (this will often form lifelong allergies and colic); mother's tension and acidity during breast feeding; mineral deficiency in the milk formula; enzyme deficiency; Candida Albicans yeast overgrowth; poor food absorption; chronic constipation.

124

COLITIS ✧ SPASTIC COLON

FOOD THERAPY

❧ **Go on a mono diet for 2 days with fresh apples. Then eat a low fat** gentle soluble fiber diet: fresh fruits, green leafy salads with olive oil and lemon dressing, whole grain cereals, (esp. oatmeal), brown rice, steamed vegetables (esp. potatoes and cabbage), fruit fiber from prunes, apples and raisins.

❧ Eat cultured foods, such as yogurt and kefir for friendly flora.

❧ Avoid nuts, seeds and citrus while healing.

❧ Have a glass of fresh carrot juice 3x a week.

❧ Eat smaller more frequent meals.

VITAMINS/ MINERALS

❖ Liquid and chewable supplements are best for colitis problems.

❖ Enzymatic Therapy CHEWABLE DGL TABS and
IBS CAPSULES ♂ with
Royal Jelly 2 t. daily.

❖ High Omega 3 Flax seed oil 3 x daily.

❖ **Country Life Bromelain with 2000GDU.**

❖ Chewable papaya enzymes as needed.

❖ Chlorophyll liquid 3t. daily before meals. with
Schiff EMULSIFIED VIT. A 50,000IU daily.

❖ Nature's Life LIQUID PHOS. FREE CAL/MAG. ♂

HERBAL THERAPY

❧ **Yerba Prima ALOE VERA JUICE WITH HERBS morning and evening.**

❧ **Peppermint oil drops in water 2 x daily.**

❧ Crystal Star BWL TONE CAPSULES with comfrey tea 2 cups daily. and/or

❧ CHO-LO FIBER TONE 1 heaping teasp. in water morning and evening.

❧ Effective teas:
Slippery Elm
Pau de Arco
Chamomile

❧ Comfrey/Pepsin tablets.

❧ Sonne BENTONITE LIQUID 1 teasp. morning and evening to clean out wastes.

BODYWORK

❖ Effective gentle enemas:
Peppermint tea
White Oak Bark
Slippery Elm
Chamomile

❖ **Apply warm ginger compresses to spine and stomach.**

❖ ACUPRESSURE HELP:
Stroke the abdomen up across and down.

❖ RELAX.

❖ Avoid antacids. They often do more harm than good by neutralizing the body's HCl needed for good assimilation of food.

❖ **If there is appendicitis-like sharp pain, seek medical help immediately.**

COMMON SYMPTOMS: Abdominal cramps and pain; recurrent constipation, usually alternating with diarrhea; ulceration and rectal bleeding; rectal abscesses and inflammation; passing of blood and mucous; dehydration and mineral loss.

COMMON CAUSES: Excess refined foods and sweets; lack of dietary fiber; anemia and electrolyte imbalance; stress, depression and anxiety; too many anti-biotics.

AN UNREFINED, HIGH FIBER DIET IS BOTH PREVENTION AND CURE. SEE CONSTIPATION RECOMMENDATIONS IN THIS BOOK.

CONSTIPATION ✧ COLON AND BOWEL HEALTH

FOOD THERAPY	VITAMINS/ MINERALS	HERBAL THERAPY	BODYWORK

FOOD THERAPY

☙ **Start with a short easy colon cleansing juice fast (Pg. 26) to rid the bowel of current wastes.** Then, follow a mild food, low fat, largely vegetarian diet, with plenty of high fiber fruits, whole grains, cereals, salad greens and cultured foods like yogurt and kefir to establish friendly flora.

☙ Take plenty of liquids daily; at least 6-8 glasses of juice or water.

☙ Avoid all refined foods, saturated fats, fried foods, and caffeine.

☙ To restore peristaltic action, mix equal parts of Flax seed and Oat bran in water over-night. Take 2 T. daily.

VITAMINS/ MINERALS

❖ **Prevent constipation by adding some or all of these supplements to the diet:**
 ◆ Acidolphilus liquid
 ◆ Garlic capsules
 ◆ Brewer's yeast
 ◆ Cod Liver Oil
 ◆ Omega 3 Flax seed oil
 ◆ Guar Gum

❖ Apple pectin or HCl tablets at meals.♂

❖ Chlorophyll liquid 3t. daily before meals.
 or
 Sun CHLORELLA or BARLEY GREEN MAGMA.

❖ **Laci LeBeau SUPER DIETER'S TEA as needed.**

❖ Alta Health CANGEST for better assimilation and liver activity.

HERBAL THERAPY

☙ **Crystal Star FIBER & HERBS COLON CLEANSE CAPSULES 2, 3x daily.** and/or LAXATEA to flush wastes gently and quickly the first few days.

☙ **Psyllium husks or Sonne LIQUID BENTO-NITE to gather up colon waste and flush it out.**
 or
 Crystal Star CHO-LO FIBER TONE DRINK in water 1 heaping teasp. morning and evening.

☙ Aloe Vera juice with herbs 8oz. daily.

☙ **Milk Thistle Seed extract to enhance bile output and soften stool.**

☙ Effective laxatives:
 ◆ Senna leaf & pods ♀
 ◆ Cascara sagrada
 ◆ HERBALTONE CAPS ♀
 ◆ Solaray REFRESH
 ◆ Flax seed tea

BODYWORK

❖ Take a colonic irrigation to start your program. A catnip enema once a week to keep cleansing well.

❖ Avoid drugstore antibiotics, antacids, and milk of magnesia. They kill friendly G.I. flora.

❖ Chew food well, and eat smaller meals. No large heavy meals.

❖ **Take a brisk walk daily.**

❖ Stroke and press each of the REFLEXOLOGY POINTS for 3-5 minutes:

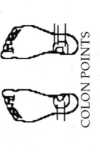

COLON POINTS

COMMON SYMPTOMS: Infrequent bowel movements: fatigue, nausea and depression; nervous irritability; coated tongue; headaches; bad breath and body odor; mental dullness; sallow skin.

COMMON CAUSES: Poor diet with too many refined carbohydrates, and deficient fiber; autotoxemia from too much red meat, pasteurized dairy, fried foods, caffeine and alcohol; overeating; overuse of drugs and laxatives; hypothyroidism; lack of exercise.

See brief CONSTIPATION DIET on the next page; complete program in "COOKING FOR HEALTHY HEALING" by Linda Rector-Page.

DIET SUGGESTIONS FOR CONSTIPATION

A high fiber, unrefined foods diet is of course the key to both cure and prevention of most waste elimination problems. Most poor health conditions that we endure extend from poor body cleansing in one way or another. Even a gentle and gradual improvement from low fiber, low residue foods will help almost immediately. In fact, graduated change is often better than a sudden, drastic about-face, especially when the colon, bowel or bladder are painful and inflamed. Constipation is usually a chronic problem, and while waste elimination progress can be felt fairly quickly with a diet change, it takes from three to six months to rebuild bowel and colon elasticity with good systol/diastol action. There is no easy route, but the rewards of a regular, energetic life are worth it.

The following diet should be used, after the initial cleansing juice fast, for 1-2 months for best results.

ON RISING: take a glass of aloe vera juice with herbs, **or** Sonne's LIQUID BENTONITE with 1t. acidolphilus liquid; **or** Crystal Star CHO-LO FIBER TONE DRINK in apple or orange juice.

BREAKFAST: soak a mix of dried prunes, raisins and figs, blackstrap molasses and water til soft. Take some daily; **or** take a mix of oat bran raisins, pumpkin seeds, yogurt and brewer's yeast (or Lewis Labs FIBER YEAST); **or** have some oatmeal or whole fiber cereal, granola or muesli with yogurt or apple juice.

MIDMORNING: have a green drink, (Pg.34) or one such as Sun CHLORELLA or Crystal Star ENERGY GREEN; **or** a small bottle of mineral water; **or** a small bottle of apple juice.

LUNCH: have a fresh green salad every day with lemon/oil dressing, and yogurt or kefir cheese; **or** some steamed vegies with tofu or a baked potato with soy cream cheese; **or** a fresh fruit salad with yogurt topping.

MIDAFTERNOON: have some fresh raw vegetables with a vegie or kefir cheese dip; **or** a fresh carrot juice or apple juice; **or** a cup of comfrey or slippery elm tea, **or** Crystal Star LICORICE MINTS TEA.

DINNER: have a large dinner salad with a black bean or lentil soup; **or** an oriental vegetable/seafood stir fry with miso soup; **or** a steamed or baked vegetable casserole with a yogurt or soy cream cheese sauce; **or** a whole grain or vegetable pasta dish with broiled chicken or fish, and a light lemon sauce.

BEFORE BED: have a glass of apple or papaya juice, or another glass of aloe vera juice with herbs; **and** another Crystal Star CHO-LO FIBER TONE DRINK

The protective level of fiber in the diet can be easily measured: <u>the stool should be light enough to float.</u>

There are three other ways to guage dietary fibery use in the body:
◆ **Bowel movements should be regular daily, and effortless.**
◆ **The stool should be almost odorless (signalling decreased transit time in the bowel with no fermentation.)**
◆ **There should be no gas or flatulence.**

COUGH

CHRONIC ✦ DRY AND HACKING

FOOD THERAPY	VITAMINS/ MINERALS	HERBAL THERAPY	BODYWORK
🍃 Take 2T. honey and 2T. lemon juice in water or cider vinegar to stop the tickle.	✤ **Enzymatic Therapy ORALZYME LOZENGES** or other low dose (about 10-30Mg.) lozenges under the tongue til dissolved.	🌿 Crystal Star COFEX TEA, especially at night. Usually works within 24 hours.☺ and/or 🌿 OPEN UP TEA as an expectorant.	❖ Avoid smoking and secondary smoke.
🍃 Drink cleansing fruit juices. Eat high vitamin C foods, such as sprouts, green peppers, broccoli, and cherries.	✤ **Bioforce SANTASAPINA or DROSINULA COUGH LIQUIDS. or Hylands COUGH SYRUP.**☺	🌿 **Horehound, Licorice, and Wild Cherry drops, syrups, or teas.**	❖ Effective gargles: ◆ **Tea Tree oil drops in water.** ◆ **Slippery Elm tea** ◆ **Aloe Vera juice**
🍃 Take a cup of hot black tea with the juice of 1 lemon and 1t. honey.	✤ Ascorbate vitamin C or Ester C powders: 1/4t. every half hour to bowel tolerance.	🌿 Effective teas or steams: Eucalyptus Peppermint Pleurisy Rt. Slippery Elm	❖ Steam Eucalyptus or Tincture of Benzoin in a vaporizer at night.
🍃 Take a cup of hot water with 2T. brandy and 2T. lemon juice.	✤ **Propolis tincture or lozenges.**♂	🌿 Crystal Star ANTI-SPAZ CAPSULES, 4 at a time as needed.	❖ Effective lozenges: ◆ **Zand HERBAL INSURE** ◆ **SANTASAPINA**
🍃 Avoid pasteurized dairy products during acute stages.	✤ N.F. HERBALSEPTIC ☺	🌿 Natures Way ANTI-SPASMODIC TINCTURE.	❖ Avoid commercial cough and over-the-counter medicines. They often make the problem worse by suppression, and forcing infection deeper into the tissues.
	✤ **BioForce BIOTUSSIN DROPS AND TABLETS.**	🌿 **Sage or rose hips tea with lemon juice, honey, and fresh ginger root.**	
	✤ **B.&T. COUGH SYRUP**	🌿 **BioForce DROSINULA or SANTASAPINA SYRUPS.** ☺	
	✤ Ricola lozenges/pearls.		
	✤ Standard Homeopathic HYLAVIR TABLETS.☺		

COMMON SYMPTOMS: Hacking, dry or chronic coughing with no phlegm or mucous eliminated.

COMMON CAUSES: Low grade chronic infection of throat and sinuses; mucous-forming diet; allergies; smoking.

CROHN'S DISEASE
REGIONAL ILEITIS

FOOD THERAPY	VITAMINS/ MINERALS	HERBAL THERAPY	BODYWORK
❧ **Diet improvement is the key:** 1)**Start with an alkalizing liquid diet for 3 days;** ◆ Carrot and apple juice, ◆ Grape juice ◆ Pineapple green drinks. 2) **Then add mild fruits & vegetables for a week;** ◆ Carrots, potatoes, yams, apples, papayas, bananas, etc. 3)**Add steamed and raw vegetables, brans, cultured foods for 2 weeks.** ◆ Yogurt, kefir, miso, etc. ◆ Salads, broccoli, cabbage. ◆ Oat bran, rice bran, etc. 4)**Finally add rice, whole grains, wheat germ, tofu, fish, and seafood for healing protein.**	❖ Sun CHLORELLA or chlorophyll liquid in water 3 x daily. ❖ Enzymatic Therapy IBS and/or DGL tablets as needed. ❖ Zinc 15-30Mg. daily. with Vit. E 1000IU daily.♂	🌿 Crystal Star BWL TONE CAPSULES for 3 months. with Aloe Vera juice daily to gently aid bowel recovery. 🌿 Evening primrose oil caps 500Mg. 2 x daily.♀ 🌿 Crystal Star CHO-LO FIBER TONE DRINK or Sonne LIQUID BENTO-NITE to gently clean out toxins.	❖ **Peppermint tea enemas once a week for the first month of healing.** ❖ Apply wet ginger compresses to stomach and lower back. ❖ REFLEXOLOGY POINTS:
	❖ Natren LIFE START 2, 1/4t. 3x daily. ❖ Chewable Bromelain 40Mg. or papaya enzymes after meals.♂	🌿 Effective anti-oxidants: Spirulina Pau de Arco Fenugreek	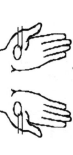 STOMACH & COLON AREA
❧ Avoid nuts, seeds, and citrus while healing. ❧ **Drink only bottled water.** Over treated tap water can often cause inflammatory bowel diseases.	❖ Take Lewis Labs FIBER YEAST each morning.♀ ❖ Niacinimide up to 1500Mg daily.♂ and Biotin 600Mcg. ❖ **B Complex liquid with** extra B$_2$, B$_6$, and pantothenic acid.	🌿 Avoid commercial antacids. They eventually make the inflammation worse by causing the stomach to produce more acids.	❖ Remember that there **must** be diet correction for there to be permanent success. **Avoid red and fatty meats, saturated fats, and fried foods. Increase high fiber and fresh foods.**

COMMON SYMPTOMS: Inflammation and soreness along the entire G.I. tract; distention and pain from food residue and gas.

COMMON CAUSES: Low dietary fiber and excess refined and acid-forming foods, leading to serious a inflammatory condition forming deep ulcers along the digestive tract from rectum to mouth; multiple food intolerances, particularly to wheat and dairy; emotional, acid-causing stress; Zinc deficiency.

See CONSTIPATION DIET and DIVERTICULITIS PAGE in this book for more suggestions and information.

CUTS ✧ SCRAPES ✧ WOUNDS

FOOD THERAPY	VITAMINS/ MINERALS	HERBAL THERAPY	BODYWORK
Apply wheat germ oil directly.	**Apply Vit. E oil. Take 400IU daily.**	Apply Aloe Vera gel as needed.	Place ice packs on the area immediately to stop bleeding and reduce trauma.
Squeeze a fresh lemon on the area to clean and disinfect.	Ester C w/ bioflavs. and **Rutin, 3-5 grams daily.** with Pantothenic acid 500Mg. for collagen/protein formation.	Apply Yarrow compresses to aid clotting ability.	**Apply a green clay poultice.**
Eat plenty of fresh greens every day for faster healing.	**Zinc 50Mg. 2 x daily.**	Deva RESCUE REMEDY.	**Clean with H$_2$O$_2$ and apply tea tree oil drops every 2 to 3 hours.**
	Nature's Plus GERMAN-IUM PLUS 25Mg. daily for a month if wound is slow healing.	Crystal Star ANTI-BIO CAPSULES OR EXTRACT to overcome infection and inflammation.	**Apply DMSO for bruising. Apply morning and evening for 2-3 days for best results.**
	Vit. K 100Mg. 3 x daily for clotting ability.♀ with	**Apply B & T CALIFLORA, or other good CALEN-DULA GEL.**	Apply alternating hot and cold witch hazel compresses.
	Cal/Mag/Zinc 4 daily for faster healing. ♂	**Apply Country Comfort** GOLDEN SEAL/ MYRRH SALVE.	**Apply Royal Jelly as needed. Take 2t. daily.**
	Apply propolis extract Take 1/2 dropperful 2x daily.	Apply a mix of St. John's Wort/Cayenne and Marshmallow.	**Prick open and apply a vitamin A&D capsule.**
	Natra Bio INJURIES TINCTURE.	Apply Country Comfort COMFREY / ALOE SALVE.	
	Enzymatic Therapy DERMAZYME OINTMENT for slow healing cuts.	**Apply cayenne tincture to stop bleeding, and take drops internally as needed for shock.**	

CYSTS ✧ POLYPS ✧ BENIGN TUMORS ✧ WENS

FOOD THERAPY	VITAMINS/ MINERALS	HERBAL THERAPY	BODYWORK
✿ Avoid red meats, caffeine, pasteurized dairy products and acid-forming foods from the diet.	✤ Beta carotene 25,000IU every 4 hours for a month. <u>with</u> Natures Plus VIT. E 800IU daily.	✿ Echinacea extract 4x daily to clear lymph nodes. and/or Crystal Star ANTI-BIO EXTRACT as an anti-infective.	❖ NO smoking. Nicotine aggravates gland imbalance that allows these deposits to form.
✿ Eliminate saturated fats (mostly animal fats), fried foods, chocolate, margerine, shortening and other refined fats.	✤ High omega 3 fish or flax oils 3 x daily.	✿ Pau de Arco tea 4 cups daily for a month. with Comfrey compresses on the affected area.	❖ Massage into affected area daily, H_2O_2 PEROXY GEL for 3 weeks, for noticeable reduction without pain.
✿ Add more fish, seafoods, sea vegetables and unsaturated oils (such as Flax and sun-flower oil) to the diet.	✤ Ascorbate C crystals with Bioflavonoids 1/4t. 4x daily for a month.	✿ Chaparral caps 6 daily, <u>or</u> extract 4 x daily.	❖ Scrub skin with a loofa or dry skin brush regularly to keep sebaceous glands unblocked.
	✤ Organic Germanium 25-50Mg. daily, with Sun CHLORELLA 1 PACKET daily in water.	✿ Evening Primrose oil 500Mg. 6 daily, <u>with</u> Nature's Plus Vit. E 800IU. ♀	
	✤ Zinc Picolinate 50Mg. 2x daily for a month. Then a maintenance dose of 30Mg. daily. ♂	✿ Apply Nutrition Resource NUTRIBIOTIC LIQUID directly 2x daily.	
	✤ Vit. B$_6$ 250Mg. 2x daily til condition clears. ♀		

COMMON SYMPTOMS: A lump or bulge seen or felt under the skin; in the case of vaginal cysts, there is often bleeding during intercourse.

COMMON CAUSES: Internal toxicity and infection; diet contains excess acid or mucous forming foods; poor assimilation/digestion of fats; for sebaceous cysts, gland outflow blocked with sebum deposits; accumulation of dead skin cells, local cosmetic irritants.

DANDRUFF ✧ DRY SCALING SCALP

FOOD THERAPY	VITAMINS/ MINERALS	HERBAL THERAPY	BODYWORK
Make sure the diet is low in sugars, salt and animal fats. No fried foods. They clog the body so it cannot eliminate wastes properly.	B Complex 100Mg. daily with extra B₆ 100Mg. and Folic acid 400Mcg. and PABA 1000IU Niacin TR 500Mg. for increased circulation.	Alta Health SIL-X SILICA CAPSULES for 1 month.	Use jojoba, aloe vera or biotin shampoos.
Add sulphur-rich foods to the diet: Lettuce, oats, green pepper, onions, cucumber, eggs, fish, cabbage, wheat germ.	Schiff EMULSIFIED A & D or Cod Liver oil 1t. daily.	Effective herb minerals: ◆ Crystal Star MEGA-MINERAL CAPSULES ◆ Crystal Star MIN-ZYME-MINOS DRINK MIX ◆ Crystal Star HIGHLY ABSORBABLE MINERAL EXTRACT ◆ Kelp tabs 8 daily	Get some mild circulation-stimulating exercise every day.
Eat lots of green salads, steamed vegetables, and whole grains to nourish the glands.	Zinc Picolinate 50Mg. 2x daily.♂ with Beta Carotene 25,000IU 4x daily.	Effective mineral rinses: Rosemary/Yarrow Nettles Chaparral	Add drops of tea tree oil to hair rinse. Use daily. Or use tea tree oil shampoo.
Take 2T. each daily: Lecithin Brewer's yeast Wheat germ	Evening primrose oil caps 4 daily. or Enzymatic Therapy E F COMPLEX CAPS.	Steep Bay leaves in olive oil til fragrant. Rub on scalp before shampoo. Leave on 30 minutes and shampoo out.	Massage head with both hands and all the fingers at once, for 5 minutes every day to stimulate scalp circulation and slough dead skin cells.
Rinse the hair with cider vinegar and water to keep sebum deposits from clogging pores.	Biotin 600Mcg. daily. ♂	Massage jojoba oil into scalp. Leave on 1 hour. Shampoo out.	Add a few drops Nutrition Resource NUTRIBIOTIC LIQUID to shampoo, and use daily.
	Vit. E w/ Selenium, 400IU daily.	Steep cider vinegar and peppermint oil drops in 1 cup water. Rinse hair.	

COMMON SYMPTOMS: Scaling flakes on scalp and eyebrows; itching scalp.

COMMON CAUSES: Sebaceous gland malfunction; too much alcohol, saturated fat, sugar and salt in the diet; essential fatty acid deficiency; lack of green vegetables; excessively strong or harsh hair dyes.

DEPRESSION ✧ ANXIETY ✧ PARANOIA

FOOD THERAPY	VITAMINS/ MINERALS	HERBAL THERAPY	BODYWORK
Have a glass of carrot juice 2-3 x a week with a pinch of sage and Bragg's liquid aminos.	Relief from depression: ◆ DLPA 750Mg. as needed. ◆ Tyrosine 500Mg. with B_6 ◆ Country Life RELAXER ◆ Natrol SAF CAPSULES♀ ◆ GABA caps with Glycine.	Ginkgo Biloba extract drops as needed.	Exercise worry and anxiety away. Give yourself plenty of body oxygen. Exercise is a nutrient in itself.
Take 2T. each daily: Brewer's yeast Lecithin Wheat germ	Niacin Therapy 500Mg. 2x daily.♂ or Solaray CHROMIACIN.	Crystal Star MENTAL CLARITY CAPS for mental energy, RELAX CAPS for nerve repair.	Sunlight therapy; get some on the body every day possible for Vit. D.
Eat plenty of vegetable protein with lots of fresh foods. Keep tissue oxygen high for red blood cell formation. (See healthy heart diet in this book). Make sure there is good soluble fiber in the diet.	ENER B Vit. B_{12} nasal gel every other day.	Crystal Star CREATIVI-TEA Step 1 oz. tea in brandy for 3 days. Add cherry juice and steep for 24 hours. Take 3T. daily.	Do brain breathing exercises. (See Bragg's book) Yoga or a shiatzu massage can also clear the mind and refresh the body.
	Country Life Maxi-B Complex with Taurine.	Premier 1 or YS ROYAL JELLY 2t. daily.♀	
	Country Life MOOD FACTORS as needed.	Evening primrose oil	AROMATHERAPY: essential oils of Jasmine, Geranium, Ylang Ylang and Basil.
Omit all preserved, refined and junk foods. Avoid sweets, alcohol and drugs.	Enzymatic Therapy THYROID/TYROSINE ♀ OR NEUROPLEX CAPS	Bach Flower RESCUE REMEDY as needed.	
Drink bottled water.	Brain Oxygenators: ◆ Germanium w/Suma ◆ COQ 10 10Mg. ◆ Biotec EXTRA ENERGY ENZYMES SOD 6 daily. ◆ Glutamine 1000Mg. ◆ Wheat germ oil	For depression relief: ◆ Deva Flowers ANXIETY ◆ Medicine Wheel SERENE ◆ St. John's Wort extract ◆ Astragalus capsules	Remember that Vitamin C with bioflavs is a natural tranquilizer, and helps withdrawal from drugs or chemical dependencies.
		Solary EUROCALM CAPS as needed.	

COMMON SYMPTOMS: Feelings of sadness and hopelessness; uncontrollable grief; paranoia; withdrawal from social and family communication; too much worry, anger and guilt.

COMMON CAUSES: Hypoglycemia or other sugar imbalance; allergies; glandular imbalance with high copper levels; drug abuse; Hypothyroidism; sugar or alcohol dependency; prescription drug addiction or intolerance; negative emotions discharging hormonal secretions into the bloodstream.

133

DERMATITIS

FOOD THERAPY	VITAMINS/ MINERALS	HERBAL THERAPY	BODYWORK
Go on a short 3 day juice cleanse to clear acid waste from the system. Then eat a diet full of leafy greens, and other mineral-rich foods, such as sea vegetables for rebuilding healthy tissue and good adrenal function.	**Biotin 600Mcg. daily. ♂**	Ginkgo Biloba extract 3-4x daily <u>with</u> Suma caps 3-4 daily. ♀	Avoid perfumed cosmetics.
	Collagen tabs 6 daily. and/or Ascorbate vitamin C 3-5000Mg. daily for collagen/connective tissue growth.	**Apply Calendula Gel.** ☺	Use **Zia** PAPAYA PEEL to smooth skin after inflammation is gone.
	Alta Health SIL-X SILICA for healthy new growth.	Crystal Star ◆ADRN EXTRACT for adrenal cortex formation. ◆SILICA SOURCE for collagen formation. ◆THERADERM CAPSULES or tea as an anti-inflammatory.	Use tea tree oil or castile non-irritating soap.
Use only poly or mono-unsaturated oils. Keep the diet very low in fats and calories.	Anti-inflammatories: ◆Quercetin Plus with Bromelain 500Mg. 2 daily. ◆Germanium Plus 30Mg.	Crystal Star BEAUTIFUL SKIN TEA applied as a wash to neutralize acids coming out through the skin.	Get early morning sunlight on the skin every day possible for healing vitamin D.
Take 2T. <u>each</u> daily: Molasses Brewer's yeast Wheat germ oil	**Zinc 50Mg. 2 x daily. ♂**	Solaray Turmeric caps.	Apply and use Aubrey Organics collagen therapy cream.
	Apply Enzyme Therapy DERMAZYME CREAM.	**Apply aloe vera gel or ALOE ICE GEL.**	**Apply an ascorbate vitamin C with <u>bioflavs</u> solution in water to the affected areas.**
Particularly avoid **caffeine, chocolate, and acid-forming refined carbohydrates.**	Apply A D & E oil, <u>and</u> Take Schiff emulsified A & D or dry A & D. <u>and</u> Vit. E with Selenium.	Essential fatty acids: ◆Evening Primrose oil ◆Omega 3 Flax oil ◆Enzymatic Therapy EFA	Apply directly Nutrition Resource NUTRIBIOTIC LIQUID til improvement begins.
	Beta Carotene 100,000IU with Omega 3 Flax oil.		

COMMON SYMPTOMS: Inflamed dry skin; scaly, lumpy skin; itching skin.

COMMON CAUSES: EFA deficiency; alleric reaction to cosmetics; emotional stress; over-acid diet with too many refined foods and saturated fats; poor liver activity resulting in non-metabolism of fats; over-use of prescription or pleasure drugs.

DIABETES

FOOD THERAPY

❧ Diet improvement is absolutely necessary to overcoming Diabetes. See DIABETES DIET SUGGESTIONS on the following page.

❧ The diet should be high in fiber and complex carbohydrates, to reduce insulin requirements; low in calories, sugars, and fats; and alkalizing.

❧ Eat plenty of chromium-rich foods: whole grains, brewer's yeast, string beans, eggs cucumbers, soy foods, liver and organ meats, onions and garlic, fresh and dried fruits, shiitake mushrooms, wheat germ, etc.
Have a green salad for vegetable fiber each day

❧ Avoid sugars, all fried, fatty and high cholesterol foods. Omit refined foods, caffeine, & alcohol from the diet.

❧ Drink only spring water with plenty of minerals.

VITAMINS/ MINERALS

✣ GTF Chromium or Chromium picolinate 200Mcg. daily for sugar balance.

or

Solaray CHROMIACIN.

✣ Guar Gum caps daily to flatten sugar curve.♀

✣ To normalize Pancreatic activity:
◆ Alta Health CANGEST
◆ Manganese 5 Mg.
◆ Twin Lab LIQUID K
◆ Glutamine 500Mg.
◆ Raw Pancreas glandular

✣ Ener B B₁₂ INTERNASAL GEL or B₁₂ sublingual with Carnitine 500Mg.♂

✣ Enzymatic Therapy LIQUID LIVER / GINSENG

✣ B Complex 100Mg. daily with Pantothenic acid 500Mg. to encourage adrenal activity. Niacin 250Mg. to stimulate circulation, and Zinc 30Mg.

✣ Omega 3 fish or flax oils. or Vit. E 400IU w/ Selenium 2 daily.

✣ Magnesium/Potassium/ Bromelain 3 daily.

HERBAL THERAPY

❧ Gymnema before meals to block sugar uptake.

❧ Crystal Star INSULFORM CAPSULES to encourage insulin formation. PANCRAID to balance pancreatic activity.

❧ Crystal Star BODY REBUILDER CAPS for stablized energy. ADRN-ALIVE CAPS OR ADRN EXTRACT for cortex support. ♀

❧ Sun CHLORELLA 15-20 tabs daily for absorbable germanium.

❧ Effective teas:
Dandelion/Licorice ♂
Comfrey/Lemon Balm
Siberian Ginseng

❧ Insulin forming herbs:
Pau de Arco
Garlic oil capsules
Bilberry
Astragalus

❧ Use Stevia instead of sugar for sweetening. It does not have sugar's insulin requirements.

BODYWORK

✣ Exercise every day to increase metabolic processes and reduce need for insulin.♂

✣ A regular deep therapy massage is effective in regulating sugar use.

✣ Don't smoke. Nicotine increases sugar desire.

✣ Avoid phenalalanine. No Nutra-Sweet, etc. (Check labels on colas, diet drinks, etc.)

✣ Lose weight. Poor biochemistry often results from overweight. A fiber weight loss drink is effective here.

✣ Alternating hot and cold hydrotherapy to stimulate circulation.

✣ REFLEXOLOGY POINTS:

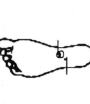

PANCREAS & ADRENALS

DIET FOR DIABETES CONTROL

Diabetes is a chronic degenerative disease, proneness is often hereditary, and is often caused when a diabetic-liable person regularly eats a diet with excess sugars and refined carbohydrates. Pancreatic activity is damaged, the body loses its ability to form enough insulin, and raised blood sugar results. As less and less insulin is produced, simple carbohydrates and sugars, which require a large secretion of insulin for metabolism, keep accumulating in the body and **are stored as fat.** The following diet, in addition to reducing insulin requirements and balancing the action of sugars in the bloodstream, has the nice "side effect" of healthy weight loss.

The key to this diet is in supplying slow-burning complex carbohydrate fuels to the body that do not need much insulin for metabolism. Meals should be small, frequent, vegetarian, and low in fats of all kinds. Proteins should be from soy foods, low fat or cultured dairy products, and whole grains rich in lecithin and chromium. At least 50% of the diet should be in fresh and simply cooked vegetables for low calories and high digestibility.

All sugars, refined, fried and fatty foods must be excluded.

ON RISING: take 2 lemons in a glass of water with 1t. spirulina or 2t. chlorella granules added.

BREAKFAST: take a heaping teasp. of Crystal Star CHO-LO FIBER TONE DRINK or other natural fiber drink mix, in water or apple juice, to regulate and balance sugar curve;
and/or make a mix of 2T. **each:** brewer's yeast, wheat germ, lecithin granules and oat or rice bran.
Sprinkle some daily on your choice of breakfast foods: ◆poached eggs on whole grain toast, ◆muesli, granola or whole grain cereal with apple juice or soy milk, ◆buckwheat or whole grain pancakes with barley syrup or molasses, ◆or simply mix into yogurt with fresh fruit.

MID-MORNING: have a green drink such as Crystal Star ENERGY GREEN or Sun CHLORELLA;
or a refreshing herb tea such as Licorice, Roasted Dandelion Rt. or Pau de Arco tea;
or some whole grain crackers or muffins with soy cream cheese or kefir cheese.

LUNCH: have a fresh green salad, with celery, sprouts, green pepper and tofu, and a mushroom or chicken soup;
or baked tofu or roast turkey with steamed vegetables and brown rice or cornbread;
or a baked potato with yogurt or kefir cheese, and a cup of miso soup;
or a whole grain sandwich with avocado, low fat or soy cheese and a low fat sandwich spread.

MIDAFTERNOON: have a fresh carrot juice, and/or fruit-juice sweetened cookies with a bottle of mineral water.

DINNER: have a baked or broiled sea food dish with brown rice and peas;
or a Chinese stir fry with rice, vegetables and miso soup;
or a spanish beans and rice dish with onions and peppers;
or a light Italian polenta with a hearty vegetable soup or whole grain pasta salad;
or a mushroom quiche with a whole grain crust.

BEFORE BED: **take another teasp. of** CHO-LO FIBER TONE DRINK MIX in apple juice;
or a VEGEX yeast broth drink (1 teasp. in a cup of hot water)

A little white wine is fine occasionally at dinner for relaxation and suprisingly high Chromium content.

CONTROLLING OTHER PROBLEMS ASSOCIATED WITH DIABETES

Diabetic sugar imbalance often leads to other disease conditions. CATARACTS, GLAUCOMA, OBESITY, ULCERS AND FOOD ALLERGIES.

FOR CATARACTS, GLAUCOMA, DIABETIC RETINOPATHY AND IMPAIRED VISION RESULTING FROM DIABETES:

◆ **Quercetin Plus with Bromelain and vitamin E 400IU 3 x daily.**
◆ **Kal PYCNOGENOL**
◆ Take raw Thyroid glandular (N.F. Factors, Enzymatic Therapy or Natra-Bio).
◆ B Complex 150Mg. (Nature's Plus).
◆ Ascorbate vitamin C or Ester C powder with bioflavonoids, 1/4t. at a time, **4-8 x** daily.
◆ Extra Strength digestive enzymes (Rainbow Light DOUBLE STRENGTH ALL-ZYME, Alta Health CANGEST)
◆ Chaparral tea.

FOR CHRONIC OBESITY RESULTING FROM DIABETES:

◆ Lewis Labs FIBER YEAST daily.
◆ **Lewis Labs WEIGH DOWN DIET DRINK with chromium picolinate.**
◆ Gymnema Sylvestre sugar blocking herb 2-3 before each meal.
◆ **Carnitine 500Mg. daily.3**

FOR DIABETIC ULCERS:

◆ Take emulsified vitamin A & D 25,000/1,000IU (Schiff, Solaray). Apply vitamin E oil squeezed from capsules.
◆ Take Zinc 30Mg. 2x daily.
◆ Clean ulcer of necrotic tissue and apply a comfrey poultice or B & T CALIFLORA GEL.
◆ Country Comfort GOLDEN SEAL/MYRRH SALVE.

FOR FOOD ALLERGIES CAUSED BY DIABETIC SUGAR IMBALANCE:

◆ Keep the diet high in fresh raw fruits and vegetables, with lots of soluble vegetable and grain fiber.
◆ Avoid all acid-forming foods, refined carbohydrates, and preserved foods.
◆ **When being tested for glucose tolerance, be sure to take food tolerance tests also, to determine food allergies.**

❖ **Never stop or reduce insulin without monitoring by your physician.**

COMMON SYMPTOMS: High blood sugar; constant hunger with rapid weight change; dry, itching skin; excessive thirst; lack of energy; kidney malfunction leading to bladder and prostate problems and excessive urination; high sugar in the urine.

COMMON CAUSES: Poor diet with too many refined foods and carbohydrates; insulin deficiency; chromium deficiency; metabolic breakdown leading to poor assimilation of fats leading to obesity; pancreas and liver malfunction from caffeine, alcohol and stress overloads; inherited proneness usually accompanied by several allergies; HCl deficiency; Hyperthyroidism.

DIARRHEA

FOOD THERAPY

- Go on a short juice fast for 24 hours (Pg. 27) to clean out harmful bacteria. Then take daily for 3 days: Miso soup with sea vegetables, papaya juice, a fresh green salad, and brown rice with steamed vegetables.

- Eat plenty of yogurt, kefir and cultured foods for friendly flora.

- Take a potassium broth or mineral drink such as Crystal Star MIN-ZYME-MINOS to alkalize, replace lost electrolytes and stimulate enzyme activity.

- Take 2 t. roasted carob powder in water with 1t. of cinnamon.

- Take 2T. cider vinegar in a cup of hot water with honey 2-3x daily.

VITAMINS/ MINERALS

- Natren MEGADOLPHILUS POWDER 1/2t. 3x daily.

- Niacin Therapy 250Mg. 3x daily with Twin Lab Liquid K. ♂

- Chlorophyll liquid 1 t. 3x daily before meals.

- Source of Life FOOD SENSITIVITY SYSTEM.

- Natra-Bio DIARRHEA TINCTURE. ☺

- Lewis Labs FIBER YEAST daily as directed.

- Pancreatin 1400Mg. with meals for better metabolism of fats and oils.

- Activated charcoal tabs with Cal/Mag/Zinc at night.

- Raw Pituitary glandular for chronic diarrhea.

HERBAL THERAPY

- Crystal Star BWL TONE CAPSULES for gentle bowel rebalance.
  or
  FIBER & HERBS COLON CLEANSE CAPSULES if rebuilding is needed.

- Myrrh tincture drops. ♀

- Black orange pekoe tea with 1 lemon and a pinch of cloves.

- Kukicha twig tea with 1/4t. ginger powder and 1t. tamari daily.

- Effective teas:
  Motherwort
  Peppermint
  Bayberry/Barberry
  Slippery Elm
  Calendula
  Catnip ☺

- Yerba Prima ALOE VERA JUICE WITH HERBS 3x daily. ♀

BODYWORK

- **Mix psyllium husk, Flax seed, Chia seed, and Slippery Elm in water. Let soak for 30 minutes. Take 2T. at night before bed.**

- Use mild catnip enemas to rid the body of toxic matter if no inflammation is present.

- **Apply ice packs to the middle and lower back to stimulate nerve force.**

- Eat only small meals. Chew food well.

COMMON SYMPTOMS: Loose, watery, frequent stools , often with abdominal pain and dehydration.

COPMMON CAUSES: Poor food absorption, and lack of fiber in the diet; intestinal parasites; too many anti-biotics; viral infection; enzyme deficiency; adrenal and pancreas exhaustion; lactose intolerance; allergic reaction to certain chemicals.

DIVERTICULITIS

FOOD THERAPY	VITAMINS/ MINERALS	HERBAL THERAPY	BODYWORK
Diet improvement is the main solution: **Start** with a short juice diet for 3 days(Pg.26). Use Carrot, apple, grape or carrot/spinach juice. **Then** add mild fruits and vegetables, such as carrots, bananas, potatoes, yams, papayas, broccoli, etc. for a week. **Finally** add whole grains, rice, tofu, baked fish or sea food for healing protein.	Liquid and chewable supplements are preferable for ease and gentleness.	**Crystal Star BWL TONE CAPSULES 2-3x daily for 3 months to heal and re-tone bowel tissue. with** ENERGY GREEN DRINK with sea vegetables for iodine therapy 3x a week.	Avoid fats, red meats and fried foods.
	Food source multiple (Living Source or New Chapter) to curb gas & rumbling as fiber combines with minerals.		Avoid drugstore antacids. They eventually make the problems worse by causing the stomach to produce more acids.
	Natren LIFE START 2 - 1/2t. 3x daily with meals.	Enzymatic Therapy DGL CHEWABLES as needed.♂	Take peppermint or catnip enemas for bowel cleansing and rebalancing.
See CONSTIPATION DIET in this book for more information.	Chlorophyll liquid or Barley green magma granules before meals.	Aloe Vera juice to soothe pain and gently aid bowel action.	A chiropractic manipulation can often help.
Add oat or rice bran to the diet. Take 2T. Molasses with a banana and plain yogurt daily.	Whey complex powder after meals for bowel rebalance. ♂	Pau de Arco tea 3 cups daily.	Apply wet hot compresses to abdomen and lower back to stimulate systol/diastol action.
	Natures Plus CHEWABLE BROMELAIN 40MG. or papaya enzymes at each meal.	**Psyllium husks, liquid bentonite or Crystal Star CHO-LO FIBER TONE to clean the bowel.**	
Eat cultured foods for healthy G.I. flora; yogurt, kefir, miso, etc.	Twin Lab B COMPLEX LIQUID WITH IRON.	Effective teas: Slippery Elm Comfrey/Fenugreek	
	Solaray REFRESH CAPS.		

COMMON SYMPTOMS: Inflammation and soreness in the colon area from unpassed food residues and gas; chronic constipation; abdominal pain and distention.

COMMON CAUSES: Fiber deficiency from too many refined foods, leading to weakening of the colon wall, and formation of pockets like worn tire bulges; thyroid deficiency; emotional stress causing colon spasms; obesity.

DRUG ABUSE ✧ REHABILITATION ✧ WITHDRAWAL

FOOD THERAPY

☙ Keep plenty of complex carbohydrates and vegetable protein in the diet. Nutritional support is the key to recovering from addiction.

☙ Avoid refined sugars, alcohol and carbohydrates. They aggravate the craving for drugs.

☙ Take 2T. each daily:
Wheat germ
Brewer's yeast

☙ See HYPOGLYCEMIA DIET in this book for more information. See "COOKING FOR HEALTHY HEALING" by Linda Rector-Page for a complete program.

☙ No program will be successful against drug abuse without continued, consistent therapy and awareness.

VITAMINS/ MINERALS

✤ Take 2 each daily:
Glutamine 500Mg.
Tyrosine 500Mg.

✤ Vitamin C crystals up to 10,000Mg daily with

✤ Niacin 1000Mg 3x daily.

✤ Cysteine 500Mg. with Evening Primrose capsules 4-6 daily.

✤ Country Life RELAXER (GABA with taurine)

✤ Excel ENERGY FORMULAS as natural non-addictive energizers. Use on a temporary basis to let the body rebuild ♂

✤ Lexon B BLEND as an "inositol cocktail" for liver detoxification.

✤ Methionine for heroine, Tyrosine for cocaine CO Q 10 for prescription drug overuse.

HERBAL THERAPY

☙ Crystal Star ANTI-HST CAPSULES or EXTRACT to open up veins and HEAVY METAL or DETOX CAPSULES 4 daily.

☙ Sun CHLORELLA TABS for detoxification with Chaparral caps as an anti-oxidant.

☙ Crystal Star RELAX CAPSULES or STRESS RELIEF EXTRACT to relieve tension and nervousness.♀

☙ High potency aged ginseng, especially sages ginseng to uphold energy levels and reduce desire. ♂

☙ Effective teas/extracts:
◆ Ephedra to dilate veins
◆ Echinacea/Myrrh
◆ Chamomile for relaxation
◆ Gotu Kola for energy

BODYWORK

✤ It takes a year or more to detoxify the blood of drugs.

✤ Avoid smoking. It increases craving for drugs.

✤ Apply tea tree oil or B&T califlora gel to ulcers in the nose.

✤ REFLEXOLOGY POINT:

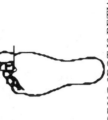

DRUG SPOT IS BETWEEN THE 2ND AND 3RD TOE ON TOP OF THE FOOT.

COMMON SYMPTOMS: Low blood sugar; irritability; fatigue and unusual drowsiness, shakiness, nervousness, trembling; disorientation; memory loss; wired feeling; anxiety and paranoia; headaches; sweating, cramps; palpitations; poor food absorption even when meals are good.

COMMON CAUSES: Too much and too many drugs, both pleasure and prescription; severe metabolic and nutritional deficiencies; underactive thyroid ; exhausted liver and adrenal glands; malnourishment from using drugs as food for energy.

140

DYSENTERY

ACUTE ✦ AMOEBIC

FOOD THERAPY	VITAMINS/ MINERALS	HERBAL THERAPY	BODYWORK
❧ Take carrot/beet/cucumber juice once a day for a week to clean the kidneys, so they can rid the body of the infestation as efficiently as possible.	❖ Natren MEGA-DOLPHILUS or LIFE START 2, 1/2t. 6x daily.	❧ Cayenne/Garlic capsules 6-8 daily.	❖ Take a garlic enema every other day to combat organisms. and/or
❧ Take a lemon juice and egg white drink every morning.	❖ Homeopathic remedy IPECAC as directed.	❧ Tea Tree oil, 4 drops in water 4x daily. with	❖ A high colonic irrigation to clean the colon fast.
❧ Take 2T. epsom salts in a glass of water to purge the bowel.	❖ Alta Health CANGEST ♀ or Enzymatic Therapy MEGA-ZYME CAPSULES.	❧ Crystal Star VERMEX CAPSULES as directed.	❖ See page on INTERNAL PARASITES in this book for more information.
❧ Amaranth is used successfully in South America to remove parasites and strengthen the system.	❖ Chlorophyll liquid 1 t. 3x daily with meals. or Sun CHLORELLA GRANULES 2 PKTS. in water daily.	❧ Black Walnut extract or Myrrh tincture 10 drops under the tongue every 4 hours.	
	❖ Yerba Prima Aloe Vera juice with herbs, one glass daily. ♀	❧ Red Raspberry extract ☺	
		❧ Effective teas: Slippery Elm Strawberry Leaf ☺ Calendula flwrs. Wild Cherry Bark	
		❧ Witch Hazel tea, bark and leaf, 4 cups daily.	
		❧ Psyllium husks, or Sonne BENTONITE #7 LIQUID, 2T. morning and evening to clean the colon and bowel.	

COMMON SYMPTOMS: Frequent and often uncontrollable running of the bowels; irritation, pain, and dehydration; inflammation and infection.

COMMON CAUSES: Parasite infestation from bad water, usually contracted in tropical countries; extreme nutritional deficiency from rancid or unsanitary food.

EARACHES

EXCESSIVE EARWAX ✦ INFECTIONS

FOOD THERAPY	VITAMINS/ MINERALS	HERBAL THERAPY	BODYWORK
If earaches are chronic, keep the diet low in fats and mucous forming dairy products.	Vitamin C 3-5000Mg. daily with Bioflavs and Rutin.	Mullein oil ear drops as needed. ☺	Use ice packs on the ear to relieve pain instead of hea. ♂
Use castor oil drops in the ear, and hold in with cotton. ☺	Use a small dropper and flush ear gently with a food grade dilute solution of 3% H_2O_2 to clear infection.	Warm garlic oil ear drops. Also take garlic tabs 4x daily.	Massage ear, neck and temple region. Pull lobe 10 times on each ear. Fold ear shell over and back repeatedly til blood suffuses the area.
Press out and strain onion juice onto a small cotton plug. Place in the ear for fast, effective relief and infection fighting.	Natra-Bio EARACHE homeopathic tincture. ☺	Crystal Star ANTIBIO CAPSULES 4-6 daily, followed by COLD SEASON DEFENSE CAPSULES to take down swelling and inflammation. (Use ANTI-BIO EXTRACT as ear drops morning and evening)	Have the ear flushed for earwax or infection by a doctor.
	Beta carotene 25,000IU 4x daily. with	Crystal Star ANTI-HST CAPSULES to shrink swollen membranes. ASPIRSOURCE CAPSULES, 4 at a time for pain.	For earwax: Press firmly but gently behind, then in front of the ear. Pull lobe up and down to work wax out. Fold ear shell in half. Open and fold repeatedly to bring up circulation.
	Zinc Lozenges 30Mg. under the tongue til dissolved.	Drop warm Lobelia extract in the ear for pain as needed.	Put 2-3 drops of warm olive oil in each ear to soften wax, and flush with warm water.
	Enzymatic Therapy ORAL-ZYME as needed.	Effective teas: Chamomile for pain Yarrow	
	Mix warm vegetable glycerine and witch hazel. Soak a piece of cotton and insert in the ear to draw out infection.		

142

COMMON SYMPTOMS: Pain in the mastoid, eustacion and ear area; swelling, inflammation and thickness in the ear area.

COMMON CAUSES: Residue of a cold or flu; bronchial settling in the ear; viral infection; too many mucous forming and fatty foods; excess dairy products and carbohydrates.

ECZEMA ✧ PSORIASIS

FOOD THERAPY	VITAMINS/ MINERALS	HERBAL THERAPY	BODYWORK
❧ A high fiber, high mineral diet with lots of vegetable protein is the key to clearing and preventing these conditions.	❖ High omega 3 fish or flax oils 3 daily.	❧ Crystal Star THERADERM CAPSULES for 3 months. Take THERADERM TEA internally 2 cups daily, and apply to lesions with soaked cotton balls.	❖ Apply hot ginger or fresh comfrey leaf compresses.
❧ Go on a short 3 day cleansing diet (Pg. 26) to release acid wastes. ◆ Take 1T. psyllium husk in water morning and evening. ◆ Take a green drink daily (BARLEY GREEN MAGMA, CHLORELLA, or CRYSTAL STAR ENERGY GREEN) ◆ Take 3 glasses of cranberry or apple juice daily. Then eat a low fat, sugar and milk free, alkaline diet with 60-70% fresh foods, whole grains and sea vegetables for iodine therapy.	❖ Alta Health SIL-X TABS with Evening primrose oil 4 x daily for 3 months. ♀	❧ Use Crystal Star ADRN EXTRACT DROPS daily to help form adrenal cortex with MILK THISTLE DROPS for better liver function.	❖ Take a Catnip or chlorophyll enema once a week to release acid toxins faster.
	❖ Ester C w/ bioflavonoids 3000Mg. daily for tissue and collagen re-growth. with Emulsified A 100,000IU daily. and Vit. E 400IU 2 x daily.	❧ Bioforce ECHINAFORCE or ECZEMA EXTRACT and ECHINACEA CREAM. ♀	❖ Effective applications: ◆ ALOE ICE ◆ Tea Tree oil ◆ Calendula gel ◆ Jojoba oil (to scalp)
	❖ High potency ACT CLEAR PANCREATIN to process fats and oils better.	❧ Effective topical solutions: ◆ Myrrh/ Golden Seal Rt. tea ◆ Black Walnut Lf. tea ◆ Dandelion/ Burdock tea ◆ ComfreyLeaf tea ◆ Crystal Star SILICA SOURCE	❖ Expose affected areas to early morning sunlight every day possible for healing Vit. D.
❧ NO refined fatty or fried foods, red meats, sugars.	❖ Zinc picolinate 50Mg. 2x daily. with Glutamine 500Mg. daily and Lecithin 1900Gr. 8 daily. ♂	❧ Apply H₂O₂ PEROXY GEL to affected areas daily.	❖ Relax more. Tension and emotional stress often cause and aggravate flare ups.
❧ Take 2T. each daily: ◆ Lecithin granules ◆ Brewer's yeast ◆ Unsulphured Molasses	❖ B Complex 100Mg. with extra Panto. Acid 500Mg. and PABA 1000Mg.	❧ Apply Aloe Vera gel and drink aloe vera juice 2 glasses daily.	❖ Swim or wade in the ocean, or take Kelp foot baths for iodine therapy.

COMMON SYMPTOMS: Silvery red, scaly, irritating skin patches on knees, elbows, scalp or chest that flare up irregularly.

COMMON CAUSES: Overuse of drugs and anti-biotics; associated with diabetes and candida allergies; hypothyroidism; EFA deficiency; liver malfunction; thin bowel walls allowing too much acid waste in the system that is eliminated through the skin; too many refined foods in the diet

Natural therapies have had notable achievement in these skin conditions because they get to the root of the problem. Natural methods take several months to produce consistent improvement, but they offer lasting recovery. Drugs can produce dramatic short term results, but the problem reappears after they are discontinued.

EMPHYSEMA

FOOD THERAPY	VITAMINS/ MINERALS	HERBAL THERAPY	BODYWORK
Go on a short mucous cleansing juice fast for 3-5 days (Pg. 25) Then, eat a largely fresh foods diet with lots of vegetable protein from whole grains, tofu, nuts, seeds and sprouts. Have a green salad every day and add vitamin B rich foods such as brown rice and eggs frequently.	B Complex 150Mg. daily with Panto. Acid 500Mg. and Vitamin C crystals 1/4t. every hour to bowel tolerance, for a month. This is an ascorbic acid body flush to neutralize lung poisons and encourage tissue growth.	Crystal Star RESPIRCAPS AND RESPIRTEA 2 x daily.	Avoid smoking and secondary smoke. (Use Enzymatic Therapy NICOTABS).
		Crystal Star SUPER LICORICE EXTRACT to encourage adrenal activity. OPEN UP TEA to expel mucous congestion.	Do deep breathing exercises for 3 minutes every morning when rising to clean the lungs.
Have a glass of fresh carrot juice every day for a month.	Enzymatic Therapy LUNG~THYMUS COMPLEX and ADRENAL COMPLEX or LIQUID LIVER CAPS.	Effective Lung teas: Comfrey/Fenugreek Mullein/Lobelia extract Pleurisy root	Take a brisk deep breathing daily walk to increase oxygen uptake.
	Liquid Chlorophyll or Sun CHLORELLA DRINK 3x daily with meals.	High potency Y S or Premier ROYAL JELLY 2t. for pantothenic acid. ♀ with Aloe Vera juice, 2 glasses.	Emphysema is a wasting disease. Get some early sunlight on the body every day possible.
Avoid all mucous-forming foods such as pasteurized dairy, red meats, and caffeine.	Effective anti-oxidants: ◆ CO Q10 30Mg. ♂ ◆ Germanium 30-50Mg. ◆ Vit. E with selenium ♂ ◆ B15 with extra folic acid ♀ ◆ Beta carotene 100,000IU	Crystal Star HEAVY METAL CAPS if the cause is chemical pollutants.	Steam head and nasal passages with Eucalyptus and wintergreen steams.
Take 1T. each daily: Brewer's yeast Lecithin granules Unsulphured Molasses Wheat germ	Food grade H_2O_2 3% solution, 1T in 8oz. water internally, and in the vaporizer at night.	Natures Plus GARLITE Garlic/Onion caps 6 daily to dissolve mucous, act as an anti-infective.	REFLEXOLOGY POINT: LUNG
See MUCOUS CLEANSING DIET under ASTHMA in this book for more information.	BioForce ASTHMASAN DROPS or TABLETS. ♂	Take 5 drops anise oil in a teasp. brown sugar 3x daily before meals.	Use 1t. H_2O_2 and water in the vaporizer at night.

COMMON SYMPTOMS: Bronchitis; frequent colds; coated tongue; bad breath; shortness of breath; lack of energy and vitallity.

COMMON CAUSES: Smoking and secondary smoke; air and environmental pollution; excess refined foods and dairy produts; allergies; heavy metal pollution from industry; poor circulation and elimination of poisons by the body.

♀ ENDOMETRIOSIS ✧ PELVIC INFLAMMATORY DISEASE ♀

FOOD THERAPY	VITAMINS/ MINERALS	HERBAL THERAPY	BODYWORK
● Omit caffeine in all forms from the diet permanently. Avoid refined sugars, alcohol, salt, acid-forming foods, red meats and dairy foods during healing. *Keeping animal fats and cholesterol low, prevents excess estrogen production. (a cause of endometriosis)*	❖ Enzymatic Therapy RAW OVARY and RAW PANCREAS 3x daily. and/or NUCLEO-PRO F for pain relief. Chew tablets for faster results.	❧ Evening Primrose oil caps 6-8 daily. <u>with</u> Crystal Star WOMAN'S BEST FRIEND CAPSULES <u>and</u> burdock tea 2 cups daily for 3 months.	❖ Remember, before you jump into surgery or any drastic treatment decision, endometriosis fibroids often go away when glands and hormones <u>rebalance</u>, such as after pregnancy and birth, or menopause.
	❖ Nature's Plus Dyna-Mins CALCIUM/ MAGNESIUM 1000Mg/ 1000Mg, daily.	❧ Crystal Star ANTI-BIO CAPS OR EXTRACT for 1-2 weeks until inflammation is relieved.	❖ Keep weight down through lower dietary fats, but make sure you are not Anorexic, because this affects hormone and lipo substances balance.
● A short 24 hour juice diet (Pg. 27) will clear out acid wastes. Then eat plenty of cultured foods, fresh fruits and salads, whole grains and cereals until condition clears.	❖ Twin Labs LIQUID K POTASSIUM 3t. daily. with B Complex 100Mg. and extra Folic acid and B₆.	❧ Crystal Star SUPER LICORICE EXTRACT or ADRN EXTRACT for estrogen and adrenal cortex balance.	❖ Get mild exercise and some early morning sunlight on the body every day.
	❖ Beta carotene 100,000IU	❧ Sarsaparilla tincture under the tongue as needed for progesterone stimulation.	❖ Effective douches: ◆ Garlic ◆ Mineral water
● Take a low fat protein drink each morning, such as Nature's Plus SPIRUTEIN.	❖ Nature's Plus VITAMIN E 800IU 2 daily. with Solaray LIPOTROPIC COMPLEX.	❧ Echinacea extract and Milk Thistle extract 3x daily.	❖ Avoid all IUDs. They have been a major contributor to endometriosis.
● See HYPOGLYCEMIA DIET suggestions in this book, or "COOKING FOR HEALTHY HEALING" by Linda Rector-Page for more information.	❖ Effective oils: ◆ Shark Liver oil, a superior anti-infective. ◆ Omega 3 Flax oil ◆ Borage or Black currant oil ◆ Omega 3 fish oil	❧ Golden Seal/Chaparral caps, 2 every 4 hrs., and Floradix LIQUID IRON.	◆ REFLEXOLOGY POINT: Press both sides of the foot just below the ankle bone, 2x daily for 10 seconds each.

COMMON SYMPTOMS: Mislocation and overgrowth of uterine tissue (normal tissue growing in abnormal places), and attachment of this tissue to other organs; extreme pain during menses, ovulation and sex; fluid retention; swelling of the abdomen; excessive menstruation.; infertility.

COMMON CAUSES: Excess estrogen, deficient progesterone, and general hormone imbalance; stress; magnesium deficiency; hypoglycemia; EFA deficiency; chlamydia; X-Ray consequence; too much caffeine and alcohol.

ENERGY ◇ STAMINA ◇ ENDURANCE

FOOD THERAPY	VITAMINS/ MINERALS	HERBAL THERAPY	BODYWORK
☙ The basic diet should consist of 65-70% **complex carbohydrates,** fresh fruits, vegetables, grains and legumes; 20-**25% protein,** from nuts, seeds, whole grains, legumes, soy and dairy products, sea foods and poultry; **10-15% fats** from quality sources, like unrefined vegetable, nut and seed oils, eggs and dairy products.	❖ **B Complex 100Mg. with extra Pantothenic acid 500Mg. 2x daily.** ♀	❧ **Bioforce GINSAVENA EXTRACT.** ♂	❖ Take a brisk walk or other aerobic exercise every day for tissue oxygen.
	❖ Ener B$_{12}$ INTERNASAL GEL every 3-4 days. or **Dibencozide** ♂	❧ **Effective Ginseng combinations: Sages Ginseng Ginseng/Gotu Kola Ginseng/Damiana Siberian Ginseng Chinese Red Ginseng** ♂	❖ Get some early morning sunlight on the body every day possible.
☙ **Take a high protein drink every morning (Pg. 39) Add spirulina or bee pollen if desired.**	❖ Effective anti-oxidants: ◆ Country Life B$_{15}$ DMG ◆ Germanium 25-30Mg. ◆ CO Q10 10Mg. ◆ **Sun CHLORELLA TABS.**	❧ Crystal Star energizers: **SUPERMAX** ♂ **FEEL GREAT CAPS & TEA HIGH PERFORMANCE** ♂ **DONG QUAI/ DAMIANA** ♀ **ZING** ♂ **HIGH ENERGY TEA BODY REBUILDER/ ADRN-**	❖ Have a full spinal massage for increased nerve force.
	❖ Glutamine 1000Mg. daily.	**ALIVE CAPSULES** ♀ or **ADRN EXRACT**	❖ Alternating hot and cold hydrotherapy to increase circulation.
☙ Effective food additions: **Alacer HI-K KOLA Braggs LIQUID AMINOS ALL 1 Nature's Plus SPIRUTEIN** Brewer's yeast **Vegex YEAST EXTRACT WHEAT GERM**	❖ Zinc Picolinate 50-75Mg. ♂	❧ **Country Life ENERGIX VIALS.** 1 daily.	❖ Acupressure procedure to restore energy: Squeeze point between the eyes where brows come together.
	❖ **Rainbow Light** ULTRA ENERGY PLUS 3 daily. ♀		❖ Use a Shiatzu exercise and stretching program for 5 minutes daily to release energy blocks.
	❖ **Biotec EXTRA ENERGY ENZYMES SOD** 6 daily.	❧ **Enzymatic Therapy SIBERIAN GINSENG EXTRACT caps 2000Mg.**	
☙ Avoid tobacco, drugs and caffeine. Reduce sugar and alcohol intake.	❖ **Enzymatic Therapy LIQUID LIVER W/ GINSENG.** ♂		❖ Energy factors for supplement addition: **adrenals, thyroid, liver, minerals.**
	❖ Floradix **HERBAL IRON.** ♀	❧ Royal jelly / Ginseng vials.	

COMMON SYMPTOMS: Lack of energy for even everyday tasks; mental depression; lethargy.

COMMON CAUSES: Poor eating habits and lack of nutrition; Protein deficiency caused by "new age" eating beliefs; too much sugar; Poor thyroid , liver and adrenal activity; anemia; stress; Chronic Fatigue Syndrome; Candida Albicans.

EPILEPSY ✧ PETIT MAL

FOOD THERAPY	VITAMINS/ MINERALS	HERBAL THERAPY	BODYWORK
✦ There must be a diet and lifestyle change for there to be permanent control and improvement. Go on a 3 day liquid diet (Pg.25) to release mucous from the system. Then follow a diet with at least 70% fresh raw foods for a month. Have a green salad every day. Add cultured foods such as yogurt and kefir, tofu, brown rice and other whole grains frequently. After a month, add eggs, small amounts of low fat and raw dairy, legumes and seafoods.	✦ Evening Primrose caps 4-6 daily for 2 months, then 3-4 daily for 1 mo. with ✦ Raw Thyroid glandular Country Life MAXI-B W/ TAURINE & B$_6$ as an anti-convulsant. and Magnesium 500Mg. daily.	✦ Crystal Star RELAX CAPS and ANTI-SPAZ CAPS as needed. ✦ Nature's Way ANTSP TINCTURE or LOBELIA TINCTURE under the tongue as emergency measures.	✦ Take lemon juice or catnip enemas once a month to keep the body pH balanced and toxin-free. ✦ Get some outdoor exercise every day for healthy circulation.
	✦ Country Life RELAXER with GABA and Taurine and Glutamine 500Mg. daily.	✦ Effective teas: Catnip ☺ Scullcap 3 cups daily. Siberian Ginseng	✦ Squeeze the little finger *very firmly* during a seizure. Let the person lie down and get lots of fresh air. Do not put anything in the person's mouth or throw water on the face. Turn head to let excess saliva drain out.
	✦ Alta Health sublingual Manganese with vit. B$_{12}$. and Cysteine 500Mg.	✦ Crystal Star ANEMI-GIZE CAPSULES to strengthen spleen for tissue oxygen and red blood cell formation.	
✦ See HYPOGLYCEMIA DIET in this book, "COOKING FOR HEALTHY HEALING" by Linda Rector-Page, or Airola's ROTATION DIET for more information.	✦ Carnitine 250Mg. ☺ with Folic acid 400Mcg. esp. if taking Dilantin.	✦ Mezotrace MINERAL COMPLEX to resupply against deficiencies.	
	✦ Phosphatidyl choline 2-4.	✦ Floradix LIQUID MULTIPLE VIT/MIN. COMPLEX for body balance. ☺	
✦ Avoid all refined foods sugars, fried and canned foods, red meats, pork, alcohol, and pasteurized dairy products.	✦ Niacin therapy: 100-250Mg 3x daily.		
	✦ Tryptophane 500Mg. ☺	✦ Solaray EUROCALM CAPS.	

COMMON SYMPTOMS: Brief seizures, often with motor disability; loss of memory, and often loss of consciousness; falling down and jerking with foam at the mouth. Seizures are usually short, and there is usually immediate recovery of consciousness.

COMMON CAUSES: inability of the body to eliminate wastes properly with a resultant overload on the nervous system; heavy metal toxicity; allergies; magnesium and other mineral deficiency; hypoglycemia; deficient metabolic function and prostaglandin formation.

147

EXHAUSTION ✧ FATIGUE ✧ MENTAL BURNOUT

FOOD THERAPY	VITAMINS/ MINERALS	HERBAL THERAPY	BODYWORK

FOOD THERAPY

❧ Make sure you are eating for optimum nutrition. The brain requires almost every known nutrient for maximum function. Start each day with a protein drink (Pg. 39) or ALL 1 VITAMIN DRINK. Include plenty of protein building foods such as whole grains, brown rice, nuts, seeds, soy products, sea vegetables and sprouts.

❧ Take 1 Tblsp each daily:
Wheat germ
Bee Pollen
Brewer's yeast
Spirulina

❧ Have a little white wine at dinner for mental relaxation, good digestion, and minerals.

❧ Take 2T. cider vinegar and honey in water daily for nerve health.

❧ Avoid caffeine foods.

VITAMINS/ MINERALS

✧ Ener B₁₂ INTERNASAL GEL every 3 days.

✧ Country Life ENERGIX VIALS every 2 days. ♂

✧ Mezotrace MINERALS
or
White Birch Min. water

✧ Living Source MASTER NUTRIENT SYSTEM CAPS.

✧ Effective anti-oxidants:
◆ B₁₅ DMG with Tyrosine
◆ CO Q 10 10Mg. daily
◆ Vitamin. E w/Selenium
◆ Vitamin C 3000Mg. daily
◆ Sun CHLORELLA

✧ Effective glandulars:
◆ Raw Adrenal complex
◆ Raw Pituitary ♂
◆ Raw Thyroid w/ Tyrosine ♀
◆ Raw Brain

✧ B Complex 100M. daily.
Extra Niacin Therapy
250-500Mg. daily
with
Twin Lab LIQUID K ♀

HERBAL THERAPY

❧ Crystal Star energizers:
◆ BODY REBUILDER CAPS W/
◆ ADRN-ALIVE CAPS OR EXT.
◆ SUPERMAX
◆ FEEL GREAT CAPS & TEA
◆ HIGH ENERGY TEA
◆ HYPO BLUES CAPS & TEA
◆ ENERGY GREEN DRINK
◆ MIN-ZYME-MINOS DRINK

❧ Effective Ginseng capsule combinations:
◆ Ginseng/Gotu Kola ♂
◆ Ginseng/Damiana
◆ Dong Quai/Damiana ♀
◆ Ginseng/Cayenne
◆ Floradix HERBAL IRON

❧ Ginseng/Royal Jelly vials.

❧ Effective extracts:
◆ Hawthorne Lf. & Flwr.
◆ Siberian Ginseng in Sage tea.
◆ Ginkgo Biloba
◆ CYCLONE CIDER

❧ Excel ENERGY FORMULAS

❧ Rainbow Light ULTRA
ENERGY PLUS CAPSULES. ♀

❧ Enzymatic Therapy
LIQUID LIVER W/
SIBERIAN GINSENG.

BODYWORK

❖ Get some aerobic exercise every day to stimulate endorphins and replenish oxygen in the blood, brain and tissues.

❖ See a massage therapist or reflexologist for a total foot and body massage. Chiropractic adjustment and Shiatzu are also effective.

❖ Alternate hot and cold hydrotherapy to stimulate circulation.

❖ Avoid smoking as circulation constricting. Relax more. Quiet meditative time every day is like a "brain" vacation.

❖ See HYPOGLYCEMIA and CANDIDA ALBICANS diets in this book for more suggestions.

❖ If symptoms are chronic for more than 6 months, get a test for EBV or Candida.

148

COMMON SYMPTOMS: Abnormal tiredness and weakness; mental dullness and depression; lethargy; avoidance of family, friends and co-workers; resentment towards authority and defensiveness; loss of confidence; constant anxiety and mood swings; low sex drive; boredom; insomnia; fatigue.

COMMON CAUSES: Stress; anemia; exhausted adrenal glands;allergies; hypothyroidism; constipation; hypoglycemia; candida albicans; poor circulation; poor food and mineral absorption; toxicity from drugs, tobacco, caffeine and lack of tissue oxygen; Epstein Barr virus; B ₁ and B ₁₂ deficiency.

EYESIGHT

FOOD THERAPY

❧ Keep plenty of protein in the diet from sea and soy foods, whole grains, low fat dairy foods, eggs sprouts and seeds.

❧ Include lots of vitamin A and high mineral foods in the diet, such as leafy greens, endive, carrots, broccoli, sea vegetables and parsley.

❧ Take a good eyesight drink twice a week: Mix 1 cup carrot juice, 1/2 cup eyebright tea, 1 egg, 1T. wheat germ, 1t. rose hips powder, 1t. honey, 1t. sesame seeds, 1t. brewer's yeast, 1t. kelp.

❧ Reduce sugar intake. Avoid refined foods, pasteurized dairy, and red meats. All of these cause the body to metabolize slowly, use sugars badly, and form clogging crystallizations.

VITAMINS/ MINERALS

❖ Beta Carotene up to 150,000IU daily. with GTF Chromium 200Mcg. to regulate sugar use.

❖ Effective Bioflavonoids to strengthen eye vessels:
◆ Quercetin Plus w/ Bromelain
◆ Kal Pycnogenol with Vit. D.

❖ For dry eyes; non-tearing:
◆ Vit B 6 500Mg. daily.
◆ Evening Primrose oil caps
◆ Aloe Vera Juice washes

❖ For floaters:
◆ Bioflavonoids 500Mg. daily
◆ Vit. K 100Mg. 2x daily.
◆ Choline/Inositol

❖ For spots before the eyes:
◆ Vit. B 6 250Mg. 2x daily,
◆ Pantothenic acid 500Mg.
◆ Ascorbate vit. C or Ester C

❖ For retinitis pigmentosa:
◆ Pycnogenol
◆ Zinc picolinate 50Mg.

❖ For Myopia:
◆ Ascorbate C powder 5000Mg.

HERBAL THERAPY

❧ Effective eyewashes:
◆ Crystal Star EYELIGHT TEA
◆ Aloe Vera juice
◆ Chaparral tea.
◆ Calendula tea for scleroderma.

❧ Crystal Star VISI-CARE CAPSULES 4-6 daily with LIVA-ALIVE CAPSULES, LIV-TONIC EXTRACT, and/or LIV-FLUSH TEA.

❧ Parsley Root capsules 4 with kelp tabs 6 daily.♀

❧ For night blindness:
◆ Crystal Star Bilberry extract
◆ Marine Carotene
◆ Enzymatic Herbal Flavonoids

❧ For Floaters:
◆ H₂O₂ PEROXY GEL rubbed on the feet at night.

❧ Enzymatic Therapy SILYMARIN CAPS as a liver cleanser.

❧ For myopia/ eye fatigue:
◆ Bilberry extract
◆ Solaray VIZON CAPS.
◆ Pycnogenol capsules

BODYWORK

❖ Palm each eye 3 x daily for 10 seconds per time. See THE BATES METHOD BOOK for more exercise and information.

❖ Massage temples; pinch skin between the brows to relieve strain.

❖ Bad substances for eyes:
Cocaine
Aspirin
Phenalalanine
Hydrocortisone

❖ Bathe eyes in a Witch Hazel/ Rosemary solution, or Chamomile tea, for clarity and to relieve strain. (Better than Visine)

❖ REFLEXOLOGY POINT:

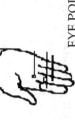

EYE POINTS

COMMON SYMPTOMS: Poor, often degenerating vision; easily strained eyes, blurring more as the days goes on; frequent headaches over the eyes; spots and floaters before the eyes.

COMMON CAUSES:Liver malfunction is the most common cause. Keep it clean and active. SEE LIVER CLEANSING DIET IN THIS BOOK. Environmental pollutants; allergies; poor diet deficient in usable proteins and minerals, excessive in sugars and refined foods; serious illness; drug abuse.

FEVERS AS CLEANSERS AND HEALERS

A slight fever is often the body's own way of clearing up an infection or toxic overload quickly. The body temperature is naturally raised to literally "burn out" the poisons, to throw them off through heat and then through sweating. The heat from a fever can also de-activate viruses, so unless a fever is exceptionally high or long lasting, it is sometimes a wise choice to let it run, even with children. Often they will get better faster. Administer lots of liquids during a fever - juices, water, broths. Bathe frequently. Infection and toxic waste from the illness are largely thrown off through the skin. If not regularly washed off, these substances will just lay on the skin and be partially reabsorbed into the body. As there is usually substantial body odor during a cleansing fever when the toxins are being eliminated, frequent baths and showers help you feel better, too.
A cup of hot Bayberry Bark or Elder Flower tea, or Cayenne and Ginger capsules or extracts will noticeably speed up the cleansing process, by encouraging body temperature to rise, and stimulating circulation.

FOOD THERAPY

🌿 Stay on a liquid diet during a fever to maximize the cleansing process: bottled water, fruit juices, broths and herb teas.

🌿 Carrot/Beet/Cucumber juice is a specific to clean the kidneys and help bring a fever down.

🌿 Sip on lemon juice with honey all during the morning grapefruit juice during the evening.

🌿 After the fever breaks, take strengthening hot tonics (Pg. 36).

VITAMINS/ MINERALS

❖ Beta carotene 10,000IU ☺ or 25,000IU ♂♀ every 6 hours as an anti-infective.

❖ Vitamin C crystals 1/4t. per 1/2 hour in juice or water to bowel tolerance as an ascorbic acid flush.

❖ Bioforce FIEBRESAN DROPS
Natra-Bio FEVER TINCTURE
Hylands HYLAVIR TABLETS ☺

❖ No aspirin to children to reduce fever. Give herb teas instead; chamomile, peppermint, or catnip.

HERBAL THERAPY

🐚 Lobelia tincture drops in water every few hours if fever is severe. ☺

🐚 Crystal Star CRISIS CAPS til sweating occurs, usually within 24 hours.

🐚 Crystal Star ANTI-BIO CAPS or DROPS as an anti-infective. Then, COLD SEASON DEFENSE CAPS.

🐚 Effective teas:
◆ Catnip/Peppermint/Ginger
◆ Elder flower/Sage
◆ Boneset/White Willow

🐚 Take 2 cups daily, fenugreek or sassafras tea with lemon and honey.

BODYWORK

❖ Take a catnip enema to cleanse the elimination channels.

❖ Use cool water or alcohol rubs downs to reduce a fever. Add lots of extra water to the diet.

❖ Take echinacea tincture to encourage lymph gland to throw off toxins. Then sponge off with cool water, and follow with a brisk towel rub.

❖ Crystal Star DRAWING & SWEATING WRAP.

❖ Take a sauna to sweat toxins out.

COMMON SYMPTOMS: Hot, dry, flushed skin; lethargy.

COMMON CAUSES: Bacterial or viral infection in the system that the body is trying to throw off.
Remember: Fevers are a <u>result</u> of the problem and a <u>part</u> of the cure.

150

♀ FIBROID BREAST GROWTHS ♀

FOOD THERAPY

❧ Follow a <u>low fat</u> vegetarian diet to guard against fibroid formation. High fats mean high estrogen production (too much estrogen is a common cause of fibroids).

❧ Avoid caffeine and caffeine-containing foods, such as chocolate, cooked rhubarb or spinach and sodas.

❧ Reduce sugars and salt intake. Omit smoked or preserved meats and fish.

❧ No fried foods, esp. during the menstrual cycle.

❧ Take 4t.wheat germ oil daily for a month.

❧ Add Miso , sea vegetables, and other alkalizing foods to the diet to neutralize toxins.

VITAMINS/ MINERALS

✣ Nature's Plus Vitamin E 800IU during healing.
with
Schiff EMULSIFIED A 25,000IU 3x daily.

✣ High Omega 3 oils or Shark Liver oil as an anti-infective.

✣ Ascorbate Vitamin C or Ester C powder with Bioflavonoids 5000Mg.
with
Alta Health SIL-X SILICA for collagen regrowth.

✣ Food grade H_2O_2 PEROXY GEL rubbed on the fibroids. Noticeable reduction in 3-6 weeks.

✣ Sun CHLORELLA 20 daily
with

✣ Germanium 30-100Mg. daily as anti-oxidants.

✣ Enzymatic Therapy RAW MAMMARY CAPS <u>or</u> NUCLEOPRO F CAPS.

HERBAL THERAPY

❧ Crystal Star WOMAN'S BEST FRIEND CAPSULES **4** daily or 3 months.
<u>with</u>
Evening Primrose oil or Borage capsules 6 daily.
then

❧ Crystal Star FEMALE HARMONY CAPSULES **2** daily as a hormone balancer to prevent return.

❧ Iodine Therapy: often effective in 3-4 months. ATOMODINE or MIODIN DROPS 2-3x daily, or Crystal Star IODINE THERAPY EXTRACT (Take <u>with vitamin E for best results)</u>

❧ Dong Quai/Damiana caps or <u>extract</u> 4 x daily.

❧ Apply a fresh Comfrey leaf poultice. Drink 4 cups comfrey tea daily.

❧ Crystal Star SILICA SOURCE EXTRACT for collagen regrowth.

BODYWORK

✣ No smoking. Avoid secondary smoke.

✣ Get some exercise every day for tissue oxygen.

✣ Do not take synthetic estrogen compounds if possible. They keep fibroids growing even after menopause .

✣ Try to avoid mammagrams and X-rays. We have seen lumps grow significantly and sometimes appear after even small X-Ray doses. Breast tissue is so sensitive to it. X-rays also cause iodine deficiency.

✣ REFLEXOLOGY POINT:

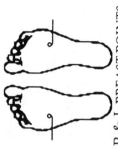

R & L BREAST POINTS

COMMON SYMPTOMS: Moveable nodules or cysts near the surface of the breasts; growths usually cease after menopause; sometimes the cause of excessive vaginal bleeding, back and abdominal pain, and bladder infections.

COMMON CAUSES: Too much caffeine and too many fats in the diet; EFA deficiency; hormone imbalance with too much estrogen production and an underactive thyroid; obesity; high dose birth control pills; X-rays; high stress lifestyle, producing acid wastes in the body.

151

FLATULENCE

FOOD THERAPY

☙ **Start with a cleansing high pectin mono diet of apples and apple juice for 2 days. Follow for 4 days with a diet of 70% fresh foods and steamed brown rice to add B vitamins and rebalance digestion.**

☙ Keep the diet high in soluble fiber foods. Include plenty of cultured foods such as yogurt and kefir.

☙ **Avoid fatty and fried foods, cooked fruits and highly spiced foods. No red meats, refined sugars, pizza, soft drinks, caffeine, etc.**

☙ Avoid the following foods until digestion is better balanced. Beans, full fat dairy products, cabbages, bagels, dried fruits, and onions.

☙ Practice good food combining.

VITAMINS/ MINERALS

✢ **Liquid chlorophyll 1t. before meals. ♂**

✢ Acidolphilus caps or liquid before meals.

✢ **Sun CHLORELLA or BARLEY GREEN on a regular basis for prevention.**

✢ Effective gas busters:
◆ **HCl capsules**
◆ **Activated charcoal tabs ♂**
◆ **Apple pectin tabs ♂**

✢ Schiff ENZYMALL ♀

✢ **Comfrey pepsin tabs**
or
Papaya enzyme chewables after meals.

HERBAL THERAPY

☙ **Turmeric capsules or Ginger capsules as needed.**

☙ **Hylands BILIOUSNESS TABS as needed. ☺**

☙ Effective teas:
Sage
Spearmint
Peppermint
Wild Yam
Catnip ☺
Alfalfa/Mint
Fennel

☙ **BioForce FLATULENCE tabs as needed.**

☙ Crystal Star HERBAL ENZYMES, 2 before a meal; or open into a small glass of water and drink down for immediate relief.

BODYWORK

❖ **Lie on the back and draw knees up to chest to relieve abdominal pressure.**

❖ Avoid over-using anti-biotics, that destroy friendly flora in the digestive tract.

❖ Apply hot ginger compresses to the abdomen.

❖ Take a catnip enema for immediate relief.

COMMON SYMPTOMS: Excess gas and abdominal distention; passing foul gas; poor food assimilation.

COMMON CAUSES: Poor food combining; eating too much, and too many refined, fatty and spicy foods; allergies to sugar, wheat or dairy; enzyme deficiency; constipation; poor food assimilation; candida yeast overgrowth; diverticulitis.

152

FOOD THERAPY	VITAMINS/ MINERALS	HERBAL THERAPY	BODYWORK
❧ For frostbite: paint on, but do not rub in, warm olive oil. Massage in for gangrene.	✤ Deva Flowers FIRST AID REMEDY or Bach Flowers RESCUE REMEDY every 5 minutes under the tongue as needed for shock.	❧ Effective compresses mixed with oil: Marshmallow Slippery Elm Comfrey/Plantain Ginger/Cayenne	✤ ◆ Get the person to a heated room immediately. ◆ Gently rub the kidneys toward the middle of the back.
❧ Give the person warm drinks or green drinks, but no alcohol. It constricts blood flow.	✤ Vitamin C powder with bioflavs and rutin, 1/4t. every half hour for 3 days for collagen and tissue rebuilding.	❧ Effective tincture: Black Walnut Myrrh Witch Hazel	◆ Cover warmly, so frostbitten areas will warm up gradually. ◆ If case is severe, wrap in gauze so blisters don't break. Elevate legs.
❧ Eat a high protein diet for the next two weeks with plenty of whole grains to speed recovery.	✤ Vitamin E 400IU. Take internally and prick and apply oil to affected areas.	❧ Effective applied oils: Cajeput Mullein Olive oil	✤ Use alternating warm and cool hydrotherapy to stimulate circulation.. No hot water bottles, hair dryers, or heating pads. Slow warming is the key.
	✤ H_2O_2 PEROXY GEL. Rub on affected area til healing begins.	or ❧ Tea Tree oil. It sloughs off old and infected tissue, and leaves healthy tissue intact.	✤ If case is very severe, immerse areas in warm water and massage under water for 5-10 minutes.
	✤ Ginkgo Biloba extract, Kukicha tea or Butcher's Broom caps to stimulate circulation.	❧ Apply Aloe Vera Gel often; several times daily.	
	✤ Oral chelation therapy 2 packets daily for 2 months.	❧ Crystal Star CARDI-STRENGTH CAPSULES 4 daily for circulation, with Sage tea 2 cups daily.	

COMMON SYMPTOMS: Freezing and its effects of redness, swelling, blistering, numbness, etc. to exposed parts of the body. Gangrene may follow if left unattended.

FUNGAL INFECTION ✧ THRUSH ✧ RINGWORM

FOOD THERAPY	VITAMINS/ MINERALS	HERBAL THERAPY	BODYWORK
Avoid pasteurized dairy products. Keep the diet low in carbohydrates - both simple carbos as in sugar and sweeteners, and complex carbos from whole grains and nuts. (vegetable carbohydrates are fine).	Maintaining healthy bowel flora is crucial to overcoming this condition. Take a dairy-free acidolphilus complex such as DDS in capsules or liquid before each meal.	Tea Tree oil as an anti-fungal: apply to affected areas; rinse mouth with a dilute solution for thrush.	Avoid alcohol, tobacco and sugars as prime culprits for this body imbalance condition.
Omit red meats, fried and fatty foods during healing.	Effective acidolphilus compounds: ◆ Nature's Plus JUNIORDOLPH.ILUS CHEWS ☺ ◆ Solaray MULTIDOLPHILUS ☺ ◆ Natren LIFE START ☺ ◆ Natren LIFE START 2 ◆ Natures Way PRIMADOLPH.	Garlic oil capsules 6 daily.	Avoid drug overuse, particularly anti-biotics.
Eat plenty of cultured foods such as plain yogurt, kefir and tofu.		Crystal Star HERBAL DEFENSE CAPSULES to stimulate better immune strength.	Get early morning sunlight on the body every day possible for healing vitamin D.
Keep dietary protein high for fastest healing: from sea foods and sea vegetables, sprouts, eggs, soy foods, poultry and vegetables.	Solaray CAPRYL CAPS. ♀	Black Walnut tincture. Apply to affected areas and take a few drops under the tongue daily.	Pat cider vinegar, or rub papaya skins on affected areas.
	Effective digestive aids: Schiff ENZYMALL Alta Health CANGEST	For bowel health and regulation: Barberry/Chaparral tea Sonne #7 BENTONITE	Use a mild non-detergent soap to clean skin.
	Stimulating and re-building healthy immunity is the second key to overcoming recurring infection: **Biotin 600Mcg,** Beta Carotene 50,000IU Nutrapathic NUTRAMUNE	Food Grade H₂O₂ peroxy gel. Rub on affected area, or take a 3% dilution, 1T. in 8oz. water for 2 weeks, til infection clears.	Take Epsom salts baths; use 1 cup saltss to bath water, and soak for 20-30 minutes.
		Shark Liver oil capsules 3x daily.♀	**Nutrition Resource** NUTRIBIOTIC LIQUID. Mix 1-4 drops in 5 oz. water and apply directly.
		Apply a Golden Seal/ Myrrh solution to area.	

COMMON SYMPTOMS: Athlete's foot; excessive belching and internal gas; loss of sexual desire; anxiety attacks and paranoia; cold hands and feet; mood swings; unexplained allergies; bronchitis; persistant headaches; acne.; diaper rash in babies; ringworm; a weeping non-healing cut.

COMMON CAUSES: Broad spectrum anti-biotic and prescription drug use; synthetic steroid use; birth control pills; low immunity; poor hygiene.

GALLSTONES ✧ GALL BLADDER PROBLEMS

FOOD THERAPY

🐌 Go on a short juice and gallbladder flush fast for 3 days. (see following page for details).
◆ In acute stage, all food should be avoided. Only pure water should be taken, until condition clears.

🐌 After this fast and flush, take a glass of cider vinegar and honey in water daily for prevention and oxygen uptake.

🐌 Take 1T. Lecithin granules before each meal to help dissolve cholesterol sediment.
◆ Take 1T. Brewer's Yeast, and 1T. Olive Oil to stimulate bile and prevent gallstone formation.

🐌 Eat small meals more frequently. No large meals. Avoid all red meats and animal fats, refined and hydrogenated fats and oils.

VITAMINS/ MINERALS

✤ Take full spectrum digestive enzymes with meals to stimulate bile such as Alta Health CANGEST or Schiff ENZYMALL.
or

✤ Take 2 acidolphilus complex caps before meals.
✤ Take 1 HCl tablet after meals if necessary.

✤ Enzymatic Therapy LIVA-TOX 4-6 daily with BIO-CALCIUM 4 daily.

✤ High Omega 3 Flax or fish oils 3 x daily.

✤ Choline/Inositol 2 daily with Vit. E 400IU and Biotin 600Mcg. daily.

✤ Ascorbate vitamin C or Ester C 550Mg. with bioflavonoids 6 daily.♂

✤ Glycine -for sugar regulation Methionine-for liver cleanse Taurine-to keep bile thinned

✤ BioForce GALLBLADDER extract ♀

HERBAL THERAPY

🐌 Chamomile or Queen of the Meadow tea 5-7 cups daily to dissolve stones.

🐌 Crystal Star STONES AWAY CAPSULES with lemon juice and water, or LIV-FLUSH TEA.

🐌 Effective Gallbladder teas:
Wild Yam
Catnip
Peppermint
Comfrey/Dandelion Rt.

🐌 Ginkgo Biloba extract drops 2x daily.

🐌 Crystal Star PANCRAID CAPS with BLDR-K TEA.♀

🐌 Yerba Prima ALOE VERA JUICE WITH HERBS daily with Millk Thistle extract drops added.

BODYWORK

✤ Take garlic or catnip enemas every 3 days til relief.

✤ Take olive oil flushes for 2-3 weeks til stones pass (see next page).

✤ Get mild regular exercise and reduce body weight to keep the system free and flowing. High saturated fats in the diet and a sedentary lifestyle are the two most conducive environments for gallstone formation.

✤ Apply cold milk compresses to the abdomen area.

✤ REFLEXOLOGY POINT:

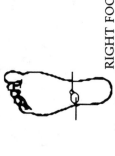

RIGHT FOOT
LIVER & GALLBLADDER

155

COMMON SYMPTOMS: Chronic gas , belching, pain, and bloating; headache and bad temper; sluggishness, nerves.

COMMON CAUSES: Too many fatty and fried foods, and lack of ability to digest them; high cholesterol sediment (coagulated serum fats that do not pass); chronic indigestion and gas from too much dairy and refined sugars; birth control pills; lack of regular exercise.

THERAPEUTIC GALLSTONE FLUSHES ✧ GALLBLADDER HEALING DIET

Gallbladder cleansing flushes have been very effective in passing and dissolving gallstones. Depending on the size of the stones and the length of time they have been forming, the programs may last from 3 days to a month. Have a sonogram before embarking on a flush to determine the size of the stones. If they are too large to pass through the urethral ducts, other surgical methods must be used.

MILD 3 DAY OLIVE OIL & LEMON JUICE FLUSH: **Repeat for 3 days.**
ON RISING: take 2T. of olive oil and the juice of two lemons in water, or 1 grapefruit juiced.
BREAKFAST: have a glass of carrot/beet/cucumber juice or a potassium broth (Pg.33).
MIDMORNING: take 1-2 cups of chamomile tea.
LUNCH: take another glass of lemon juice in water with 2T. olive oil, **and** a glass of fresh carrot, apple, or pear juice.
MIDAFTERNOON: take 1-2 cups of chamomile tea.
DINNER: have another glass of apple or pear juice, or black cherry juice.
BEFORE BED: take a cup of chamomile tea, **or** a cup of VEGEX YEAST BROTH.

4 DAY INTENSIVE OLIVE OIL FLUSH:
If olive oil is hard for you to take "straight", sip through a straw.
ON RISING, AND EVERY 2 HOURS THROUGHOUT THE DAY FOR THREE DAYS: take a glass of apple or pear juice. Take a catnip or garlic enema each day.
BEFORE BED ON THE 3 RD DAY: take 1/2 cup olive oil mixed with 1/2 cup lemon or grapefruit juice. Sip slowly. Sleep on the right side with a pillow under the hip to concentrate the remedy in the gallbladder area.
ON THE MORNING OF THE 4TH DAY: take a garlic enema. The stones will often pass during the day.
Take 6-8 glasses of bottled water throughout the day.

2 DAY ALKALIZING FOLLOW UP DIET: **to rebalance the system and build a preventive environment against gallstones.**
ON RISING: take 2T. cider vinegar or lemon juice in water, or a glass of fresh grapefruit juice.
BREAKFAST: take a potassium juice or essence (Pg. 33).
MIDMORNING: take a cup of chamomile tea and a glass of pear or apple juice.
LUNCH: have a green drink (Pg.34) or Sun CHLORELLA or BARLEY GREEN MAGMA GRANULES in water; **and** a small fresh green salad with lemon/oil dressing.
MIDAFTERNOON: take a cup of dandelion root tea, and a glass of apple, pear or black cherry juice.
DINNER: have a small green salad, and some steamed vegetables with brown rice or millet **and** a glass of apple juice.
BEFORE BED: have a cup of chamomile or dandelion root tea.
Repeat for 2 days. Include 6-8 glasses of bottled water each day.

GALLSTONE PREVENTION DIET:
Make sure the continuing diet is very low in fats of all kinds. Oils should be mono or poly-unsaturated. Eat low cholesterol foods, cultured foods such as yogurt, kefir and tofu, and alkaline foods such as miso soup, sea vegetables and whole grains. Specific beneficial foods include pears, apples, beets, soaked prunes, figs and leafy greens.
See "COOKING FOR HEALTHY HEALING" by Linda Rector-Page for a complete diet program to prevent gallstones.

GAS ◇ INDIGESTION ◇ HEARTBURN

FOOD THERAPY

🐍 Make sure you are eating an alkalizing diet, with plenty of cultured foods such as yogurt, kefir and miso soup, high fiber foods such as whole grains, fresh vegetables and fruits, and enzyme-rich foods such as papaya and pineapple.

🐍 Follow good food combining (get a good chart for help on this).

🐍 Take one of these daily:
◆ 1 tsp. cider vinegar in water
◆ 2 lemons in water
◆ a green drink (Pg.34)

🐍 Avoid fatty, spicy, and acid-forming foods. Omit fried foods, red meats, refined sugars, sodas and caffeine.

🐍 Eat smaller meals. Chew food very well.

🐍 No smoking with meals. No fluids with meals. A little white wine is OK for better absorption.

VITAMINS/ MINERALS

✣ Enzymatic Therapy MEGA-ZYME, or Living Source FOOD SENSITIVITY SYSTEM after eating.

✣ Schiff ENZYMALL TABS, ♀ Solaray MULTIDOLPHILUS CAPS, or 1 teasp. Chloro-phyll liquid before eating.

✣ If belching and burping:
◆ Betaine HCl
◆ Schiff SUPER ENZYMALL
◆ Twin Lab HISTIDINE
If gas and bloating:
◆ Pancreatin capsules 1400Mg.
◆ Act Clear PANCREATIN
If there are ulcers:
◆ Glutamine 500Mg.
◆ Enzymatic Therapy DGL
If there is diarrhea:
◆ Activated charcoal tabs
If acute indigestion:
◆ Papaya chewables
◆ Cal/Mag liquid or chewables
◆ Enzymatic Therapy DGL

✣ Hyland's BILIOUSNESS TABS after MEALS.

✣ Nature's Plus CHEWABLE BROMELAIN 40MG. after meals.♂

HERBAL THERAPY

🐍 To relieve gas quickly; put pinches of cinnamon, nutmeg, ginger and cloves in water and drink down.

🐍 Crystal Star HERBAL ENZYMES, MEAL'S END TEA or MEDITATION TEA as needed.

🐍 Crystal Star MIN-ZYME-MINOS DRINK MIX for good enzyme activity and system alkalizing.

🐍 Yerba Prima ALOE VERA JUICE WITH HERBS after meals, and Bee Pollen 2 teasp. daily. ♂

🐍 Good digestion teas:
Catnip/Fennel
Slippery Elm
Peppermint/Spearmint
Wild Yam

🐍 Effective digestive caps:
Turmeric ♀
Garlic/Parsley
Comfrey/Pepsin
🐍 Solaray ALFAJUICE CAPS.

BODYWORK

✢ Apply Ginger com-presses to abdominal area. Take 2 ginger capsules as needed to break up gas.

✢ Take peppermint oil drops in a cup of water as needed. (also helpful if there is IRRITABLE BOWEL SYNDROME).

✢ Commercial antacids neutralize stomach acid, inviting the stomach to produce even more acid, and therefore usually making the condition worse in the long run.

✢ Try to eat when relaxed. Meals eaten in a hurry and under stress all contribute to poor digestion. Life isn't going to slow down, so a conscious effort must be made to break this "vicious digestive circle". *Try a short walk before eating.*

COMMON SYMPTOMS: Gnawing, burning pain and tenderness occurring directly after food consumption.

COMMON CAUSES: Poor diet with too many refined foods, sugars, fried and spicy foods; overeating; Candida yeast overgrowth; food allergies; too much caffeine, sodas and acid-forming foods; vegetable protein deficiency; enzyme and/or HCl deficiency.

157

GASTRITIS ✧ GASTROENTERITIS ✧ GASTRIC ULCERS

FOOD THERAPY

☙ Include plenty of soluble fiber foods in the diet: whole grains, brown rice, fresh fruits and vegetables, etc. Have a leafy green salad daily.

☙ Effective juices for stomach acid balance:
Carrot
Carrot/Cabbage
Pineapple/Papaya
☙ Have a glass of mineral water every evening.

☙ Eat cultured foods for friendly G.I. flora.

☙ Avoid alcohol (except a little wine at dinner), caffeine, tobacco, aspirin and all fried foods.

☙ Eat small meals more frequently. No large meals. Chew everything well.

☙ See COLITIS AND DIVERTICULITIS pages for more diet information.

VITAMINS/ MINERALS

✤ Natren MEGA-DOLPHILUS or DDS DAIRY FREE COMPLEX before meals.
or
Liquid chlorophyll 1 tsp. before each meal.

✤ Effective aids to rebalance digestive activity:
◆ Activated charcoal for gas
◆ HCl for stomach acid
◆ Pancreatin for fat digestion
◆ Magnesium to soothe
◆ Raw Pancreas for enzymes
◆ Shiff ENZYMALL w/ ox bile

✤ Nature's Plus CHEWABLE BROMELAIN 40MG. before meals. ♂

✤ Aloe Vera juice and MAG./POTASS./BROMELAIN 2 before meals. ♂

✤ Living source FOOD SENSITIVITY SYSTEM.

✤ Ester C 550Mg. with Zinc 75Mg. daily. ♂

✤ Calcium Citrate 4 daily for low stomach acid. ♀

HERBAL THERAPY

☙ Enzymatic Therapy CHEWABLE DGL TABS.

☙ Hyland's BILIOUSNESS TABS after meals. ♀

☙ Crystal Star RELAX CAPS for nerve stress as needed. with MEGA-MINERAL CAPS 4 daily.

☙ Hops/Valerian/Scullcap tea to relax esophagus.

☙ Effective teas made with mineral water:
◆ Pau de Arco
◆ Comfrey Rt. & Lf.
◆ Slippery Elm

☙ Twin Lab Propolis tincture
or
Golden Seal/Myrrh tincture 3x daily for a month. ♂

☙ Comfrey/Pepsin tabs 2 before each meal.

☙ Ginkgo Biloba extract 2-3x daily for a month.

BODYWORK

✤ Remember that Tagamet and Zantac, both drugs prescribed regularly (one billion dollars in sales yearly) for ulcers and other gastric problems, can be addictive. They also inhibit bone formation and proper liver function. DGL normalizes these processes after drugs.

✤ Avoid cortisone drugs. They often cause ulcers.

✤ REFLEXOLOGY POINT:

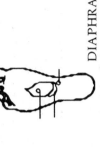

DIAPHRAGM, SOLAR PLEXUS & STOMACH

✤ Acupressure points: Pull middle toe on each foot for 1 minute.

COMMON SYMPTOMS: Chronic poor digestion, with sharp abdominal pains; heartburn and tenderness; nausea and bile reflux in the throat.

COMMON CAUSES: Poor diet with too many fried, fatty foods, sugars, and refined foods; poor food combining; drinking with meals; eating too fast, too much and too often; acidosis; intestinal parasites; food allergies; too much caffeine and alcohol; steroid use; stress.

GLANDS

HEALTH ✦ REGULATION ✦ BALANCE

FOOD THERAPY

✿ For best results in a gland balance program, start with a 24 hr. detox watermelon only diet. Then eat a high vegetable protein diet with whole grains, brown rice, nuts, seeds and sprouts.

✿ Include good gland foods in the diet: sea foods and sea vegies, fresh figs and raisins, pumpkin and sesame seeds, green leafy vegetables, broccoli, avocados, yams, and dark fruits.

✿ Drink 6 glasses of bottled water daily. The glands are affected first by poor water.

✿ Take 2T. each daily:
Brewer's yeast
wheat germ
sesame seeds

✿ Avoid red meats and all refined foods.

VITAMINS/ MINERALS

✤ Mezotrace MINERAL COMPLEX TABS 2-4 daily.

✤ White Birch Mineral Water

✤ N.F. MIODIN DROPS 2-3x daily, with Vit. E 400IU 2 daily.

✤ Nature's Plus RNA/DNA

✤ Vit. B_6 250Mg. 2x daily. with A & D 25M/1M.

✤ High potency Premier or YS ROYAL JELLY 2t. daily.

✤ Superior BEE SECRETION 1/2 dropperful 2x daily.

HERBAL THERAPY

❧ Crystal Star ENDOCRINE BALANCE CAPS 2 daily and HIGHLY ABSORBABLE MINERAL COMPLEX EXTRACT or MEGA-MINERAL CAPS twice daily.

❧ Crystal Star ENERGY GREEN and/or HEAVY METAL CAPSULES if pollutants are prevalent. The glands are very sensitive to pollutants and chemical toxins.

❧ Effective capsules:
◆ Kelp 6 daily
◆ Wild Yam 4 daily
◆ Saw Palmetto 2 daily

❧ Effective extracts:
Siberian Ginseng
Lobelia
Mullein

❧ Effective balancing teas:
Horsetail/Blue Malva
Lemon Balm
Sarsaparilla

BODYWORK

✤ Avoid air and environmental pollutants. The glands go first.

✤ Acupressure points: stroke the top of the foot on both feet for 5 minutes each to stimulate endocrine and hormone secretions.

✤ REFLEXOLOGY POINT:

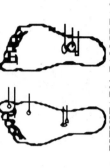

PITUITARY, PANCREAS, SPLEEN, THYROID, PARA-THYROID, ADRENALS, THYMUS.

COMMON SYMPTOMS: Poor assimilation of nutrients; adrenal exhaustion; constant tiredness; hypoglycemia.

COMMON CAUSES: Mineral deficiency; stress; hypothyroidism; environmental pollutants; too much sugar,alcohol , caffeine, tobacco and drugs.

FOOD THERAPY

🍂 Follow a fresh foods only diet for 2 weeks to clear the system of inorganic crystalline deposits. Take 1 of the following every day for 2 weeks:
  ◆ Carrot, beet, cucumber, parsley juice
  ◆ Fresh Carrot juice
  ◆ Potassium broth (Pg.33).

🍂 Effective vit.A rich foods:
  ◆ Endive and leafy greens
  ◆ Carrots
  ◆ Sea foods
  ◆ Broccoli

🍂 Effective Vit. C sources:
  ◆ Citrus juice
  ◆ Green peppers
  ◆ Cucumbers
  ◆ Carrot juice
  ◆ Beets

🍂 Avoid chemical over-the-counter cold medicines, aspirin, and cortico-steroids.

🍂 Avoid all refined sugars, caffeine and caffeine-containing foods.

VITAMINS/ MINERALS

✣ Quercitin Plus with Bromelain 6 daily.
  or
  Ascorbate Vit. C 5-10,000Mg. daily with bioflavonoids and rutin.
  and
  Wash eyes daily with a weak ascorbate C and bioflavs powder solution in water.

✣ Kal PYCNOGENOL 6 daily. with vitamin D 1000IU.♂

✣ Taurine 500Mg. daily for retinitis pigmentosa
  and

✣ Vitamin E 400IU 2x daily if retinitis is hemorrhagic.

✣ Vital Health FORMULA 1 ORAL CHELATION with EDTA 2 -3 daily.♂

✣ Beta Carotene 150,000IU daily, with Glutathione 50Mg. 2x daily.

✣ B Complex 100Mg. with extra B_2 100Mg., B_6 250Mg., Niacin 250Mg.

HERBAL THERAPY

🍃 Crystal Star VISICARE CAPSULES 4 daily to strengthen eyes, RELAX CAPS to ease tension, (a major contributor.)

🍃 Effective eye washes:
  ◆ Crystal Star EYELIGHT TEA
  ◆ Weak Golden Seal solution
  ◆ Aloe Vera juice.
  ◆ Calendula tea

🍃 Evening Primrose oil capsules 4-6 daily.

🍃 Effective herbal "greens":
  ◆ Sun CHLORELLA
  ◆ Spirulina tabs
  ◆ Crystal Star ENERGY GREEN

🍃 Kelp tabs 6 daily or Black Walnut tincture for iodine imbalance.♀

🍃 BILBERRY EXTRACT for high bioflavonoids.
  or
  Solaray VIZION CAPSULES with Bilberry.

🍃 Beet root capsules 6 daily.

BODYWORK

✣ Relax more. Cultivate a calmer lifestyle. Stop smoking. It constricts eye blood vessels and increases fluid pressure.

✣ Get a good spinal and chiropractic adjustment.

✣ Glaucoma is often the result of, and accompanied by, liver malfunction. The liver must be cleansed for there to be real advancement against glaucoma.

✣ Avoid using sunglasses whenever possible.

✣ REFLEXOLOGY POINT: Very important to break up crystalline deposits:

EYES

COMMON SYMPTOMS: Colored haloes around lights; allergies; eye and head aches; tunnel vision; inability to tear; gradual vision loss; increased eye fluid pressure.
COMMON CAUSES: Over-use of cortco-steroid drugs; Diabetes; too much caffeine and sugar; prolonged stress; allergies; adrenal exhaustion and liver malfunction; long TV watching in the dark; thyroid imbalance; over-the-counter cold prescription drugs; arterioscleriosis.

GOITER

FOOD THERAPY	VITAMINS/ MINERALS	HERBAL THERAPY	BODYWORK
❧ Go on a diet of 75% fresh foods for a month. Have a green salad at least twice a day. Eat plenty of iodine-rich foods, such as sea vegetables, sea foods, fish, mushrooms, garlic, onions and watercress.	❖ Spirulina or Chlorella 6 tablets daily.	❧ Pau de Arco tea 2-3 cups daily.	❖ Swim or wade in the ocean whenever possible.
	❖ Beta Carotene 100,000IU. and Vitamin E 400IU daily.	❧ Effective teas: Dulse Irish Moss Alfalfa/Dandelion Parsley Watercress	❖ Get some mild daily outdoors exercise.
❧ Take a green drink (Pg.34) or a potassium broth (Pg. 33) or Crystal Star ENERGY GREEN DRINK each day.	❖ N. F. MIODIN DROPS or Heritage ATOMODINE ♀	❧ Crystal Star THY-METABS 4 daily. and/or MIN-ZYME-MINOS DRINK	❖ Apply Calendula compresses to the area twice a day for a month.
	❖ Enzymatic Therapy THYROID/ TYROSINE COMPLEX CAPSULES.		❖ REFLEXOLOGY POINT:
❧ Include 2T. each daily: Brewer's yeast Wheat germ	❖ Effective Glandulars: Raw Thyroid Raw Adrenal Raw Pituitary	❧ Calendula tea 2 cups daily with Sarsaparilla caps 4 daily.	THYROID/THYMUS
❧ Use an herb salt instead of table salt.	❖ B6 100Mg. 3x daily.	❧ Black Walnut tincture: use as a throat paint, and take 1/2 dropperful 2x daily.	
	❖ Country Life ADRENAL COMPLEX WITH TYROSINE 2-3 daily. ♀		

COMMON SYMPTOMS: Enlargement of the thyroid gland. This is usually a woman's problem.

COMMON CAUSES: Iodine deficiency; Vitamin E and A deficiency; too many iodine-depleting prescription diet pills.

GOUT

FOOD THERAPY	VITAMINS/ MINERALS	HERBAL THERAPY	BODYWORK
❧ Go on a short 3 day liquid cleansing diet (Pg. 26) to rid the body of acid wastes quickly. Then follow a diet of 75% fresh foods for the rest of the month to rebalance uric acid formation.	❖ Ascorbate vitamin C powder with bioflavs. and rutin, 1/4t. every 4 hours daily for a month.	❧ Solaray ALFAJUICE TABS. with Enzymatic Therapy CHERRY JUICE EXTRACT TABS 6 daily. ♂	❖ Keep weight down to ease pressure on feet and legs.
	❖ Enzymatic Therapy ACID-A-CAL CAPSULES. ♂		❖ Keep the kidneys clean and working so uric acid is easily released. (See KIDNEY MALFUNCTION page in this book)
❧ Drink 2-3 glasses of black cherry juice daily. Eat high potassium foods: fresh cherries, bananas, strawberries, celery, broccoli, potatoes, greens to put crystals in solution. Drink 6-8 glasses daily of water and citrus juices to flush them out.	❖ B Complex 100Mg. with extra B₆ 250Mg. and pantothenic acid 1000Mg	❧ Crystal Star R™ EASE CAPSULES as directed. with ADRN EXTRACT 2x daily.	❖ See ARTHRITIS DIET suggestions in this book for more information.
	❖ Biotec EXTRA ENERGY ENZYMES SOD, 6 daily.	❧ Crystal Star ENERGY GREEN DRINK 2-3x weekly for absorbable potassium and greens.	❖ Check your high blood pressure medicine. Several of them cause formation of inorganic crystal sediments.
❧ Avoid high purine foods that form uric acid: red meats, red meat extracts, gravies, broths and bouillon, organ meats, mushrooms, dry beans, cooked spinach and rhubarb, sardines and anchovies, etc.	❖ Apply DMSO for pain. ♂	❧ Effective teas: Dandelion/Yarrow Horsetail Queen of the meadow White Willow/Scullcap	❖ Crystal Star ALKALIZING ENZYME HERBAL BODY WRAP to neutralize acids and balance body pH right away.
	❖ Twin Lab Liquid K 3t. daily with vitamin E 400IU and Niacin 500Mg. to increase circulation. ♂	❧ Apply Plantain, Ginger, or Comfrey compresses.	
	❖ Vital Health FORMULA 1 ORAL CHELATION WITH EDTA to help dissolve heavy metal, inorganic calcium and cholesterol build-up.	❧ Drink Aloe Vera juice 1 glass daily. or White Birch mineral water. ♂	
❧ Reduce alcohol, caffeine, fried foods, animal fats. ❧ Low fats and low grains are the diet key	❖ Glycine 500Mg. daily.		

COMMON SYMPTOMS: A disease of adult males with arthritic symptoms;extremely painful joints in the foot and toe; tenderness, redness and swelling; gradual joint destruction with longer and longer attacks.

COMMON CAUSES: Excess uric acid condition due to overeating too much red meat, refined food, alcohol, sugar, caffeine, etc.; overuse of drugs, such as thiazide diuretics causing potassium deficiency; obesity; hypoglycemia.

162

GRAVES DISEASE ✧ HYPERTHYROIDISM

FOOD THERAPY	VITAMINS/ MINERALS	HERBAL THERAPY	BODYWORK

🐍 For the first month of healing, follow a diet of at least 75% fresh foods, Include plenty of vegetable proteins from sprouts, sea vegetables soy foods and whole grains. Add B vitamins and complex carbo-hydrates from brown rice and vegetables, for stable energy.

🐍 Have a potassium broth or green drink frequently (Pg.33, 34).

🐍 Take 2T. each daily:
Brewer's yeast
Wheat germ
Lecithin

🐍 Eat plenty of cultured foods for friendly G.I. flora.

🐍 Nature's Plus SPIRUTEIN PROTEIN DRINK daily for increased energy level.

✤ Living Source MASTER NUTRIENT SYSTEM food source multiple daily.

✤ Ester C with bioflavs. 550Mg. 6 daily.
with
Zinc picolinate 50-75Mg. daily.

✤ Stress B Complex with extra B_2 100Mg. and B_6 100Mg.
with
Marine Carotene daily.

✤ CO Q 10, 10 Mg daily.

✤ Twin Lab LIQUID K 2t. daily.

✤ Enzymatic Therapy THYROID/ TYROSINE COMPLEX 4 daily.

✤ For Thyroid storms:
◆ Calcium Citrate 4 daily
◆ Lecithin 1900Gr. daily
◆ Vitamin E 800IU daily

🍃 Crystal Star THY-METABS CAPSULES 2-4 daily.
with
LIV-FLUSH TEA or MILK THISTLE EXTRACT for 2 months.

🍃 Effective extracts:
◆ Ginkgo Biloba
◆ Echinacea
◆ Mullein/Lobelia
◆ Hawthorne

🍃 Astragalus capsules 4 daily.

🍃 Evening Primrose oil caps 4 daily.

🍃 Effective potassium sources:
◆ Crystal Star POTASSIUM SOURCE CAPSULES
◆ Crystal Star Min-ZYME-MINOS DRINK

✤ Exercise daily to the breathless and mild sweating point.

✤ Get some early morning sun on the body every day possible, and wade and swim in the ocean frequently for balancing thyroid minerals.

✤ Acupressure points: press points on both sides of the spinal column at the base of the neck, 3 times for 10 seconds each.

✤ REFLEXOLOGY POINT:

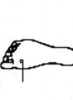

THYROID/ THYMUS

COMMON SYMPTOMS: Bulging eyes and blurred vision; fatigue; restlessness and irritability; insomnia; nervous tension; sweating and tremors; weight loss from increased metabolic rate; systolic hypertension, mood swings, and sometimes mental psychosis during a "thyroid storm".

COMMON CAUSES: Stress; overuse of diet pills; mental burnout and fatigue; zinc deficiency; anorexia syndrome.

163

GUM DISEASE ✧ GINGIVITIS ✧ PYORRHEA

FOOD THERAPY

🌱 Avoid acid-forming foods, such as tomatoes, sugars, refined foods, colas and carbonated drinks.

🌱 Eat raw crunchy foods to stimulate the gums; apples, celery, Grape Nuts cereal, seeds, high fiber grains. Have a green salad every day.

🌱 Eat high vitamin C foods, such as broccoli, green peppers, papaya, cantaloupe, and citrus fruits.

🌱 Rub gums with halved fresh strawberries, or honey or lemon juice.

🌱 Eat cultured foods for friendly digestive flora.

VITAMINS/ MINERALS

❖ Ascorbate vitamin C powder with rutin and bioflavonoids. Make into a solution with water. Rub directly onto gums, and take 1-2t. daily.

❖ COQ 10 30Mg. daily for almost immediate relief. Continue for prevention.

❖ Quercetin Plus with Bromelain to control inflammation.
with
Lysine 500Mg. 2x daily.

❖ Chlorophyll liquid 3t. daily before meals. Make into a solution with water and apply directly to gums daily.

❖ B Complex 100Mg. daily with Betaine HCl 600Mg.

❖ Vitamin E oil caps 400IU. Take internally and prick to rub directly on gums.

❖ Nature's Life LIQUID CAL-CIUM PHOS. FREE. W/ D.♀

HERBAL THERAPY

🌿 Effective solutions to apply to the gums to stop bleeding and counter infection:
◆ Golden Seal/Myrrh
◆ Tea Tree oil
◆ Witch Hazel
◆ Comfrey tincture
◆ Cayenne extract
◆ Aloe vera/Myrrh

🌿 Use propolis toothpaste. Rub on propolis tincture.

🌿 Crystal Star MEGA MINERAL CAPSULES to strengthen gums.
and
open up an ANTI-BIO CAPSULE, or use ANTI-BIO EXTRACT and rub directly onto gums to counter infection.

🌿 Siberian ginseng extract 2-3x daily.♂

🌿 Evening Primrose oil caps as an effective EFA source, 4 daily.

BODYWORK

❖ Chew propolis lozenges. ♂

❖ Effective gum massages to control pain and soothe inflammation:
Clove oil
Sea salt
Eucalyptus oil
Sage oil
Baking soda
Lobelia extract

❖ REFLEXOLOGY POINT:

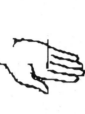

TEETH & GUMS

❖ Put 4-5 drops of Nutrition Resource NUTRIBIOTIC LIQUID in a Water Pik for recurring gum infections.

❖ Floss well every day.

COMMON SYMPTOMS: Red, swollen, bleeding gums; bad breath, and bad taste in the mouth; loose teeth; hot and cold sensitivity in the mouth.

COMMON CAUSES: Too much red meat, refined foods, sugar and soft drinks in the diet; poor tooth brushing; diabetes; vitamin A,C, and D deficiencies; lack of fresh foods in the diet. Low intake od dietary calcium and other minerals shows first depletions in the gums and jawbone.

HAIR GROWTH ✧ SCALP ✧ GRAY HAIR

FOOD THERAPY

- Feed your hair a high vegetable protein diet. Make a mix of the following hair foods and take 3T. daily:
  Wheat germ
  Lecithin granules.
  Blackstrap molasses
  Brewer's yeast
  Sesame seeds

- Avoid saturated fats, sugars, refined foods.

- Good hair foods:
  Carrots, green peppers, lettuces, bananas, strawberries, apples, peas, green peppers, cucumbers and sprouts.

- Sea vegetables are excellent for hair health. Try Crystal Star MINZYME-MINOS DRINK MIX.

- Poor liver function is often the cause of unhealthy hair. See LIVER HEALTH pages in this book.♂

- For dry hair shine; rub drops of coconut oil between palms. Apply.

VITAMINS/ MINERALS

- For color and growth, take together daily:
  PABA 1000Mg.
  Molasses 2T.
  Pantothenic acid 1000Mg.
  Folic acid 800Mcg.♂

- Alta Health SIL-X SILICA CAPSULES 2 daily for growth.
  with
  raw thyroid extract

- Mezotrace MINERAL COMPLEX 3 daily with Boron 3 Mg. for mineral uptake.

- Biotin 600Mcg. daily with
  Choline/Inositol capsules

- B Complex 100Mg. daily with extra B6 100Mg. and Folic acid 800Mcg.♀

- Ener B B12 INTERNASAL GEL every 3 days.

HERBAL THERAPY

- Take Rosemary tea steeped in wine for maximum uptake of minerals.

- Effective extracts to blend through hair and scalp:
  ◆ CamoCare concentrate for dazzle.
  ◆ New Moon HAIR RUSH for shine and elasticity.
  ◆ Jojoba oil to dissolve sebum deposits.

- Crystal Star MEGA-MINERAL CAPSULES or MASTER BUILDER CAPS 2x daily for a month for strength and growth.
  ◆ HEALTHY HAIR & NAILS TEA as a rinse and shine.
  ◆ ADRN-ALIVE CAPS and ADRN EXTRACT to prevent graying.

- Effective teas and rinses:
  ◆ Horsetail for strength
  ◆ Nettles for shine and to darken graying hair.
  ◆ Japanese green tea

BODYWORK

❖ Massage the head and scalp every morning for 2 or 3 minutes to waken the brain and stimulate hair growth.
  Take 6 Kelp tablets.

❖ Use mousse gel as a style holder, not hair sprays.

❖ Wash hair in warm, not hot water. Rinse in cool water for scalp circulation.
  Condition regularly.

❖ Effective shampoos:
  Aloe vera
  Jojoba♂
  Premier 1 PREM ROYAL

❖ Effective hair rinses:
  ◆ Nettles to darken
  ◆ Rosemary/Sage to shine dark hair.
  ◆ Kelp or sea water for strength and body.
  ◆ Cider Vinegar for acid/alkaline pH balance
  ◆ Calendula/Lemon to tint blonde hair
  ◆ Chamomile to brighten hair
  ◆ 1 egg yolk with the 2nd shampoo for bounce/protein.

COMMON SYMPTOMS: Too dry or too oily hair; lots of falling hair; flaky deposits on the scalp; brittle hair with split ends; poor bounce and elasticity.

COMMON CAUSES: Poor diet with several mineral deficiencies; lack of usable protein; poor circulation; recent illness and drug residues; liver malfunction resulting in jaundice and loss of hair.

HAIR LOSS ✧ MALE PATTERN BALDNESS ✧ ALOPECIA

FOOD THERAPY

🍃 Take daily: 2 T.
Blackstrap Molasses
with
PABA 1000Mg. and
Pantothenic acid
1000Mg. for 2 months.

🍃 Diet is very important.
Avoid caffeine, refined
and preserved foods.
Reduce salt, sugar, fat.

🍃 Eat foods rich in silica,
sulphur, and iodine;
onions, garlic, sprouts,
horseradish, green leafy
vegies, carrots, bell
peppers, cucumbers,
rice, seeds, <u>sea vegies</u>.

🍃 Take 2 T. each daily:
Wheat germ
Brewer's yeast
Chopped dulse.

🍃 6 glasses of water daily.

VITAMINS/MINERALS

❖ Biotin 1000Mcg. daily
with
Choline/Inositol 500-
1000Mg. daily.

❖ B Complex 150Mg daily
with
Pancreatin 1400Mg at
meals. ♀

❖ Mezotrace MINERAL
COMPLEX 2 x daily.
and
Ester C with Bioflavs
and Rutin 1000Mg.

❖ High Omega 3 fish or
flax oils 3 daily.
or
Vit. E 400IU daily as an
anti-oxidant.

❖ Niacin 500Mg. 3 x daily.

❖ Cysteine 500Mg. daily
<u>with Zinc 75Mg. daily.</u> ♂

HERBAL THERAPY

🌿 Crystal Star SILICA
SOURCE EXTRACT daily.
and / or
🌿 HEALTHY HAIR & NAILS
TEA both as a drink and
hair rinse.

🌿 Effective teas:
Comfrey / Alfalfa
Nettles
Horsetail
Rosemary / Dulse

🌿 Crystal Star MEGA-
MINERAL CAPSULES OR
HIGHLY ABSORBABLE
MINERAL EXTRACT.

🌿 Alta Health SIL-X CAPS.

🌿 Cayenne extract: take 2x
daily, Rub directly onto
scalp before sham-
pooing. Leave on for
30min.

BODYWORK

❖ Effective shampoos:
Biotin
Jojoba
Aloe Vera

❖ **Good circulation is the
key. ◆ Massage scalp
vigorously. ◆ Brush
well. ◆ Rinse with
alternating hot and
cold water. ◆ Use a
slant board.**

❖ Get mild exercise every
day for oxygen.

❖ REFLEXOLOGY POINT:

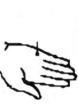
CRANIUM

❖ Rinse hair with sea
water when possible.

COMMON SYMPTOMS: Thinning or complete loss of hair.

COMMON CAUSES: Poor circulation; poor diet with excess salt and sugar; gland imbalance; plugs of sebum, cholesterol, testosterone; overproduction of male sex hormones; dandruff or seborrhea; B vitamin deficiency; stress and anxiety; anemia; mineral deficiency; raised copper levels.

<u>REMEMBER:</u> **Your therapy choice must be vigorously followed. Occasional therapy will have little or no effect. Two months is usually the minimum for really noticeable growth.**

HANGOVER ✧ ALCOHOL TOXICITY

FOOD THERAPY

❧ Eat vitamin B-rich and high fiber foods to give stability and soak up blood alcohol.

❧ No sugar or "hair of the dog". Both may seem to make you feel better, but really drag out a hangover.

❧ Effective tonics:
#1) Brewer's yeast, raw egg, orange juice, cayenne. Drink all at once straight down.
#2) Tomato juice, mixed green and yellow onions, celery, parsley, hot pepper sauce, rosemary leaves, fennel seeds, basil, water, bragg's liquid aminos. Drink straight down.

VITAMINS/ MINERALS

❖ Vitamin C powder 1/2t. in water with 2 vitamin B Complex capsules before drinking.
or

❖ Cysteine 500Mg. with 2 Evening Primrose oil capsules before drinking and before retiring.

❖ Glutamine 500Mg. with vitamin E 400IU with Selenium to reduce oxygen loss.
or

❖ B₁₅ DMG sublingual before drinking.

❖ Biotec EXTRA ENERGY ENZYMES SOD.

❖ Ener B INTERNASAL B₁₂ .

❖ Vitamin B₁ Thiamine 500Mg.

HERBAL THERAPY

❧ Crystal Star ASPIRSOURCE CAPSULES before drinking, with a B₂ capsule.♀

❧ Cayenne / Ginger capsules to settle stomach and relieve headache.

❧ Scullcap tea to soothe nerves and oxygenate the brain.

BODYWORK

❖ Apply cold compresses to the head before and after a long hot shower, or take alternating hot and cool showers, to stimulate circulation and eliminate blood alcohol.

❖ Take a spa or sauna for 20 minutes.

❖ Rub H₂O₂ PEROXY GEL on the feet, or take a teaspoonful of 3% dilute solution in a glass of water.

COMMON SYMPTOMS: Sensitivity to light, headache, eyeache; weakness; debility; shakiness; dull mind and senses; lethargy.

COMMON CAUSES: Alcohol poisoning from too much alcohol; liver exhaustion and consequent malfunction.

167

HAYFEVER ✧ POLLEN & ENVIRONMENTAL ALLERGIES

FOOD THERAPY	VITAMINS/ MINERALS	HERBAL THERAPY	BODYWORK
❧ During an attack or high risk seasons: ◆ Change your diet to include at least 75% fresh raw foods. ◆ Take 2 teasp. raw honey in cider vinegar or a glass of lemon water every morning. ◆ Take a green drink (Pg. 34) or fresh carrot juice daily.	✤ Beta carotene 100,000IU with Zinc 50Mg. 2x daily.♂	❧ Preventive herbs before an attack: ◆ Crystal Star ADRN-ALIVE CAPSULES or ADRN EXTRACT. ◆ Twin Lab Propolis tincture. ◆ Unsprayed Bee Pollen ◆ Garlic tabs 6 daily. ◆ Evening Primrose oil caps	✤ Acupressure points: During an attack: press tip of nose hard as needed for relief. Press hollow above the center of upper lip as needed.
❧ Preventive measures include 2T. wheat germ and 2T brewer's yeast on a regular basis.	✤ Ascorbate vitamin C crystals with Bioflavonoids, 1/4t. every hour to bowel tolerance during an attack. and Pantothenic acid 1000Mg. with extra B_6 100Mg.	❧ Effective herbs during an attack: ◆ Crystal Star ALRG CAPSULES or POLLEN-EX TEA. ◆ Crystal Star ALRG-HST EXTRACT♂ ◆ Hyland's HAYFEVER SYMPT. ◆ BioForce POLLINOSAN TABS ◆ BioForce SINUSAN TABS ◆ Lobelia extract	✤ Avoid smoking and secondary smoke.
❧ Good non-mucous-forming foods: "stone" fruits (apricots, cherries, peaches, etc.), green salads, steamed vegetables, low fat foods	✤ Enzymatic Therapy AIR POWER or AS COMP.	❧ Effective teas: Ephedra Rose Hips Black Cohosh Mullein/Wild Cherry Comfrey Rt.and Lf.	
❧ Avoid junk foods, pasteurized dairy, red meats, bread and sugars.	✤ Raw Thymus or Raw Adrenal extracts regularly during high risk seasons to build immunity.♀	❧ Take some fresh grated horseradish in a spoon with lemon juice. Hang over a sink to release great quantities of excess mucous fast.	
❧ See MUCOUS CLEANSING DIET (Pg.25) and ASTHMA SECTION for more information.	✤ Premier 1 or YS ROYAL JELLY (highest potency) 1 tsp. as needed during an attack.		
	✤ Stress B Complex 100Mg. with extra B_6 100Mg. for anti-body formation; with B_12 sublingual tabs.		

COMMON SYMPTOMS: Inflamed lungs; difficulty breathing, resting, sleeping; coughing; wheezing; sneezing; red, runny nose and eyes; stuffiness.

COMMON CAUSES: pollen reaction; stirred up body toxicity and excess accumulation of mucous waste in the system which harbors pollen irritants; environmental chemical reactions against pollutants that are too much for the body to cope with.

HEADACHES ✧ TENSION & SINUS HEADACHES

FOOD THERAPY

- Go on a short 24 hour juice fast (Pg. 27) to remove body clogs. Drink lots of water, lemon and green drinks (Pg. 34) and potassium broth.(Pg. 33).

- Follow the next day with a very alkaline diet: apples and apple juice, cranberry juice, sprouts, and salads and some brown rice.

- **Take 2T. each daily to restore body balance:**
  Brewer's yeast
  Lecithin granules
  Cider vinegar and honey

- **Avoid refined foods, salty, sugary foods, and chemical foods.**

- See LIVER CLEANSING and HYPOGLYCEMIA DIET suggestions in this book.

- Apply cold black tea bags to the eyes for 15 minutes.

VITAMINS/ MINERALS

- ✤ **Stress B Complex as needed**
  and
  Ester C 550Mg. with Bioflavs and Rutin 3 -4 daily.

- ✤ Niacin Therapy 100Mg. or more as needed daily to keep blood vessels and circulation open.

- ✤ DLPA 500-750Mg or a GABA compound such as Country Life RELAXER CAPS for brain relief.

- ✤ Bromelain 500Mg. as needed. Acts like aspirin without the stomach upset.

- ✤ Magnesium 800Mg. daily.

- ✤ **Nature's Plus Germanium 25Mg. with SUMA ♂**
  and
  Evening Primrose caps 3-4 daily.

- ✤ Hylands Homeopathic remedy HYLAVIR.

HERBAL THERAPY

- ❧ Crystal Star RELAX CAPS 2 as needed to rebuild nerve sheath, ASPIRSOURCE CAPSULES, HEADACHES DEFENSE, or STRESS RELIEF EXTRACT ♂ for pain relief.

- ❧ Effective extracts:
  ◆ Valerian/Wild Lettuce
  ◆ Feverfew
  ◆ Ginkgo Biloba

- ❧ Effective teas:
  ◆ St. John's Wort
  ◆ White Willow
  ◆ Chamomile
  ◆ Catnip/Sage

- ❧ Use Rosemary as a tea, or mix the essential oil in hot water and inhale as an effective steam; or take the extract under the tongue as an anti-oxidant.

- ❧ **Apply Peppermint oil to the temples. ♀**

- ❧ **Dong Quai/Damiana caps for prevention. ♀**

BODYWORK

- ✤ Take a brisk aerobic walk. Breathe deeply for oxygen. The more brain oxygen, the less headaches.

- ✤ REFLEXOLOGY POINT:

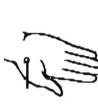

  Apply an ice cube on the above point for fast relief.

- ✤ Lie down with the head higher than the body.

- ✤ An ice massage on the back of the neck and upper back will **dramatically reduce pain.**

- ✤ Have a chiropractic adjustment or shiatzu massage if headaches are chronic.

- ✤ Aromatherapy: Lavender essential oil.

COMMON SYMPTOMS: Pain over the eyes, forehead and temples; food sensitivities; eyestrain; muscle tension; constipation; too much caffeine; salt, sugar or MSG intake; hypoglycemia; allergies; edema; poor circulation; sluggish liver; jawbone misalignment; arthritis; Candida Albicans; drug toxicity. TENSION HEADACHES: muscle contractions of the scalp and back of the head. SINUS HEADACHES: congestion and inflammation of the nasal sinuses.

COMMON CAUSES: Emotional stress; inability to sleep; irritability.

HEARING LOSS

FOOD THERAPY

❧ Keep the diet low in fats, cholesterol and mucous-forming foods. See HEALTHY HEART DIET in this book.

❧ Avoid refined sugars, heavy starches and concentrated foods.

❧ Eat light to hear better; plenty of vegetable proteins, sprouts, whole grains, fruits, and cultured foods .

❧ Garlic and fresh horseradish are excellent for clearing head passages.

VITAMINS/ MINERALS

✤ Take together, one of each 2 x daily:
◆ Emulsified A 25,000IU
◆ Ester C with Bioflavonoids
◆ Mezotrace MULTIMINERAL
◆ Methionine
◆ Glutamine 500Mg.

✤ For ringing in the ears: Beta Carotene 150,000IU

✤ Mega C therapy: Use Ascorbate or Ester C crystals 1/4t. every half hour to bowel tolerance.

✤ Nature's Plus Germanium w/ Suma 30Mg. daily. ♂

✤ Health Plus ORAL CHEL-ATION 2 packs daily ♂ with pantothenic acid 500Mg.

✤ Use dilute hydrogen peroxide to gently clean out excess ear wax or obstructions.

HERBAL THERAPY

❧ Ginkgo Biloba extract 2-3x daily under the tongue.

❧ Mullein oil drops in the ears for 2 weeks. ☺

❧ Crystal Star ANTI-HST CAPS to relieve pressure in ears and sinus canals.

❧ Echinacea extract liquid and Siberian Ginseng extract capsules 4 daily.♂

❧ Put 6 drops garlic oil and 3 drops Golden Seal extract in the ear. Hold in with cotton. Repeat daily for a week. Flush out with vinegar and water.

❧ Take fresh grated horseradish in a spoon with lemon juice. Hang over a sink to release excess mucous and clear head passages.

BODYWORK

✤ Massage neck, ear and temples. Pull ear lobes; top front and back to clear passages.

✤ Lose excess body weight. Fat clogs the head, too.

✤ Acupressure point: Squeeze the joints of the ring finger and the 4th toe, covering all sides for several minutes each day.

✤ REFLEXOLOGY POINT:

EARS

COMMON SYMPTOMS: Degenerative hearing loss; clogged ears; obstructed ear passages.

COMMON CAUSES: Arteriosclerosis; thickening of the passages and tubes in the ear so that there is no vibration; excess ear wax or other obstruction; mucous clog; infection or inflammation; swelling and congestion; chronic bronchial infection; swollen glands.

HEART ARRYTHMIA ✧ TACHYCARDIA

FIBRILLATION ✦ PALPITATIONS

FOOD THERAPY

𝇋 Keep your diet low in fats, salt and calories. Have a fresh green salad and some whole grain protein every day.

𝇋 Add sunflower and sesame seeds, miso soup, rice and oat bran, green leafy vegetables, or a green drink frequently.

𝇋 Take a low fat protein drink every morning such as NaturesPlus SPIRUTEIN as a preventive measure.

𝇋 Take 1/4 cup mineral water and/or a Crystal Star MIN-ZYME-MINOS DRINK daily for potassium.

𝇋 Avoid hard liquor, caffeine and tobacco.

𝇋 Take 2T. each daily:
Lecithin granules
Wheat germ
Brewer's yeast

VITAMINS/ MINERALS

❖ Twin Lab LIQUID K or WHITE BIRCH MINERAL WATER 3 t. daily.
<u>and</u>

❖ Liquid chlorophyll 3t. daily before meals.

❖ Country Life RELAXER CAPSULES as needed, and/or
CALCIUM/ MAGNESIUM/ POTASSIUM CAPSULES.

❖ Effective preventives:
◆ Vit. E w/Selenium ♂
◆ Stress B Complex   150Mg.
◆ Carnitine 500Mg. daily ♀
◆ Cal/Mag/Bromelain ♂
◆ Taurine 2 daily ☺

❖ CO Q 10 30Mg. daily. with Sun CHLORELLA TABS 10 daily.

❖ Rainbow Light CALCIUM PLUS CAPS 4 daily ♀

❖ Omega 3 fish or Flax oils.

❖ Solaray CHROMIACIN CAPS 3x daily.

HERBAL THERAPY

𝇋 Crystal Star CARDI-STRENGTH CAPSULES as a preventive measure.
<u>and</u>
HAWTHORNE LEAF & FLOWER EXTRACT as needed to regulate.

𝇋 Cayenne/Ginger capsules 2 daily regularly.

𝇋 Ginkgo Biloba extract as needed 2-3x daily.

𝇋 Emergency measures:
◆ Cayenne extract drops
◆ Tansy tea
◆ Hawthorne extract drops

𝇋 Effective capsules:
◆ Siberian Ginseng 2 daily
◆ Garlic oil capsules 6 daily.
◆ Bee Pollen 2 daily

𝇋 Evening Primrose oil caps.

𝇋 Effective teas:
◆ Butchers Broom
◆ Rosemary
◆ Wild Cherry
◆ Peppermint/Sage

BODYWORK

❖ Plunge the face into cold water when arrhythmia occurs to stop palpitations.

❖ Avoid soft drinks. The phosphorus binds up magnesium and makes it unavailable for heart regularity.

❖ REFLEXOLOGY POINT:

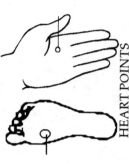

HEART POINTS

❖ See HEALTHY HEART DIET in this book for more information.

COMMON SYMPTOMS: Irregular heartbeat; shortness of breath, and a feeling that you cannot breathe.

COMMON CAUSES: Poor diet with too many saturated fats and refined sugar; lack of exercise and aerobic strength; obesity; smoking; stress; high blood pressure; diabetes.

HEART DISEASE

ANGINA ✦ CORONARY ✦ STROKE ✦ ARTERIOSCLEROSIS

FOOD THERAPY

🐾 See HEALTHY HEART DIET on the following pages.

🐾 A healthy heart diet has plenty of magnesium and potassium rich foods: fresh greens, sea vegetables, pitted fruits, sea food and fish, tofu, brown rice and whole grains, garlic and onions.

🐾 Take 2T. each daily:
Lecithin granules
Brewer's yeast
Wheat germ
Molasses

🐾 Pay conscious attention to omitting red meats, caffeine and caffeine - containing foods, refined sugars, fatty, salty and fried foods, prepared meats and soft drinks. The rewards are worth the effort.

🐾 Drink at least 1 cup of mineral water daily. (Remember that chlorinated/fluoridated water destroys vitamin E in the body).

VITAMINS/ MINERALS

❖ Vital Health ADVANCED CHELATION FORMULA 1 W/ EDTA 2 packs daily.

❖ Effectivity anti-oxidants for aerobic action:
◆ COQ 10, 10Mg. daily
◆ Inosine 150Mg.
◆ Carnitine 250Mg. ♀
◆ DMG B₁₅ 125Mg.
◆ Vitamin E with Selenium

❖ Carnitine 500Mg. daily (use LIQUID CARNITINE for myocardial infarction during an attack)

❖ Ascorbate or Ester C with bioflavonoids, up to 5000Mg. daily.
with
Chromium picolinate or Solaray CHROMIACIN to control arterial plaque.

❖ Biotec EXTRA ENERGY ENZYMES to decrease free radical activity.

❖ Germanium 1 gm. in 1 qt. water, take 2-3T. daily.♂

❖ Omega 3 fish and flax oils 3x daily for prevention.

HERBAL THERAPY

🐾 In an emergency; 1t. cayenne powder, or several drops of cayenne tincture in water will often bring a person out of a heart attack or coronary.

🐾 Effective emergency aid: 1/2 dropperful Hawthorne extract every 1/2 hour.
Take 1/2 dropperful daily as preventive support.

🐾 Crystal Star CARDI-STRENGTH CAPSULES, POTASSIUM SOURCE CAPS, or HEMA CLEANSE TEA.

🐾 Effective heart tonics:
◆ Cayenne/Ginger capsules
◆ Liquid chlorophyll
◆ Chaparral caps
◆ Garlic oil capsules
◆ Wheat germ oil caps

🐾 Evening Primrose oil caps 2-4 daily.♀

🐾 Siberian Ginseng extract caps 2000Mg. or tea 2 cups daily.♂

BODYWORK

✦ Apply hot compresses and massage chest of the victim to ease a heart attack.

✦ Take alternate hot and cold showers frequently to increase circulation.

✦ Stop smoking.

✦ Take some mild regular daily exercise. Do deep breathing exercises every morning for body oxygen, and to stimulate brain activity.

✦ Consciously add relaxation and a good daily laugh to your life. A positive mental outlook does wonders for stress.

✦ REFLEXOLOGY POINTS:

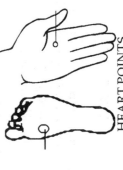

HEART POINTS

DIAGNOSING HEART PROBLEMS

ANGINA: Recurring, sudden, intense chest pains, lasting 1/2 to 1 minute, with a vise-like grip across the chest. Angina is usually brought on by emotional stress, exposure to cold, or overexertion. The usual cause is degeneration of the major artery walls.

ARTERIOSCLEROSIS: Hardening and loss of elasticity of the arteries resulting from degeneration of the artery walls.

CONGESTIVE HEART FAILURE: A condition resulting from a heart weakened by arteriosclerosis or other disease such as hypothyroidism. Circulation is inefficient and organs and tissues become clogged with blood. Early symptoms include abnormal fatigue, and shortness of breath, ankles and feet usually swell, breathing is impaired, and there is nausea and gas.

ATHEROSCLEROSIS: Degeneration of the major arteries resulting from multiple fat and cholesterol plaque lesions, causing narrowing and possible embolism when these break loose into the bloodstream.

MYOCARDIAL INFARCTION/ CORONARY OCCLUSION/ CORONARY THROMBOSIS: Conditions resulting from fatty plaque obstructions, and narrowing of the artery walls from atherosclerosis, impairing and cutting off oxygen to the heart. The pain experienced can be excruciating, starting in the lower chest and spreading throughout the upper half of the body. The pulse is weak and rapid, with perspiring skin, blood pressure drops and the skin pales. A fever usually follows this kind of attack.

STROKE: Impaired or fluctuating state of consciousness, tingling sensations and visual disturbances, headache and stiff neck, dizziness, nausea, vomiting, and the inability to speak or move the limbs. The condition is a result of blood vessels blocked by atherosclerosis, clotting or hemorrhaging. The process is similar to that of a coronary, the difference being cell death in the brain during a stroke.

QUICK HEART REHABILITATION CHECK PROGRAM

This program is especially for those of you who have survived a heart attack or major heart surgery. Coming back is tough. Beginning and sticking to a new lifestyle that changes almost everything about the way you eat, exercise, handle stress, and even the smallest details of your life is a challenge. The following mini-rehabilitation program is a blueprint that you can use with confidence. It has proven successful against heart disease recurrence.

♠ **Reduce fats to 15% of your diet; less if possible. Limit polyunsaturates (margerine, oils) to 10%. Add mono-unsaturates (olive oil, avocados, nuts, seeds)**

♠ Take some regular daily exercise. To be effective for heart, circulation and artery health, the heart rate and respiration must rise to the point of mild breathlessness for 5 minutes each day.

♠ Have several servings of cold water fish or seafood every week for high omega 3 oils.

♠ Have a fresh green salad every day.

♠ **Add Miso and Oat or Rice bran to your diet regularly.**

♠ Eat plenty of complex carbohydrates, such as broccoli, peas, whole grain breads, vegetable pastas, potatoes, sprouts, tofu and brown rice.

♠ Have a glass of white wine before dinner for relaxation and better digestion.

♠ Eat potassium-rich foods for cardiotonic activity: fresh spinach and chard, broccoli, bananas, sea vegetables, molasses, canteloupe, apricots, papayas, mushrooms, tomatoes, yams. OR take a high potassium drink regularly, such as POTASSIUM BROTH (Pg. 33), Crystal Star MIN-ZYME-MINOS DRINK,or WHITE BIRCH MINERAL WATER. (a serving of high potassium fruits or vegetables offers about 400Mg. of potassium; a serving of the above drinks offers approx. 1000-1250Mg. of potassium)

♠ Eat magnesium-rich foods for heart regulation: tofu, wheat germ, bran, broccoli, potatoes, lima beans, spinach, chard.

♠ Eat copper-rich foods for clear arteries: oysters,clams, crab, fish, brewer's yeast, fresh fruit and vegetables, nuts, seeds.

♠ Eat high fiber foods for a clean system and alkalinity: whole grains, fruits and vegetables, legumes and herbs.

♠ Choose several of the following supplements as your individual daily micro-nutrients:
- ◆ Anti-oxidants: Wheat germ oil raises oxygen level 30%; vitamin E 400IU with Selenium; CO Q 10, 30Mg.; Rosemary.
- ◆ Regulation & stability: Sun CHLORELLA; Magnesium; Selenium; Omega 3 flax or fish oils; advanced oral chelation.
- ◆ Clear arteries: Solaray CHROMIACIN; Selenium; Carnitine 500Mg.; Evening Primrose oil.
- ◆ Cardiac tonics: Hawthorne extract; Cayenne; Garlic; Niacin 500Mg.TR.
- ◆ Anti-cholesterol/blood thinning: Ginger; Butcher's Broom; Taurine; oral chelation with EDTA.
- ◆ Healthy blood chemistry: Chromium picolinate; Ester C 500Mg. with bioflavonoids

173

DIET FOR A HEALTHY HEART

Diet is the single most influential key to heart health. In general, refined, high fat and high calorie foods create cardiovascular problems, and natural foods relieve them. Fried foods, salty foods, sugar, low fiber foods, pasteurized dairy products, red meats and processed meats, tobacco, hard liquor and caffeine all contribute to clogged and reduced arteries, LDL cholesterol, high blood pressure and heart attacks. **Almost all circulatory disease can be treated and prevented with improvement in diet and nutrition.** You can carve out health with your own knife and fork. **The following diet** is for long term heart and circulatory health. It emphasizes fresh foods, high fiber and mineral foods, and oxygenating foods.

ON RISING: take a protein drink such as Nature's Plus SPIRUTEIN, or a vitamin mineral drink such as ALL 1.

BREAKFAST: make the following mix with 2T. <u>each</u>: lecithin granules, wheat germ, brewer's yeast, honey, sesame seeds.
Sprinkle on fresh fruits, or mix with yogurt;
and have a whole grain cereal with apple juice, **or** a poached egg with bran muffins or whole grain toast.

MIDMORNING: have a green drink (Pg. 34) or high potassium drink such as Crystal Star MIN-ZYME-MINOS;
and crunchy raw vegies with kefir cheese or yogurt cheese, **or** a cup of miso soup with sea vegetables.

LUNCH: have a fresh salad with sprouts, leafy greens, and a lemon/oil dressing;
and/or a whole grain sandwich with vegetables, low fat cheeses and spreads;
or a light vegie or tofu omelet, with a brown rice or whole grain pasta salad.

MIDAFTERNOON: have a cup of mint, fenugreek, or other herbal tea; or Crystal Star ROYAL MU tonic tea;
or a glass of fresh carrot or "Personal V-8" juice (Pg. 39);
and/or a cup of miso soup with rice cakes or crackers.

DINNER: have a vegetable casserole with brown rice or other whole grain, and Tofu or seafood;
and a hearty vegetable protein dinner salad;
or a vegetable souffle or quiche with a whole grain crust, and a cup of onion, lentil or black bean soup;
or baked or broiled fish, with a baked potato and salad;
or an Oriental stir fry with brown rice or light noodles;
A glass of white wine at dinner is often good for reducing stress and allowing relaxation.

BEFORE BED: have another cup of Miso soup, a cup of VEGEX yeast paste broth, apple juice, or chamomile tea.

DAILY PREVENTION SUPPLEMENTATION SHOULD INCLUDE: Vitamin E 400IU, Solaray CHROMIACIN, CO Q 10, 10Mg., Sun CHLORELLA, and Flax oil.

PREVENTIVE BODYWORK SHOULD INCLUDE: a regular daily walk, or other aerobic exercise to strengthen the heart muscle.

See"COOKING FOR HEALTHY HEALING" **by Linda Rector-Page for a complete heart diet and healing program.**

174

HEEL & BONE SPURS ✧ PLANTAR WARTS

FOOD THERAPY

- Avoid oxalic acid forming foods that produce crystals in the body, and bind up organic calcium: red meats, caffeine, carbonated drinks, cooked spinach, chocolate, etc.
- Avoid sugars, hard liquor, fried foods and saturated fats.
- Drink black cherry juice daily. Take a potassium drink or green drink often to keep the body alkaline and kidney function good.
- Rub cut papaya skins on affected areas.
- See other diet suggestions on ACIDOSIS and GOUT pages in this book.
- Effective alkalizing foods:
  - Miso soup
  - Fresh vegetables
  - Brewer's yeast
  - Cranberry juice

VITAMINS/ MINERALS

- Ener B INTERNASAL GEL OR B$_{12}$ sublingual tabs.
- Enzymatic Therapy ACID-A-CAL CAPSULES. ♀
- Vitamin C with Rose Hips, up to 5000Mg. daily with extra bioflavonoids 500Mg daily, for collagen and interstitial tissue formation. with Pantothenic acid 500Mg. or
- Mix Vitamin C crystals with water to a paste and apply to spur, and secure with tape. Leave on all day for several weeks for improvement.
- Cal/Mag/Zinc 4 daily.♀
- Country Life LIGA-TEND
- Magnesium/Potassium/Bromelain capsules ♂ or
- Quercitin Plus w/ Bromelain 2 daily. ♀

HERBAL THERAPY

- Apply a mixture of wintergreen oil, witch hazel, and black walnut tincture.
- Take Betaine HCl for better assimilation.
- Apply propolis tincture.
- Apply Tea Tree oil.
- Apply a paste mixture of green clay and liquid chlorophyll
- Apply Swedish Bitters
- Take Echinacea fresh plant extract internally 2x daily, and apply several times daily.
- Apply BioForce ECHINACEA CREAM.
- Enzymatic Therapy CHERRY FRUIT CAPSULES.

BODYWORK

- Apply Epsom salts compresses.
- Soak feet in the hottest water you can stand for as long as you can.
- For Plantar warts: apply dandelion stem juice 3x daily. Let dry each time.
- Rub H$_2$O$_2$ PEROXY GEL directly on the wart or spur twice daily. Removal takes about 2 months.
- Apply DMSO for pain and to help dissolve crystalline deposits.
- Crystal Star ALKALIZING ENZYME BODY WRAP to rebalance body chemistry.

COMMON SYMPTOMS: Inflammation and infection; great pain from ingrown nodules on the feet.

COMMON CAUSES: Acid-forming diet with liver congstion and poor or irregular kidney function; constipation and toxemia from excess fats and refined carbohydrates; too little vegetable protein.

HEMORRHAGING ✧ INTERNAL BLEEDING

EXCESSIVE BLEEDING ✦ BLOOD CLOTTING DIFFICULTY

FOOD THERAPY	VITAMINS/MINERALS	HERBAL THERAPY	BODYWORK
● Make a variety of sprouts a regular part of your diet for natural Vitamin K.	❖ Solaray CALCIUM CITRATE CAPS 4 daily. ♀	❧ Capsicum, take 1 teasp. in a cup of hot water to stop bleeding.	❖ ACUPRESSURE POINT: Press the insides of the thighs with the fingers just above the knees, for 10 seconds at a time.
● Have a glass of Carrot/Spinach juice frequently.	❖ Vitamin C therapy for collagen and interstitial tissue formation: use Ester C or ascorbic acid crystals with bioflavs. and rutin. Take up to 5000Mg. daily. and/or	❧ External clotting agents: ◆ Plaintain and water paste ◆ Witch Hazel ◆ Cayenne powder ◆ Buckthorne tincture	❖ Hold arm in the air on the side of the bleeding to decrease pressure. ◆ Pull knuckle of the middle finger on either hand til it pops, to lower blood pressure and tension.
● Eat plenty of papayas.	❖ Quercetin Plus with Bromelain 4 daily.	❧ Internal bleeding control: ◆ Pau de Arco tea ◆ Turmeric capsules ◆ Comfrey Root ◆ Shepherd's Purse ♀	❖ Apply direct pressure to a vein or artery. Get a doctor and treat for shock. See SHOCK TREATMENT PAGE in this book for more information.
● Take green drink (Pg. 34), or use Crystal Star ENERGY GREEN DRINK at least once a week to build healthier blood.	❖ Vitamin K 100Mg. 3x daily.	❧ Herbal astringents to tighten and strengthen veins and capillaries. All may be used both externally and internally: ◆ White Oak bark ♂ ◆ Comfrey Root ◆ Cranebill ◆ Golden Seal extract	
	❖ Propolis tincture; apply directly, and take internally 4x daily. ♂	❧ Clotting agent tea: Licorice/Comfrey Rt./ Shepherd's Purse/ Golden Seal/Cranesbill.	
	❖ Enzymatic Therapy HEMTONE CAPSULES to stop rectal bleeding. ♀		
	❖ Liquid chlorophyll 3tsp. daily with vitamin E and Selenium for blood building.		

COMMON SYMPTOMS: Inability to clot even small wounds; internal pain as with a rupture or ulcer; easy bruising and ulcerations; broken blood vessels; black stools when there are stomach ulcers.

COMMON CAUSES: Broken blood vessels; weak vein and vessel walls; internal wounds as from a blow or accident; lack of vitamin K in the body, from heredity or sometimes from eating irradiated foods which deplete vitamin K in the system.

HEMORRHOIDS ✧ PILES ✧ ANAL FISSURE

FOOD THERAPY

❦ Take 1 T. olive oil before each meal. Include plenty of soluble fiber foods in the diet, particularly lots of vegetable cellulose, such as stewed and dried fruits, brans, vegetables.

❦ Include a variety of sprouts for vitamin K.

❦ Take 2T. cider vinegar mixed with honey each morning.

❦ Keep meals small, so the bowel and sphincter area will not have to work so hard.

❦ Apply papaya skins or lemon juice directly to inflamed area to relieve itching.

❦ Avoid refined, low fiber foods, and acid forming foods, such as caffeine and sugar.

❦ See DIET FOR CONSTIPATION AND COLON HEALTH in this book.

VITAMINS/ MINERALS

❖ Ascorbate Vitamin C with bioflavonoids and rutin. Take up to 500Mg. daily, and make a solution in water to apply directly.

❖ Vit. K 100Mg. 2x daily with Vit. B$_6$ 250Mg. daily.

❖ NatureAde SOFT-EX stool softener. ♀

❖ Enzymatic Therapy HEMTONE CAPSULES.

❖ Vitamin E 400IU daily. Also apply to inflamed area for healing.

❖ BioForce HEMORRHOID HOMEOPATHIC REMEDY.

❖ Bromelain 500Mg. with Lecithin caps 1900Gr. ♂ daily.

❖ Apply aloe vera gel.

❖ Evening Primrose oil caps 4 daily for a month.

HERBAL THERAPY

❧ Apply Calendula ointment. Take Stone root tea, 3 cups daily for a month. ♂

❧ Crystal Star HEMRR-EZE CAPSULES for 2 weeks to relieve inflammation and encourage healing. (May also be used as a suppository) Add LIV-FLUSH TEA to clear sluggishness, and/or LAXA TEA and BWL TONE CAPSULES for gentle healing.

❧ Effective suppositories and compresses:
◆ Golden Seal/Myrrh
◆ Slippery Elm in Cocoa Butter
◆ Garlic/Comfrey
◆ White Oak/Yarrow ♂

❧ Hemorrhoid tea: mix equal parts Comfrey root, wild yam, and cranesbill. Take internally and apply directly.

❧ For anal fissure: use Crystal Star ANTI-BIO CAPS and YSK WAKASA CHLORELLA EXTRACT.

BODYWORK

❖ Apply Mullein oil or Witch Hazel.

❖ Effective enemas:
Nettles
Chlorella

❖ Bee Pollen 1000Mg. tablet suppository. Insert 1-2x daily.

❖ Effective compresses: alternating hot and cool water to stimulate circulation.

❖ Apply Hylands PILE OINTMENT as needed.

❖ Take a good 1/2 hour walk every day.

❖ REFLEXOLOGY POINTS:

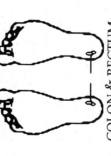

COLON & RECTUM

COMMON SYMPTOMS: Pain, itching and rectal bleeding with bowel movements; inflamed anal fissure; protruding swellings.

COMMON CAUSES: Too many refined , fried, fatty, and low residue foods; constipation; overeating; lack of exercise, too much sitting; Vit. B$_6$ deficiency; acid/alkaline imbalance; liver exhaustion and malfunction.

HEPATITIS ✧ JAUNDICE ✧ LIVER MALFUNCTION

FOOD THERAPY

🐚 **Hepatitis Healing Diet:**
For 2 weeks: Eat only fresh foods; salads, fruits, juices, bottled water.
Take a glass of carrot/beet/cucumber juice every other day.
Take a glass of lemon juice and water every morning.

🐚 **Then for 1-2 months:**
Take carrot/beet/ cucumber juice every 3 days, and papaya juice w/2t. spirulina each morning.
Eat a high vegetable protein diet, with steamed vegetables, brown rice, tofu, eggs, whole grains and yogurt. Avoid meat protein.

🐚 **Then for 1 more month:**
Take 2 glasses of tomato juice/wheat germ oil/ brewer's yeast/lemon juice every day.
Take a daily glass of apple/alfalfa sprout juice.
Continue with vegetable proteins, cultured foods, fresh salads and complex carbohydrates for strength.

🐚 Avoid all refined, fried and fatty foods, sugars, heavy spices and caffeine during healing.

VITAMINS/ MINERALS

✤ Beta Carotene 150,000IU daily, with B Complex 150Mg. and Ener B INTERNASAL B₁₂ GEL daily for 1 month.
Then reduce Beta Carotene to 50,000IU, and B Complex to 100Mg. daily.

✤ Alta Health CANGEST if detection is early:
Take 1t. powder in water 2-3x daily for 7 days; then 1t. 4x daily at meals and bedtime for 7 days.

✤ Natren LIFE START 2 daily for 1 month.

✤ Sun CHLORELLA GRANULES daily, or liquid chlorophyll 3t. daily at meals.

✤ Ascorbate Vit. C crystals, up to 10,000Mg. daily in water to bowel tolerance for 1 month.

✤ Enzymatic Therapy LIVATOX capsules.

HERBAL THERAPY

❧ Crystal Star LIV-ALIVE CAPSULES 4-6 daily, with LIV FLUSH TEA 2 cups daily for 1 month.
Reduce dose to 1/2 the 2nd month.
Add ANEMIGIZE CAPS for blood building, and ANTI-HST CAPS as needed to control histimine reactions.

❧ Enzymatic Therapy LIQUID LIVER with SIBERIAN GINSENG.♂

❧ Liver detoxifiers:
Oregon Grape
Dandelion Rt.
Pau de Arco/Calendula
Lobelia/Red Clover

❧ Comfrey tea 4 cups daily with Spirulina 6 tabs daily.♀

❧ Nutricology germanium sublingual or powder (1gm. to 1 qt. water) Shake before each use. Take 2t. daily.

BODYWORK

✤ Get plenty of bed rest.

✤ **Count on 2 weeks for emergency detox measures; 1-3 months for healing the liver and rebuilding blood and body strength.**

✤ NO alcohol, amphetamines, cocaine, barbiturates, or tobacco AT ALL.

✤ REFLEXOLOGY POINT:

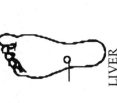

LIVER

✤ Overheating Therapy has been effective for Hepatitis. See P. Airola, "How To Get Well".

✤ See LIVER CLEANSING DIET in this book for more information.

COMMON SYMPTOMS: Great fatigue and exhaustion; enlarged liver with congestion and sluggishness; loss of appetite; gray stools; skin pallor and histimine itching; depression, cirrhosis.

COMMON CAUSES: TYPE A HEPATITIS: a viral infection passed through blood and feces.
TYPE B HEPATITIS: viral infection passed through dirty needles and sexual contact.
A STRONG IMMUNE DEFENSE SYSTEM IS ABSOLUTELY NECESSARY TO OVERCOME AND PREVENT RECURRING HEPATITIS.

HERPES GENITALIS

FOOD THERAPY

❧ Go on a short 3 day cleanse (Pg. 26) to alkalize the body. Have plenty of fruit juices, and a carrot/beet/cucumber juice or potassium broth (Pg. 33) each day. Take 2t. sesame oil daily.

❧ Then keep the diet consciously alkaline with miso soup, brown rice and vegetables frequently. Add lots of cultured foods for friendly G.I. bacteria.

❧ Avoid all sweets, alcohol, refined foods, and argenine-forming foods, such as nuts, corn, caffeine, cereals, and legumes.

❧ Avoid citrus fruits during healing.

VITAMINS/ MINERALS

✤ Apply Lysine cream. Take Lysine 500Mg. capsules 4-6 daily until clear.

✤ Natren MEGADOLPHILUS 1t. 6x daily.

✤ Quercitin Plus with Bromelain for instant action against inflammation. with

✤ B Complex 100Mg. 2x daily. Add extra pantothenic acid 500Mg. and B$_{12}$ 2000Mcg.

✤ Ascorbate vit. C or Ester C powder 1/4t. every hour in water up to 10,000Mg. or bowel tolerance daily during an attack.

✤ Emulsified Vitamin A 50,000IU daily. with Vit. E 400IU 3x daily. Also apply vitamin E oil directly. ♂

HERBAL THERAPY

❧ Crystal Star HERPEACE CAPSULES 4 daily. ♀ and/or ANTI-VI EXTRACT for 7 days to overcome virus.

❧ Locally, pat on sores Crystal Star THERADERM TEA or CALENDULA GEL. ♀

❧ Effective applications:
◆ Black Walnut tincture
◆ Myrrh tincture
◆ Comfrey extract
◆ Aloe Vera/Golden Seal solution.

❧ Enzymatic Therapy ACID-A-CAL CAPSULES.

❧ BioForce Echinacea cream.

❧ Open a Crystal Star ANTI-BIO CAPSULE and apply directly to sores. ♂

❧ St. John's Wort extract capsules as an anti-viral.

BODYWORK

✤ Apply ice packs for pain and inflammation relief.

✤ Get some early morning sunlight on the sores every day for healing Vit. D.

✤ Take hot baths frequently for overheating therapy.

✤ Wear only cotton underwear so sores won't fester.

✤ Remember, that cortisone taken over a long period of time for herpes greatly weakens both the immune system and bone density.

COMMON SYMPTOMS: A contagious viral infection, with recurring fluid-filled rupturing blisters that leave red inflamed painful lesions on thighs, genitals, and face.

COMMON CAUSES: Transmitted from kissing or sexual contact; an opportunistic disease taking over a low immune system; stress and nervous tension; excess arginine in the body; too many drugs; an acid-forming diet.

179

HIATAL HERNIA

FOOD THERAPY

🍃 Eat only raw or steamed soluble fiber foods from vegetable sources during healing. Drink 2 glasses of fresh carrot or apple juice every day.

🍃 Avoid nuts, seeds, acidic juices and gas-producing foods during healing.

🍃 Eat smaller meals more frequently. No large meals. No liquids with meals.

🍃 When digestion has normalized, keep to a low fat, low salt, high fiber diet. Avoid all stimulant foods, such as caffeine, red meats, fried and spicy foods, and carbonated drinks.

🍃 Remember that commercial antacids often do more harm than good as they upset stomach pH causing it to produce even more harmful acids.

VITAMINS/ MINERALS

❖ Quercitin Plus 3 daily for inflammation
   with
   Enzymatic therapy Chewable bromelain or DGL as needed.

❖ Schiff Emulsified A 25,000IU 2x daily.

❖ Liquid Chlorophyll 3t. daily at meals. ♂

❖ Take 1-2 glasses of mineral water daily.

❖ Chewable enzymes as needed.

❖ Alta Health CANGEST CAPS OR POWDER 3x daily. ♀

❖ Zinc Gluconate lozenges under the tongue as needed.

❖ Pancreatin 1400Mg. with meals.

HERBAL THERAPY

🌿 Crystal Star ANTI-BIO CAPS 4 daily, and ANTI SPAZ CAPS 2 with each meal.

🌿 Aloe Vera juice or Slippery Elm tea daily as needed to soothe inflamed tissue.

🌿 Psyllium husk 1-2T. morning and evening to provide gentle cleansing fiber.
   or
🌿 Crystal Star CHO-LO FIBER TONE DRINK.

🌿 Crystal Star CRAMP CONTROL EXTRACT 1/2 dropperful at a time as needed for pain and spasms.

🌿 Propolis extract 1/2 dropperful every 4 hours during an attack. ♂

🌿 Chewable comfrey pepsin tabs.

🌿 Pau de Arco tea daily. ♀

BODYWORK

❖ No smoking. Avoid all tobacco.

❖ Lose weight. Tone the abdomen with exercise. Watch posture to avoid slouching.

❖ Wear loose comfortable, non-binding clothing.

❖ Apply a green clay pack to the area.

❖ REFLEXOLOGY POINT:

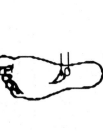

STOMACH & DIAPHRAGM

COMMON SYMPTOMS: Chest pains and heartburn; belching, excess gas and bloating; difficulty swallowing and a full feeling at the base of the throat; hiccups and regurgitation; raised blood pressure; diarrhea; inflammation and gastrointestinal bleeding; mental confusion and nerves.

COMMON CAUSES: Stomach protruding through the esophagus wall, causing reflux of stomach acid in the throat; short esophagus; overeating; obesity; enzyme deficiency; constipation from a low residue diet; too many refined and acid-forming foods; tobacco; too tight jeans.

HIGH BLOOD PRESSURE ✧ HYPERTENSION

FOOD THERAPY	VITAMINS/ MINERALS	HERBAL THERAPY	BODYWORK
❧ Go on a liquid juice diet for 1 day every week for 2 months to alkalize the body and reduce excess blood fats: ◆ Have some citrus juices or a Potassium Essence (Pg. 33) in the morning; ◆ a green drink (Pg. 34) V-8, or carrot juice at mid-day; ◆ apple, pear or papaya juice at dinner; ◆ Chamomile tea or VEGEX broth at bedtime.	✦ Vitamin E therapy: Take 1 100IU. capsule daily for 1 week, then 4 capsules daily for 1 week, then 2 400IU capsules daily for 2 weeks.	❧ Crystal Star HI PRESSURE CARE CAPSULES daily, with POTASSIUM SOURCE CAPS and HAWTHORNE EXTRACT daily.	✚ Keep body weight down. Avoid tobacco in all forms.
❧ Then follow the HIGH BLOOD PRESSURE DIET on the next page, including plenty of magnesium and potassium-rich foods.	✦ Add 1 selenium 100Mcg. and 1 Ester C with bio-flavonoids each time for best results. ♂	❧ Crystal Star DIURCAPS to clear edema; ADRN-ALIVE CAPSULES or EXTRACT to combat fatigue.	✚ Take a brisk 1/2 hour walk every day, with plenty of deep lung breathing.
	✦ B Complex 100Mg. daily with extra B₆ 100Mg. and Niacin 100Mg. 3x daily. ♀	❧ Crystal Star RELAX CAPS as needed for tension.	✚ Use a dry skin brush all over the body frequently to stimulate circulation.
❧ Avoid refined foods, caffeine, salty, fried and fatty foods, prepared meats, heavy pastries and soft drinks. All cause Potassium depletion and/or arterial plaque build-up.	✚ Omega 3 fish or flax oils 3 daily. or Choline 600Mg. daily.	❧ Solaray Siberian Ginseng extract capsules ♂	✚ REFLEXOLOGY POINT: Pull middle finger on each hand 3x for 20 seconds each, daily.
	✚ CO Q 10 30Mg. 2x daily and	❧ Other effective capsules: Garlic oil, 8 daily Alfalfa, 8 daily Evening Primrose 4-6 Cayenne/Ginger 4 daily	✚ Remember that most high blood pressure medicines cause potassium and often magnesium deficiency. Consciously add these mineral rich foods to your diet: Broccoli, bananas, prunes, figs, dates, raisins, potatoes, seafood, buckwheat, brussels sprouts, avocados, cauliflower, brown rice and leafy greens.
	✚ Country Life RELAXER CAPSULES with GABA.	❧ Effective products: ◆ Hyland's CALMS FORTE ◆ Solaray EUROCALM CAPS.	
❧ Take 2T. each daily: Wheat germ Lecithin Brewer's yeast Aloe Vera gel in water.	✚ Rainbow Light CALCIUM PLUS CAPSULES 6 daily.	◆ Medicine Wheel SERENE EXTRACT ◆ Pau de Arco	
	✚ Vital Health ORAL CHELATION WITH EDTA.	❧ Sun CHLORELLA 15 tabs daily to lower blood fats.	

COMMON SYMPTOMS: Headaches; irritability; dizziness and ringing in the ears; flushed complexion; red streaks in the eyes; fatigue and sleeplessness; edema; frequent urination; depression; heart arrhythmia; chronic respiratory problems.

COMMON CAUSES: Clogging arterial fats; calcium/fiber deficiency; thickened blood from mucous and waste loading down the circulatory system; obesity and lack of aerobic exercise; poor diet with too much salt and red meat, causing raised copper levels; kidney malfunction and auto-toxemia from constipation; prostaglandin deficiency.

HIGH BLOOD PRESSURE DIET

85% of high blood pressure is both treatable and preventable without drugs. The most beneficial change you can make to lower high blood pressure is a diet change. Reduce and control salt use. (See LOW SALT DIET Pg. 44) Eat smaller meals more frequently, and consciously undereat. Avoid large meals, caffeine, and red meats. Vegetarians have less hypertension and lower blood pressure problems.

ON RISING: Have a glass of lemon water and honey, **and/or** a high vitamin/mineral drink such as ALL 1 or Crystal Star MIN-ZYME-MINOS. DRINK.

BREAKFAST: Make a mix of lecithin granules, wheat germ, brewer's yeast and sesame or sunflower seeds. Sprinkle some on fresh fruit or mix with yogurt;
   and have a whole grain cereal, toast or muffins with a little kefir cheese or unsalted butter.

MIDMORNING: Have a green drink (Pg. 34) or natural V-8 juice (Pg.39) or mint tea, or a cup of miso or ramen noodle soup.

LUNCH: Have a large fresh green salad with a lemon oil dressing. Add plenty of sprouts, tofu, raisins, cottage cheese, nuts, and seeds as desired;
   or have a baked potato with yogurt or kefir cheese topping, and a light vegie omelet;
   or a seafood and vegetable pasta salad;
   or a high protein whole grain sandwich, with avocados and low fat cheese.

MIDAFTERNOON: Have a glass of mineral water, or an herb tea such as Crystal Star LICORICE MINTS, OR ROYAL MU TEA.
   and/or a cup of soup and a hard boiled egg and some whole grain crackers;
   or some dried fruits, and an apple or cranberry juice.

DINNER: Have a vegetable casserole with Tofu and brown rice, and a small dinner salad;
   or a baked fish or seafood dish with rice and peas, or a baked potato;
   or a vegetable quiche (such as broccoli, artichoke, or asparagus), and a light oriental soup;
   or some roast turkey and cornbread dressing, with a small salad or mashed potatoes with a little butter;
   or an oriental vegetable and seafood or chicken stirfry, with a light clear soup.
   A little white wine is fine with dinner for relaxation, digestion and tension relief.

BEFORE BED: Have a cup of miso soup, or VEGEX YEAST PASTE broth, apple juice, or some chamomile tea.

◆ **See "COOKING FOR HEALTHY HEALING" by Linda Rector-Page for a complete diet to control High Bood Pressure.**

Foods to avoid if you have high blood pressure: canned and frozen foods; cured, smoked and canned meats, and fish, commercial peanut butter, soy sauce, bouillon cubes and condiments, fried chips and snacks, canned and dry soups.

A lifestyle change must be made for there to be permanent control of high blood pressure. It takes time and effort, but the rewards are high; a longer and healthier life, and control of your life.

182

HORMONE & GLAND IMBALANCE

EFFECTIVE FOR MEN AFTER PROSTATE AND RELATED PROBLEMS OR SURGERY
EFFECTIVE FOR WOMEN AFTER HYSTERECTOMY, CHILDBIRTH, D & C, OR SUCTION CURRETAGE.

FOOD THERAPY	VITAMINS/ MINERALS	HERBAL THERAPY	BODYWORK
● Start with a modified macrobiotic diet for 2 weeks (Pg. 42) with seasonal fresh foods, whole grains, brown rice and vegetable protein.	❖ **For male balance:** ♂ Cal/Mag/Zinc 4 daily. or Zinc 75Mg. daily. ❖ Liquid Chlorophyll 3 tsp. daily with meals.	❦ **For male balance:** ♂ Siberian Ginseng extract caps or liquid daily. ❦ Crystal Star PROSCAPS.	❖ **Applied Kinesiology** (muscle testing) is successful in this area for determining which specific products are suitable for individual problems.
● Have a protein drink such as Nature's Plus SPIRUTEIN each morning, or a green drink (Pg. 34) or Crystal Star ENERGY GREEN DRINK daily.	❖❖ Raw Pancreas glandular Raw Orchic glandular ❖ Bee Pollen 2-4 daily.	❦ Effective capsules: Ginseng/Damiana Ginseng/Sarsaparilla Licorice/Dandelion ❦ Smilax extract 10-15 drops daily.	❖ Get morning sunlight on the body every day possible, especially on the male genitalia. ♂
● Avoid sugar, refined and canned foods.	❖ **For female balance:** ♀ Evening Primrose oil 2-4 daily.	❦ **For female balance:** ♀ Crystal Star DONG QUAI/ DAMIANA EXTRACT drops or caps.	❖ Take a good brisk exercise walk every day.
● Drink 6-8 glasses of unchlorinated bottled water daily.	❖ B Complex 100Mg daily. ❖ Pantothenic acid 1000Mg.	❦ Crystal Star FEMALE HARMONY CAPULES or ESTROMONE EXTRACT.	❖ Remember that if you are taking synthetic estrogen or progesterone for glandular problems, it often destroys vitamin E in the body, allowing greater risk for heart, cancer and other diseases. Supplementation is advisable.
● Add complex carbohydrate building foods to the diet: broccoli, peas, cauliflower, tofu, wheat germ, brewer's yeast, nuts and seeds, and whole grains.	❖ **For both sexes:** High potency YS or Premier 1 ROYAL JELLY 1tsp. daily. ❖ Vitamin E 800IU daily. ❖ **Enzymatic Therapy** STEREOPLEX MF	❦ Burdock tea 2 cups daily. ❦ **For both sexes:** Crystal Star ADRN-ALIVE CAPSULES or EXTRACT ❦ Kelp tabs 6 daily.	

COMMON SYMPTOMS: WOMEN: Painful, difficult menstruation, or absence of menstruation; spotting between periods; depression; irritability; edema. MEN: Prostate pain and inflammation; lack of abdominal tone; poor urinary and sexual function.

COMMON CAUSES: Birth control pills or vasectomy; adrenal exhaustion due to stress; severe dieting or body building; surgery or illness; protein or iodine deficiency; Calcium deficiency; B Complex or EFA deficiencies; synthetic steroid use.

CONTROLLING OTHER PROBLEMS ASSOCIATED WITH HORMONE & GLAND IMBALANCE

Erratic or deficient hormone secretions can be caused by, or can lead, to, other specific conditions: HOT FLASHES, NIGHT SWEATS, CONTRACEPTIVE SIDE EFFECTS, SYNTHETIC HORMONE SIDE EFFECTS, FRIGIDITY, and PROSTAGLANDIN DEFICIENCY.

FOR HOT FLASHES and NIGHT SWEATS:
- Crystal Star ESTR-AID CAPSULES, and IODINE THERAPY CAPSULESand/or DONG QUAI/ DAMIANA EXTRACT, or SUPER LICORICE EXTRACT.
- Black Cohosh and Kelp capsules.
- Nature's Plus vitamin E 800IU
- Evening Primrose oil capsules 4 daily.
- B Complex 100Mg. daily with Ascorbate or Ester C 1-3000Mg. daily.

TO OVERCOME SIDE EFFECTS FROM CONTRACEPTIVES and BIRTH CONTROL PILLS:
- Nature's Plus vitamin E 800IU
- Country Life MAXINE CAPSULES 2-3 daily.
- B Complex 100Mg. daily, with extra B_6 250Mg., B_{12} and Folic acid capsules, and Ester C 550Mg. with Bioflavonoids 3-4x daily.
- Emulsified A & D 25,000IU/1,000IU
- Women's Health RELEAF CAPSULES.

TO OVERCOME SIDE EFFECTS FROM SYNTHETIC HORMONES: (These substances can increase the risk of uterine, ovarian and breast cancer).
- Nature's Plus vitamin E 800IU
- B Complex 100Mg. daily
- Ester C 550Mg. with Bioflavonoids, 3-4x daily.
- SolarayCALCIUM CITRATE SUPREME CAPSULES, 4-6 daily.
- Sarsaparilla extract 2-3x daily.

FOR FRIGIDITY, PAINFUL INTERCOURSE, or DRY VAGINA: (see MENOPAUSE PAGE in this book for more information)
- High potency YS or Premier 1 ROYAL JELLY 2t daily, and/or YS Ginseng tea with honey, 1 cup daily.
- Enzymatic Therapy PITUITARY GLANDULAR, and/or NUCLEO-PRO F CAPSULES.
- Natures Plus vitamin E 800IU, or vitamin E with Selenium 400IU 2x daily.
- Evening Primrose oil, 4 daily for essential fatty acids, with extra B_6 250Mg.
- Country Life MAXINE CAPSULES FOR WOMEN, 2-3 daily.
- Crystal Star LOVE CAPS FEMALE, DONG QUAI/ DAMIANA EXTRACT, LOVE BATH FOR WOMEN, and CUPID'S FLAME TEA.
- Avoid junk and processed foods.
- Country Life ADRENAL WITH TYROSINE, or Enzymatic Therapy THYROID WITH TYROSINE CAPSULES, 4 daily.

TO ENCOURAGE AND REBALANCE PROSTAGLANDIN FORMATION: prostaglandin deficiency can lead to breast and uterine fibroids, arthritis, eczema, menstrual difficulties, high blood pressure and cholesterol, and a tendency to gain weight.
- Avoid saturated fats, especially from red meats and pasteurized full fat dairy products.
- Add high Omega 3 oils to the diet from cold water fish and flax seed oil.
- Evening Primrose or Borage oil ,or Black Currant capsules 4-6 daily for 3 months.

Note: Muscle Testing (Applied Kinesiology), is effective and useful in showing which hormonal herbs are specific to an individual problem. Once the simple technique is learned, (see a nutritional consultant, a holistic chiropractor, or a massage therapist), it can easily be done at home to determine which herbs are right for your condition.

HYPERACTIVITY ✧ HYPERKINETIC CHILDREN ✧ AUTISM

FOOD THERAPY	VITAMINS/ MINERALS	HERBAL THERAPY	BODYWORK
☙ Diet improvement has been found to be the key factor in relieving hyperactive behavior. Diet change results are almost immediately evident.	✤ Tryptophane 500Mg. daily to replace Ritalin and activate serutonin production in the brain. (also give high tryptophane foods, such as Turkey, fish, wheat germ, yogurt and eggs).	☙ Evening Primrose oil caps 4 daily to improve body "electrical connections".	✤ Hyperkinesis is the behavioral expression of the allergic reaction. It is usually caused by food allergies or Hypo-glycemia, or both, and can be successfully treated in the same way. When behavior has normalized, maintain the improved diet to prevent reversion.
☙ The diet should be high in vegetable proteins and whole grains, with plenty of fresh fruits and vegetables. Have a salad every day.	✤ Stress B Complex with extra pantothenic acid 100Mg. and B$_6$ 100Mg. with	✤ Ginkgo Biloba extract for inner ear balance problems often present.	
	✤ Vitamin C with bioflav-onoids, 1-3000Mg. daily. Best in powder form, 1/4t. every hour.	☙ Crystal Star RELAX CAPS as needed.	
☙ Omit all refined and junk foods, particularly sugar, milk products, (use soy milk) caffeine foods, sodas, and restaurant fast food.	✤ Hylands CALMS TABLETS.	☙ Planetary CALM CHILD DROPS OR CAPSULES. ☺	✤ Remember that Ritalin, Cylertor, and Atarax are short term sedative drugs that are often proving to make the condition worse over long use. Avoid them if you can. Try diet improvement first.
☙ Avoid red meats and pork (nitrates) canned and frozen foods (too many salts).	✤ Choline/Inositol for brain balance. ♂	☙ Twin Lab GABA PLUS or Country Life RELAXER CAPS as needed. ♀	
☙ Read labels carefully. Avoid all foods with preservatives, (BHT, MSG, BHA,etc.) additives or colors.	✤ Taurine 500Mg. daily. ☺	☙ Effective teas: Catnip Hops/Lobelia Scullcap	✤ Applied Kinesiology is effective in determining allergic substances.
	✤ Avoid aspirin and amphetamines of all kinds.	☙ Crystal Star CALCIUM SOURCE CAPSULES or HIGHLY ABSORBABLE CALCIUM EXTRACT.	✤ Avoid fluorescent lighting and pesticides.
☙ See HYPOGLYCEMIA DIET in this book, or Optimal Eating For Children in "COOKING FOR HEALTHY HEALING" by Linda Rector-Page.	✤ Nature's Life LIQUID CALCIUM / PHOSPHORUS FREE 2 teasp. daily.		✤ See also EPILEPSY DIET PAGE in this book.

COMMON SYMPTOMS: Extreme emotional instability; anger, over-aggressive and destructive behavior; short attention span; can't sit still; slow learning and speech problems; lack of motor coordination; accident prone; chronic liar; doesn't follow directions or listen; impatient and defiant.

COMMON CAUSES: Poor diet of refined and junk foods; mineral deficiencies, and malnutrition; food sensitivities and intolerances to preservatives and additives; hyperthyroidism; Hypoglycemia; heavy metal poisoning causing excess ammonia waste in the brain; drugs that make the condition worse.

185

HYPOGLYCEMIA ✧ LOW BLOOD SUGAR

FOOD THERAPY

❧ Sugar and refined carbohydrates must be avoided. Omit natural sugars such as honey, molasses, maple syrup, and alcohol til sugar balance is achieved. Omit refined foods, caffeine, preserved foods and red meats forever.

❧ Decrease full fat dairy foods, fried and fatty foods, fast foods and pastries, prepared meats, and saturated fats.

❧ Include some vegetable protein at every meal. Add whole grains, fresh fruits and vegetables, low fat dairy products, seafoods, soy foods and brown rice frequently.

❧ Take 2T. Brewer's yeast daily for glucose tolerance.

❧ Eat plenty of cultured foods such as yogurt and kefir for G.I. flora.

VITAMINS/ MINERALS

❖ Chromium therapy: Choose:
  ◆ GTF Chromium 200Mcg.
  ◆ Solaray CHROMIACIN
  ◆ Chromium picolinate and add
  ◆ DMG B₁₅ 125Mg.
  ◆ Niacin 500Mg. 3x daily.

❖ B Complex 100Mg. daily with extra B₆ 100Mg. and panto. acid 500Mg. and Vitamin C 3000Mg. daily. (Take C immediately during an attack).

❖ CO Q 10 30Mg. daily for 3-6 weeks, with Mezotrace minerals

❖ Country Life MOOD FACTORS CAPSULES as needed. ♂

❖ Glutamine 500Mg. daily.

❖ Enzymatic Therapy HYPO-ADE CAPSULES. ♀

HERBAL THERAPY

❧ Crystal Star HYPO-BLUES CAPSULES and TEA. with ADRN-ALIVE CAPS or ADRN EXTRACT.

❧ Crystal Star MIN-ZYME-MINOS for sugar stability.

❧ High potency YS or Premier 1 ROYAL JELLY for adrenal stimulation.

❧ Effective teas:
  Dandelion / Licorice ♂
  Juniper
  Yarrow flowers

❧ Guar Gum morning and evening as a fiber cleanse to absorb unnecessary carbohydrates and balance sugar curve. with
  2t. each:
  Spirulina granules
  Bee Pollen

❧ Sun CHLORELLA daily as a Liver nutrient.

❧ Allta Health CANGEST or HI-LO BALANCE CAPS.

BODYWORK

❖ Hypoglycemia is the biological equivalent of a race car running on empty. It is not so much a disease as a symptom of other disorders. The symptoms can be improved right away by eating something, but this does not address the cause.

❖ Eat small meals frequently throughout the day to keep blood sugar levels up. Large meals throw sugar balance way off.

❖ Eat relaxed, never under stress.

❖ Get some exercise every day to work off unmetabolized acid wastes.

❖ REFLEXOLOGY POINT:

PANCREAS

COMMON SYMPTOMS: Manic/depressive psychological states; irritability, often violence; restlessness, insomnia; anxiety and depression; dizziness, shakes, and trembling; craving for sweets; headaches; lethargy; nausea; blurry vision; great fatigue.

COMMON CAUSES: Abnormal decrease of sugar in the blood, effecting both nerves and muscles; stress and poor diet; exhausted adrenals and liver damage; hypothyroidism; too many refined foods, caffeine and sugar; too much alcohol; too much junk food; too large meals.

DIET FOR HYPOGLYCEMIA CONTROL

The two key factors in low blood sugar are stress and poor diet; both a result of too much sugar and refined carbohydrates. These foods quickly raise glucose levels, causing the pancreas to overcompensate, and produce too much insulin, which lowers glucose levels too far, and too fast. The following diet supplies the body with high fiber, complex carbohydrtaes and proteins - slow even-burning fuel, that prevents sudden sugar elevations and drops. It consists of small frequent meals, with unrefined fresh foods, to keep sugar levels more stable.

ON RISING: Have a hypoglycemia cocktail: mix 1t. of each in a glass of fruit juice to give energy and control morning sugar drop: Glycine powder, powdered milk, sugar-free protein powder, brewer's yeast;
  or a good sugar-free protein powder such as Nature's Plus SPIRUTEIN.

BREAKFAST: A very important meal for hypoglycemia. Have some oatmeal with yogurt and fresh fruit;
  or a poached egg on whole grain toast with a little butter or kefir cheese;
  or whole grain cereal with apple juice or fruit yogurt, or fresh fruit and nuts;
  or a Tofu "egg" scramble with bran muffins and a little butter.

MIDMORNING: Have a green drink (pg. 34) or Sun CHLORELLA or BARLEY GREEN MAGMA with Braggs LIQUID AMINOS;
  and/or a sugar-balancing herb tea, such as Licorice or Dandelion, or Crystal Star HYPO BLUES TEA;
  and some whole grain crackers, cornbread or muffins with kefir or yogurt cheese.

LUNCH: Have a fresh salad with cottage cheese or soy cheese, and nut noodle, or seed topping, and lemon/oil dressing;
  and/or a high protein sandwich on whole grain bread, with avocados, low fat cheese and dressed greens;
  or a bean or lentil soup with a seafood salad;
  or a vegetarian mushroom pizza on a whole grain or chapati crust with low fat or soy cheese;
  or a fresh fruit salad with yogurt, and nut and seeds toppings.

MIDAFTERNOON: Have a hard boiled egg with mayonnaise; or some yogurt with fruit and nuts;
  and a glass of mineral water or cup of herb tea, such as Licorice tea, or Crystal Star LICORICE MINTS.

DINNER: Have some steamed vegetables with tofu or baked fish and brown rice;
  or a vegetable quiche with a whole grain crust, and a small mushroom salad;
  or roast turkey with cornbread stuffing and a light soup;
  or Spanish beans and rice dish, or a paella with seafood and rice;
  or an oriental stir-fry with seafood and vegetables and a clear miso soup with sea vegetables.

BEFORE BED: Have a cup of VEGEX YEAST PASTE BROTH, or apple or papaya juice.

REMEMBER TO: 1) eat potassium-rich foods, such as oranges, broccoli, bananas, and tomatoes.
  2) eat chromium-rich foods, such as brewer's yeast, mushrooms, whole wheat, sea foods, beans and peas.
  3) eat some protein at every meal.

LOW BLOOD SUGAR SELF-TEST

The importance of correct diagnosis and treatment of sugar imbalances is essential. Hypoglycemia symptoms are often mistaken for other problems. The following questionnaire is one we often give for self-determination, reprinted from the Enzymatic Therapy Notebook. It can help you decide, in cooperation with a health care professional, whether you need low blood sugar support, and whether professional help is necessary.

Mark the following symptoms as they pertain to you: (1) for mild symptoms, occurring once or twice a year; (2) for moderate symptoms, occurring several times a year; (3) severe symptoms, occurring almost constantly.

( ) Irritability
( ) Anti-social behavior
( ) Craving for sweets
( ) Blurred vision
( ) Heart palpitations
( ) Rapid pulse
( ) Mental confusion, spaciness
( ) Forgetfulness
( ) Constant phobias, fears
( ) Constant worry and anxiety
( ) Nightmares
( ) Cold sweats and shaking
( ) Frequent headaches
( ) Faintness and dizziness
( ) Nervousness
( ) Convulsions, trembling
( ) Poor concentration
( ) Crying spells
( ) Weak spells
( ) Extreme fatigue, exhaustion
( ) Lots of sighing and yawning
( ) Insomnia; inability to return to slep after awakening
( ) Twitching, involuntary muscle jerks
( ) Digestive problems
( ) Indecisiveness
( ) Unexplained depression
( ) Nervous breakdown
( ) Suicidal intent

A score of 6 or more signifies a need for sugar balancing and nutritional support. A score of 12 -18 indicates a need for therapeutic measures several times daily.

HYPOTHYROIDISM ✧ LOW METABOLISM ✧ PARATHYROID DISEASE

FOOD THERAPY

- Follow a 75% fresh foods diet for a month to rebalance the system for better metabolism.

- Eat Iodine-rich foods: Sea vegetables, sea foods and greens.

- Eat vitamin A-rich foods: yellow vegetables, eggs, carrots, dark green vegetables, raw dairy.

- Take 2T. Brewer's Yeast and 2t. Cod Liver oil every day.

- Avoid refined foods, saturated fats, sugars, white flour and red meats.

- Avoid cabbages, brussels sprouts, etc. They have anti-thyroid substances.

VITAMINS/ MINERALS

- ❖ Emulsified A 25,000IU 3x daily, or Beta carotene 100,000IU daily.
  with
  Vitamin E 400IU daily.

- ❖ Cal/Mag/Potassium caps 2 daily, with Zinc 75Mg. daily. ♂

- ❖ Taurine 500Mg. with Lysine 500Mg. 2x daily.

- ❖ Enzymatic Therapy THYROID/ TYROSINE ♀

- ❖ Ascorbate vitamin C with Bioflavonoids 3000Mg.

- ❖ B Complex 100Mg. with extra B_2 100Mg., B_1 500Mg., and B_6 250Mg.

- ❖ CO Q 10 30Mg. daily.

- ❖ Raw Thyroid
  Raw Pituitary
  Raw Adrenal substance

HERBAL THERAPY

- ❦ Crystal Star IODINE THERAPY CAPSULES or EXTRACT 2x daily.
  or
  THY-METABS 2 daily.

- ❦ N.F. MIODIN DROPS or Heritage ATOMODINE DROPS as needed.

- ❦ Evening Primrose oil caps 3x daily.

- ❦ Effective teas:
  Rhubarb Root
  Sarsaparilla ♂
  Bayberry Bark
  Gotu Kola
  Irish Moss

- ❦ Kelp tabs 10 daily
  with
  Cayenne caps 2 daily.♂

- ❦ Crystal Star MIN-ZYME-MINOS DRINK MIX daily.

BODYWORK

- ❖ Take a half hour brisk walk daily to oxygenate the tissues and stimulate circulation.

- ❖ Sun bathe in the morning. Sea bathe and wade whenever possible.

- ❖ ACUPRESSURE POINT: Press hollow at the base of the throat to stimulate thyroid, 3x for 10 seconds each.

- ❖ REFLEXOLOGY POINT:

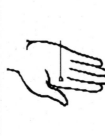

THYROID/ THYMUS

- ❖ Avoid fluorescent lights. They deplete vitamin A in the body.

TO DETERMINE YOUR THYROID CONDITION: Take your basal temperature for 10 minutes on rising in the morning. It should be between 97.8 and 98.2 for health. Below this, and a sluggish thyroid still exists. Temperature will return to normal as treatment begins to work.

COMMON SYMPTOMS: Mental depression and emotional instability; poor memory; lethargy; headaches; deep, slow speech; hoarseness; goiter; coarse hair and loss of hair; swollen hands and feet; constipation; pale and sallow skin; cold hands and feet; coarse, dry skin; swelling of the face, tongue and eyelids; excessive and painful menstruation; nervousness and heart palpitations; great fatigue; weight gain.

COMMON CAUSES: Iodine deficiency; Pituitary and Thyroid malfunction; Vitamin A, E and Zinc deficiency; air pollution; overuse of diet pills.

IMMUNITY

BUILDING IT ◆ STRENGTHENING IT

Remember that the inherited immunity and health of you, your children and your grandchildren is laid down by you. A strong immune system is absolutely necessary for prevention of modern opportunistic diseases such as Cancer, AIDS, Herpes, Lupus, Candida Albicans, and Chronic Fatigue Syndrome (EBV).

FOOD THERAPY	VITAMINS/ MINERALS	HERBAL THERAPY	BODYWORK
☙ The American diet of processed foods, 20% sugars, and 37% fat, suppresses immunity. Saturated fats, such as those in pastries, fried foods, and red meats are particular culprits. Refined food calories offer very little nutrition.	✣ CO Q 10 10Mg. daily for 3-6 weeks. **with** ◆ B Complex 100Mg. ◆ Ener B INTERNASAL GEL ◆ Mezotrace MINERAL COMPLEX. **or** ✣ Germanium 50Mg. 2x daily. **with**	☙ Crystal Star HERBAL DEFENSE TEAM CAPSULES, EXTRACT or TEA. ☙ Crystal Star FEEL GREAT TEA AND CAPS for rebuilding strength and a feeling of well-being. ♀ ☙ Zand HERBAL INSURE EXTRACT and CAPSULES.	✣ Tobacco/nicotine is a key immune depressant. The cadmium content causes Zinc deficiency. It takes 3 months to get good immune response even after you quit. ✣ Get some regular aerobic exercise every day to keep system oxygen high. Disease does not readily attack in a high oxygen, high potassium, environment.
☙ Take a sugar-free high protein drink every morning, such as Nature's Plus SPIRUTEIN.	✣ Glutathione 50Mg. **and** CO Q 10 30Mg. daily. ♂ ✣ Vitamin E 400IU with Selenium 2x daily. ♂	☙ Crystal Star SUPER LICORICE EXTRACT. ☙ Sun CHLORELLA daily.	✣ Environmental pollutants lower immunity, particularly pesticides. Eat organically grown foods whenever possible.
☙ Eat a generally cleansing/building diet, such as a MODIFIED MACROBIOTIC DIET (Pg. 42). Include lots of fresh foods, whole grains, sea foods, eggs and cultured dairy foods, such as yogurt and kefir for friendly G.I. flora.	✣ Raw Thymus extract. ✣ Vitamin C or Ester C with bioflavonoids 3000Mg. with Zinc 50Mg. daily.	☙ Effective extracts: Siberian Ginseng Propolis Echinacea Pau de Arco Ginkgo Biloba	✣ Eliminate recreational drugs. Reduce prescription drugs, especially anti-biotics and corti-coids that depress immunity.
☙ Particularly avoid junk and processed foods.	✣ Natren LIFE START #2, 1/2 t. 2x daily. ✣ Pycnogenol 2-4 daily.	☙ Effective Capsules: Echinacea/Myrrh Biotec CELL GUARD ♂ Astragalus	

COMMON SYMPTOMS: Chronic or continuing infections, colds, respiratory problems; Candida yeast overgrowth; chronic fatigue; chronic allergies.

COMMON CAUSES: Glandular malfunction, usually because of poor diet and nutrition; staph infection; prolonged use of anti-biotics and/or cortico-steroid drugs. (Long use of these drugs can depress the Immune system to the point where even minor illness can become life-threatening); some immunization shots; Candida yeast overgrowth; emotional stress; food and other allergies; environmental and heavy metal pollutants; radiation.

IMMUNE SYSTEM MAINTENANCE CHECKPOINTS

The immune defense system is the most complex in the human body. Only recently are we beginning to understand its nature and comprehensive dynamics. Primarily involving the thymus gland, lymph glands, and bone marrow, it is a wonderful autonomic, subconscious defense system that can hold off and neutralize infection so the body can heal itself. It is this quality of being a part of us, yet not under our conscious control, that manifests its greatest power. And its greatest problem. When immunity is continually involved in fighting a "rear guard" action against a constant immune-depressing overload of anti-biotics, cortisones, and antacids, etc. that destroy vital enzymes, and foods full of pesticides, chemical foods and preservatives, it gets to a point where it cannot distinguish harmful cells from healthy cells, and attacks everything (as in cases of AIDS today). In many instances, the immune system functions at its best when we just "get out of the way" by keeping the body well-nourished and clear of toxic wastes. Immune energy is then directed toward rebuilding and maintaining strength against outside invasions of harmful bacteria, viruses or pollutants,

The immune system is the body system most sensitive to nutritional deficiencies. Most disease is caused by lack of sufficient minerals, and oxygen in the vital fluids, which allows a pathogenic environment to take hold. Providing optimum nutrition at the first sign of infection or loss of health vastly improves the defense shield.
The following checkpoints can help maintain strong immunity in today's world on a continuing basis.

1) **Take some high potency, concentrated, green, "superfoods" several times a week, such as Sun CHLORELLA, Barley Green Magma, wheat grass, spirulina, alfalfa or Solaray ALFAJUICE, liquid chlorophyll, or Crystal Star ENERGY GREEN DRINK. Remember that the composition of chlorophyll is very similar to that of human haemoglobin, so these foods provide a "mini-transfusion" for your bloodstream.**

2) Include sea vegetables, such as kelp, hijiki, dulse, kombu, wakame, and sea palm, in your daily diet for their therapeutic iodine, high potassium, and sodium alginate content (See page 43); or take Crystal Star POTASSIUM SOURCE, MIN-ZYME-MINOS DRINK, or IODINE THERAPY COMPLEXES.

3) **Take a high potency lactobacillus or acidolphilus complex, such as Natren LIFE START 2, or Solaray MULTI-DOLPHILUS for friendly G.I. flora, and good food assimilation.**

4) Include one or more anti-oxidant supplements, such as vitamin E with selenium, beta carotene, zinc, CO Q 10, germanium and vitamin C. The highest potency anti-oxidants are in enzyme form from Biotec; EXTRA ENERGY ENZYMES S.O.D WITH CATALASE 1 million units, and AGELESS BEAUTY GLUTATHIONE PEROXIDASE 1.3 million units.

5) **Several herbs also have strong anti-oxidant qualities: echinacea, chaparral, golden seal, Siberian ginseng, rosemary, astragalus, suma, burdock, and pau de arco.**

6) Take anti-oxidants to protect the Thymus gland from shrinking with age, and to nourish the immune organs: vitamin E with Selenium, Beta Carotene, Raw Thymus Glandular.

7) **Regular aerobic exercise keeps system oxygen high, and circulation flowing. Remember that disease does not readily overrun a body where oxygen and organic minerals are high in the vital fluids.**

8) The immune system is stimulated by a few minutes of early morning sunlight every day. Avoid excessive sun. Sun burn depresses immunity.

See "COOKING FOR HEALTHY HEALING" by Linda Rector-Page for a complete diet to build and maintain strong immunity.

Laughter lifts more than your spirits. It also seems to boost the immune system. Laughter decreases cortisol, an immune suppressor, allowing immune boosters to function better.

♂ MALE IMPOTENCE ◇ SEXUAL PROBLEMS ◇ STERILITY ♂

FOOD THERAPY

❧ The problem can often be corrected simply by improving the diet. Junk, chemical, and processed foods are a key factor today in male impotency.

❧ Eat a high vegetable protein diet. Include a green leafy salad every day. Add plenty of potassium and selenium-rich foods.

❧ Have a POTENT-C DRINK every morning for several months:
For 4 drinks, mix in the blender:
1 cup sliced strawberries
1 sliced banana
1 cup papaya chunks
1 cup pineapple/coconut juice
1 cup Amazake rice drink
2T. honey or Barley malt
2T. toasted wheat germ
2T. Pumpkin seeds
2T. Lecithin
2T. Brewer's Yeast
1 egg
1T. sesame seeds
1 1/2t. vanilla

❧ Avoid red meats; keep dietary salt and sugar low.

VITAMINS/ MINERALS

❖ Zinc 50Mg. 2x daily.

❖ Enzymatic Therapy NUCLEO-PRO M or STEROEPLEX MF.

❖ Effective raw glandulars: Orchic w/ Arginine Pituitary Male
with
vitamin E 400IU 2x daily and Carnitine 500Mg.

❖ Smilax extract 10x strength, for increased testosterone production.

❖ Niacin (not niacinimide), up to 3000Mg. daily.

❖ B₁₅ DMG sublingual daily.

❖ Alta Health MAGNESIUM CHLORIDE 6 daily for 1 week, then 3 daily for 3 weeks.

❖ Vitamin C 3000Mg. daily if there is sperm agglutination.

❖ Country Life MAX CAPS. and ENERGIX VIALS.

HERBAL THERAPY

❧ Yohimbe capsules with Tyrosine 500Mg. daily.

❧ Crystal Star LOVE MALE CAPSULES, LOVING MOOD EXTRACT and CUPID'S FLAME TEA.

❧ Crystal Star MASTER BUILDER CAPSULES and MIN-ZYME-MINOS DRINK.

❧ Effective Ginseng formulas:
◆ Ginseng/Royal Jelly ampules
◆ Siberian Ginseng extract
◆ Chinese Red Ginseng caps
◆ Ginseng/Sarsaparilla caps
◆ Ginseng/Damiana caps
◆ Ginseng/Cayenne capsules
Remember that Ginseng is a re-generative herb. It does not make the normal body 'supernormal'.

❧ Licorice/Damiana caps to increase sperm count. Take with pineapple juice for 6 days in a row, then rest for 6 days, then resume, and etc.

❧ Highest potency ROYAL JELLY 2 teasp. daily.

❧ BioForce GINSAVENA EXTRACT as needed.

BODYWORK

❖ Take alternating hot and cool showers to increase circulation.

❖ Crystal Star LOVE BATH FOR MEN.

❖ Squeeze the testicles every day to stimulate, once for every year of your life.

❖ Breathe deeply. Get regular exercise daily. Get some early morning sunlight on the body every day possible.

❖ Hypno-therapy has been effective with this problem.

❖ REFLEXOLOGY POINT:

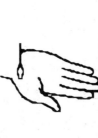

PENIS, PROSTATE, COCCYX

COMMON SYMPTOMS: Inability to have or maintain an erection during intercourse; inability to have a child.

COMMON CAUSES: Poor diet and nutrition, a problem of the dinner table, not the bedroom; psychological or emotional stress; depression; hypoglycemia; marijuana and/or other pleasure drug use; environmental or heavy metal poisoning; diabetes; gland imbalance; protein deficiency.

♂ INFERTILITY ♀

FOOD THERAPY

♋ Diet is usually an all-important key. The body does not readily allow conception without adequate nutrition. Consciously follow a healthy diet and lifestyle for at least six months before trying to conceive.

♋ Avoid tobacco, alcohol, caffeine, red meats, and refined foods.

♋ Reduce dairy products and fatty foods.

♋ Eat plenty of whole grains, cultured foods such as yogurt, sea foods and sea vegetables, fresh fruits and vegetables.

♋ See page 39 for a daily morning drink. Make sure you get 2T. each:
Brewer's yeast
Lecithin granules
Wheat germ

♋ See "COOKING FOR HEALTHY HEALING" by Linda Rector-Page for a complete diet for this condition.

VITAMINS/ MINERALS

FEMALE: ♀

❖ Enzymatic Therapy
◆ NUCLEO-PRO F
◆ STEREOPLEX MF
◆ RAW OVARIAN EXTRACT
◆ RAW FEMALE GLANDULAR

❖ Vitamin E 400IU 2x daily.

❖ A & D 25,000IU daily.

❖ B Complex 100Mg. with extra B$_6$ 100Mg. and Folic acid 800Mcg.

MALE: ♂

❖ Enzymatic Therapy
◆ NUCLEOPRO M CAPS
◆ STEROEPLEX MF

❖ Carnitine 500Mg. with Chromium picolinate for increased sperm count.

❖ Vitamin E 800Mg. with selenium 200Mcg. daily.

❖ Country Life ENERGIX VIALS and Niacin 500Mg.

❖ Zinc 75Mg. daily with vitamin C 3000Mg. daily.

HERBAL THERAPY

FEMALE: ♀

☙ Crystal Star
◆ FEMALE HARMONY CAPS
◆ WOMANS BEST FRIEND with Evening Primrose oil and

☙ High potency Premier One or YS ROYAL JELLY 2t. daily.

☙ Scullcap tea
Echinacea extract

MALE: ♂

☙ Crystal Star
◆ ADRN EXTRACT daily
◆ POTASSIUM SOURCE with highest potency YS ROYAL JELLY 2t. daily

☙ Smilax extract 2-3x daily.

☙ Effective capsules:
Damiana/Licorice
Ginseng/Damiana
Kelp tabs
Propolis tabs 2 daily.

BODYWORK

❖ Alternate hot and cold sitz baths to stimulate circulation in the reproductive area.

❖ Sun bathe in the early morning.

❖ Consciously relax your life more during this time. Get some regular mild exercise every day.

❖ Avoid areas with smog and pollutants as much as possible.

❖ REFLEXOLOGY POINTS:

UTERUS
PENIS, COCCYX, PROSTATE

❖ For vaginal pH balance right before intercourse: use baking soda/honey for over-acid, vinegar for over-alkaline.

COMMON SYMPTOMS: Inability to have a child, a condition of both man and woman.

COMMON CAUSES: FEMALE: Nutrient deficiency and hypoglycemia from too many refined foods.; emotional stress; obstruction in the fallopian tubes; pelvic infection; toxicity from drugs or environmental pollutants; birth control pill causing hormone imbalance.; chlamydia; vaginal pH imbalance.
MALE: Low sperm production; prolonged marijuana or other drug use; radiation or heavy metal poisoning; steroid use; poor nutrition and lack of protein; hypoglycemia; physical obstruction in the genital/urethral area; glandular malfunction; chlamydia.

INSECT BITES & STINGS

BEES ✦ WASPS ✦ MOSQUITOS ✦ NON-POISONOUS SPIDERS

FOOD THERAPY	VITAMINS/ MINERALS	HERBAL THERAPY	BODYWORK
❧ Food applications to take down swelling: ◆ raw onion slice ◆ raw potato slice ◆ lemon juice and vinegar ◆ wet mud pack ◆ tobacco and water paste ◆ toothpaste ◆ cologne or toilet water ◆ rubbing alcohol ◆ honey ◆ baking soda ◆ sea salt ◆ ice packs ◆ charcoal or burnt toast ◆ wheat germ oil	❖ Vitamin C therapy: Use <u>calcium ascorbate powder</u>. Take 1/4t. every 15 minutes right after the bite, then 1/4t. every few hours til pain and swelling are over. ◆ Mix some powder to a paste with water and apply directly.	❧ B&T SSSTING STOP GEL ☺	❖ Traditional preventives: ◆ Sprinkle garlic powder around the house. ◆ Sprinkle sassafras tea or dried tomato leaves around the house. ◆ Sprinkle Eucalyptus leaves around the house.
		❧ Take Comfrey extract. Apply a comfrey poultice.	
		❧ Apply Aloe Vera gel.	❖ To lessen the effect of the bite, keep quiet, and keep the affected area below the level of the heart.
	❖ Pantothenic acid as an anti-histimine for swelling.	❧ Effective compresses: Hot Parsley leaf Blue Cohosh Black Cohosh Chamomile Blessed Thistle	
❧ Avoid meats and sweets for faster healing.	❖ Quercetin Plus with Bromelain. Take every 4 hours to take down inflammation.	❧ Crystal Star ANTI-HST as needed to take down any rash or swelling.	❖ Apply cold or ice pack compresses, and see SHOCK SUGGESTIONS in this book if reaction is severe.
	❖ Take and apply chlorophyll liquid.	❧ Take a few drops of Cayenne extract in warm water every 1/2 hour to stimulate the circulatory defense mechanism.	
	❖ Dissolve PABA tablets in water and apply.	❧ Apply Witch Hazel.	
	❖ Take vitamin B₁ for a month during high risk seasons for prevention. 100Mg. for children, ☺ 500Mg. for adults.	❧ Mix and apply to exposed areas for prevention: Citronella, Pennyroyal, Eucalyptus, with safflower or sesame oil.	

INSOMNIA

FOOD THERAPY	VITAMINS/ MINERALS	HERBAL THERAPY	BODYWORK
❧ Good late night snacks about an hour before bedtime: bananas, celery and celery juice, wheat germ and wheat germ oil, brown rice, a little warm milk, lemon water and honey, brewer's yeast, VEGEX YEAST PASTE BROTH, 1 T. Bragg's LIQUID AMINOS in water.	At the time of this writing, L-Tryptophane has been recalled by the FDA, and is not available until a safe source is found. It is recommended here as an effective sleep aid with every expectation of its safe return to the public.	❧ Crystal Star RELAX AND NIGHT CAPSULES, and GOOD NIGHT TEA. ❧ Passion Flower capsules or extract, especially for weaning away from sleeping pills.	❖ Avoid commercial sleeping pills. They interfere with ability to dream, and interrupt natural sleeping patterns. They interact detrimentally with alcohol and tranquilizers. because the nervous system never really relaxes They lose their sleep promoting effectiveness in 3-7 days of use.
❧ Have a glass of wine at dinner for minerals, digestion and relaxation.	❖ Country Life RELAXER CAPSULES as needed. ❖ Alta Health MAGNESIUM CHLORIDE daily.♂	❧ Solaray EUROCALM CAPS. ❧ Make a Hops and Rosemary sleep pillow. Sprinkle with a little alcohol to enhance aromatherapy. ♀	❖ Effective sleep enhancers: Biofeedback Yoga exercises Hypno-therapy Chiropractic care
❧ Have a glass of bottled mineral water at bedtime.♂	❖ One each for sleep when there is pain: Tryptophane 500Mg. DLPA 500Mg. Calcium/Magnesium ♀	❧ Effective teas: ♀ ♦ Licorice Rt. ♀ ♦ Chamomile ♦ Catnip/Lemon Balm ♦ Hops	❖ Exercise in the morning outdoors if possible to release prostaglandins and promote sleep 12 hours later, and keep circadian rhythm regular And take a "constitutional walk" before bed.
❧ Avoid salty and sugary foods before bed.	❖ Tryptophane 500-1000Mg. with Niacin 100Mg. at bed.	❧ Effective extracts: ♦ Crystal Star HIGHLY ABSORBABLE CALCIUM ♦ Crystal Star SLEEP EASE ♦ Scullcap ♦ Wild Lettuce/Valerian	❖ Before bed: take 10 deep breaths; wait 5 minutes; take 10 more. Very effective.
❧ Eat only a light meal at night.	❖ B Complex 100Mg. with GABA or Glycine or Lexon B BLEND POWDER.	❧ For quality sleep and dream recall: Crystal Star INCREDIBLE DREAMS TEA before bed.	❖ Gaze at a lighted candle for 3 minutes before retiring as meditation.
	❧ For nightmares: B₁ 500Mg. Niacinimide 500Mg. ❖ Rainbow Light CALCIUM PLUS, 2 before bed.		

COMMON SYMPTOMS: Inability to sleep; prematurely ended or interrupted sleep; difficulty falling asleep.

COMMON CAUSES: Stress , tension, depression and anxiety; the inability to "turn your mind off"; pain; too much caffeine; overeating; too much salt and sugar; B Complex deficiency; nicotine; toxic liver overload; too high copper levels.

FOOD THERAPY

❧ Interstitial cystitis has been called the "migraine of the bladder". Many of the same foods trigger as well as benefit the problem.

❧ Cranberry juice is not beneficial for this problem.

Avoid these other trigger foods: aged proteins such as yogurt, pickled herring, cheeses, sauerkraut, citrus fruits, citrus juices and red wine until condition normalizies.

❧ Green drinks (Pg.. 34) and carrot juice during acute stages, and as a preventive.

❧ Take 2T. daily as a preventive:
Lecithin
Brewer's Yeast

❧ Increase leafy greens and fiber foods in the diet.

VITAMINS/ MINERALS

✢ Vitamin C therapy: ascorbate or Ester C powder 1/4t. every hour during acute stages to help restore normal immunity.
and

✢ Lysine 1000Mg. with Bromelain 500Mg. 6x daily.

✢ Enzymatic Therapy ACID-A-CAL CAPSULES 4-6 daily.

✢ Nature's Plus vitamin E 800IU daily.

✢ CO Q 10 10Mg. daily. with Emulsified A 25,000IU

✢ Sun CHLORELLA 15-20 tabs daily.

HERBAL THERAPY

❧ Crystal Star BLDR-K EXTRACT and/or BLADDER FLUSH TEA. and then HERBAL DEFENSE CAPS to help restore immune defense.

❧ Omega 3 Flax oil capsules 3 x daily.

❧ Effective teas:
Cornsilk
Dandelion
Uva Ursi
Astragalus
Chaparral
Watermelon seed

❧ Ginkgo Biloba extract

❧ Bilberry extract as an anti-inflammatory.

❧ Solaray ALFAJUICE as a potent anti-oxidant and green source.

BODYWORK

✢ This condition is another of today's immune system breakdown diseases, and the body will be at risk until immunity is strengthened. Attend to these symptoms immediately, not only because of the great pain, but because the infective viruses can rapidly spread in an immune deficient environment.

✢ Anti-biotics do not help and may aggravate this problem, and can actually attack the bladder lining when there is no infection.

✢ REFLEXOLOGY POINT:

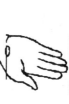

BLADDER

COMMON SYMPTOMS: Scarred , tough, atrophied bladder so that normal urination is impossible; pain goes away during urination, then immediately returns; breakdown of bladder tissue, even when infection is not present; cloudy urine with foul odor; lowered immunity; dietary "triggers" causing acidity in the system; dehydration.

COMMON CAUSES: Viral infection; environmental and food allergies; lowered immunity; dietary "triggers" causing acidity in the system; dehydration.

FOOD THERAPY

☙ Drink Lemon water in the morning to neutralize acids if the condition is chronic.

☙ Keep the Liver clean and functioning well with a carrot juice or green drink frequently.(Pg. 34).

☙ Eat cultured foods frequently for healthy G.I. flora.

☙ Effective food applications:
Wheat germ oil
Baking soda solution
Apple cider vinegar

☙ Avoid refined foods, sugar and fried foods.

VITAMINS/ MINERALS

❖ Lysine 500Mg. 3-4x daily. with
Tryptophane 500Mg. to calm the itch.

❖ Vitamin C therapy: use Ester C or Ascorbate C powder and mix with water to a solution. Apply to area, and take 1t. every hour.

❖ Vitamin E 400IU daily. Prick a capsule and apply locally.♂
and
Emulsified A&D 25M.

❖ Enzymatic Therapy HEPAZYME CAPSULES.

❖ Quercetin Plus with Bromelain as an anti-inflammatory agent.

❖ Homeopathic NAT. PHOS.

HERBAL THERAPY

❧ Crystal Star ANTI-HST CAPSULES, 4-6 daily as needed for liver stimulation to relieve a typical histamine weal rash. Very effective.
and
THERADERM TEA. Drink and pat onto affected areas with cotton.

❧ Apply Aloe Vera gel.

❧ Apply Tea Tree oil if fungus is the cause.

❧ Effective teas, for internal and topical use:
◆ Crystal Star CLEANSING & FASTING TEA to neutralize acids.
◆ Comfrey
◆ Chamomile
◆ Chickweed
◆ Red Clover/Hops

❧ Crystal Star P.O. #2 CAPSULES 2-4 daily as needed to calm the itch.

BODYWORK

❖ Apply Black Walnut tincture, and take drops internally several times daily.

❖ Avoid using detergents on the skin. Use mild castile soap.

❖ Apply fresh Comfrey Leaf compresses.

❖ Apply B & T CALIFLORA GEL, or Crystal Star CALENDULA GEL.

❖ See LIVER MALFUNCTION and ECZEMA pages in this book for more information.

COMMON SYMPTOMS: Tingling, unpleasant skin prickling; redness, rash; scaling and bumps on the skin.

COMMON CAUSES: Liver malfunction or exhaustion; allergic reaction; stress and anxiety; detergents; over-acid system; drug after-and side-effects; poor diet with too many refined and chemical foods.

197

KIDNEY MALFUNCTION ✧ NEPHRITIS ✧ BRIGHT'S DISEASE

FOOD THERAPY	VITAMINS/ MINERALS	HERBAL THERAPY	BODYWORK
❧ Go on a short 3 day kidney cleanse to clear out toxic infection: <u>each morning have 2T.</u> cider vinegar or lemon juice in water; take 1 each of the following juices daily: *carrot/beet/ cucumber, cranberry, potassium broth* (Pg. 33), *a green drink* (Pg. 34).	❖ B Complex 100Mg. daily <u>with extra B₆ 100Mg. 3x</u> daily and Magnesium 400Mg. 2x daily.	❧ Garlic/Cayenne capsules 6-8 daily.	❖ Apply WHITE FLOWER OIL or TIGER BALM to kidney area 2-3x daily.
❧ Then eat a very simple low salt vegetarian diet with 75% <u>fresh</u> foods for the next 2 weeks.	❖ Beta carotene 100,000IU and Vit. D 1000IU daily.	❧ Crystal Star ANTI-BIO CAPSULES 4 daily til infection clears; then BLDR-K CAPSULES AND TEA for a month.	❖ No smoking. Take a daily brisk walk to keep kidney function flowing.
❧ <u>Then,</u> add sea foods and sea vegetables, whole grains and vegetable proteins on a regular basis. Drink 6-8 glasses of bottled water daily.	❖ Ascorbate Vit. C powder 3-5000Mg. with bioflavs and rutin 1000Mg. daily.	❧ Crystal Star HERBAL ENZYMES CAPSULES before each meal <u>and</u> HAWTHORNE <u>OR</u> BIL-BERRY EXTRACT 2x daily.	❖ Apply <u>moist</u> heat packs on the kidney area, and/or alternating hot and cold packs.
	❖ Choline or Phosphatidyl Choline 4x daily.	❧ Evening Primrose oil caps 4 daily with Echinacea extract under the tongue several times daily.	❖ Comfrey compresses on the kidney area.
	❖ Natren LIFE START #2 1/2t. 3-4x daily.	❧ Solaray ALFAJUICE daily.	❖ REFLEXOLOGY POINTS:
❧ Avoid heavy starches, red and prepared meats, refined, salty, fatty and fast foods. They all inhibit kidney filtering.	❖ Twin Lab LIQUID K OR WHITE BIRCH MINERAL WATER for potassium. ♂	❧ Effective teas: Parsley / Cornsilk ♀ Watercress Dandelion Root & Leaf Gravel Root Burdock/Chaparral	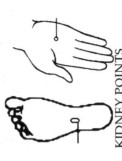 KIDNEY POINTS
	❖ Enzymatic Therapy LIQUID LIVER WITH GINSENG, 2x daily. ♂		
❧ See KIDNEY STONE DIET on the next page for more information.	❖ Activated Charcoal or liquid chlorophyll tabs with meals. ♂	❧ St. John's Wort tea if incontinent.	❖ Capsicum enemas 2-3x weekly as needed to stimulate better kidney function.
	❖ Zinc 50Mg. 2x daily. ♂		

COMMON SYMPTOMS: Painful urination, irritation and frequency; chronic lower back pain and fatigue; chills and fever as with a cold or flu; general accumulation of excess fluid.

COMMON CAUSES: Too much sugar and red meat and oxalic acid-forming foods in the diet; diabetes; EFA deficiency; adrenal exhaustion; kidney stones; overuse of prescription or pleasure drugs.

KIDNEY STONES

FOOD THERAPY

❧ Go on a 3 day intensive kidney cleansing diet til all pain clears:
◆ On rising: take 2T. Lemon juice or cider vinegar in water.
◆ Breakfast: take a glass of apple or watermelon juice.
◆ Mid-morning: take a carrot/beet/cucumber juice.
◆ Lunch: take potassium broth (Pg. 33)
◆ Midafternoon: take a green drink (Pg. 34).
◆ Dinner: take 2 cups watermelon seed tea.
◆ Before bed: take a glass of aloe vera juice.

❧ Take 2T. olive oil every 4 hours during this stage, as a kidney stone flush.

❧ Then follow the KIDNEY CLEANSING DIET on the next page for 2 more weeks to normalize kidney activity.

❧ Avoid all refined, fried and fatty foods during healing. Avoid all sugars and oxalic acid forming foods, such as red meats and caffeine.

VITAMINS/ MINERALS

✣ Ascorbate or Ester C powder in water; 1/4t. every hour to bowel tolerance daily til stones pass. (About 5-7000Mg.).

✣ Beta Carotene 100,000IU with Omega 3 Flax oil daily.

✣ Enzymatic Therapy ACID-A-CAL CAPS 2-4 daily. ♂
and/or
Solaray CALCIUM CITRATE CAPS 4 daily. ♀

✣ Vit. B Complex with extra B₆ 100Mg. and Magnesium 400Mg. 2x daily, and Vit. K 100Mg.

✣ Vital Health FORMULA 1 ORAL CHELATION/EDTA.

✣ Vit. E 400IU with Lecithin or Choline caps daily. ♂

✣ Twin Lab LIQUID K or Vital Health WHITE BIRCH MINERAL WATER if taking diuretics.

HERBAL THERAPY

❧ Crystal Star BLDR-K CAPS AND TEA as needed for both healing and preventive activity.

❧ Drink a quart daily of any of the following teas til stones dissolve:
Chamomile
Rosemary ♀
Rose Hips

❧ Other effective teas:
Watercress
Cleavors
Couchgrass ♀
Uva Ursi/Juniper ♂

❧ Apply a hot Ginger/ Oatstraw compress to kidney area.

❧ Crystal Star POTASSIUM SOURCE CAPSULES daily if taking diuretics.

❧ Aloe Vera juice or Sun Chlorella, 2 glasses daily.
or
Solaray ALFAJUICE CAPS.

BODYWORK

✣ It takes from 5-15 hours of vigorous and urgent healing attention to dissolve and pass small stones. Prevention through improved diet and exercise is the best medicine.

✣ Effective compresses:
◆ Cayenne/Ginger
◆ Mullein/Lobelia

✣ Take hot and cold, or Epsom salts sitz baths.

✣ Take a warm catnip enema daily til pain subsides.

✣ REFLEXOLOGY POINTS:

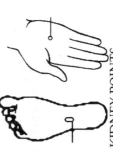

KIDNEY POINTS
In addition, press on the back, on the tops of both hip bones, 3x for 10 seconds each.

COMMON SYMPTOMS: Dull pain in the lower back and groin, increasing to sharp severe pain as the stone(s) enters the urethral canal; frequent and painful urination; nausea and vomiting.

COMMON CAUSES: B vitamin and magnesium deficiency; excess uric and oxalic acids in the elimination system from foods such as red meat, carbonated drinks, sugars and caffeine; excess aspirin, salt and chemical diuretics; potassium deficiency from too many diuretics.

KIDNEY CLEANSING & REBUILDING DIET

THIS DIET IS TO BE FOLLOWED AFTER THE 3 DAY LIQUID CLEANSE ON THE PRECEDING PAGE. INTENSE PAIN SHOULD HAVE CEASED. THE DIET IS RECOMMENDED FOR AT LEAST TWO TO THREE WEEKS AFTER ACUTE STAGES HAS PASSED, TO CONTINUE CLEANSING ACTIVITY AND TO NORMALIZE AND BALANCE KIDNEY FUNCTION.

ON RISING: take 2T. cranberry concentrate, cider vinegar, or lemon juice in water with 1/4-1/2t. ascorbate vitamin C powder and 1t. honey added.

BREAKFAST: have a glass of papaya, apple or watermelon juice, and/or fresh tropical (non-citrus) fruits, such as bananas, papayas or mangos.

MIDMORNING: have a green drink (Pg.34) or Crystal Star ENERGY GREEN DRINK, or Sun CHLORELLA;
or a kidney cleansing tea, such as dandelion, parsley, watermelon seed, or Crystal Star BLDR-K TEA.

LUNCH: have a fresh vegetable salad with plenty of leafy greens, and a lemon/oil or yogurt dressing;
or a Chinese vegetable salad with bok choy, daikon radish, pea pods, bean sprouts, and sea vegetables, and a cup of Miso or ramen noodle soup;
or baked/marinated Tofu and steamed vegies with sesame seeds and toasted wheat germ topping.

MIDAFTERNOON: have some yogurt with fresh fruit, <u>and</u> a cup of alkalizing, sediment-dissolving tea, such as chamomile, oatstraw, watermelon seed, or Crystal Star BLDR-K tea;
or some fresh carrots, celery, or apples and pears with yogurt or kefir cheese.

DINNER: have some steamed vegetables with brown rice or a baked potato, and tofu;
or broiled salmon or other fish with baked onions and peas;
or an asparagus quiche with a light clear soup.

BEFORE BED: take a kidney healing juice, such as cranberry, cranapple, aloe vera, or apple juice.

Drink at least 6 glasses of bottled water every day if you are prone to kidney problems, so that waste is continuously flushed through and out of the body.

Keep the diet low in salt and protein for at least 3 weeks. The ongoing diet should be low in cholesterol and saturated fats forever.

See "COOKING FOR HEALTHY HEALING" by Linda Rector-Page for a complete diet for kidney health.

LARYNGITIS ✧ HOARSENESS

FOOD THERAPY

🍃 Take 1t. cider vinegar and 1t. honey in a small glass of water every hour til relief.

🍃 Effective juices:
Papaya
Apple
Carrot

🍃 Effective gargles:
Lemon juice and water
Liquid chlorophyll in water or a green drink (Pg. 34).

🍃 Garlic syrup. Soak a chopped garlic bulb in 1 pt. honey and water overnight and take a teaspoonful every hour.

VITAMINS/ MINERALS

❖ Alacer EMERGEN-C. Mix in water and hold in the mouth as long as possible. ♂

❖ Zinc Gluconate lozenges. Hold in the mouth until dissolved.

❖ N.F. Factors HERBAL-SEPTIC as needed.

❖ Enzymatic Therapy ORAL-ZYME LOZENGES

❖ Vit. E 400IU daily as a preventive.

❖ Chewable Rose Hips vitamin C wafers. Take as many as needed. Hold in the mouth until dissolved.

❖ Propolis lozenges or chips as needed. Hold in the mouth as long as possible. ♂

HERBAL THERAPY

🍃 Crystal Star COFEX TEA as needed.
with
ANTI-BIO CAPS OR EXTRACT if there is infection.
or
CRISIS CAPS if the first stages of a cold or flu are evident.

🍃 Crystal Star SUPER LICORICE EXTRACT. Hold under the tongue as long as possible.

🍃 Tea Tree oil. 3 drops in water as a gargle.

🍃 CamoCare THROAT SPRAY & GARGLE as needed. ♀

🍃 Effective teas:
◆ Slippery Elm
◆ Thyme tea and gargle
◆ Crystal Star LICORICE MINTS TEA
◆ Mullein
◆ Sage tea

🍃 Aloe Vera juice.

BODYWORK

❖ Apply Ginger/Cayenne compresses to the throat.

❖ Soak in a hot mineral or Epsom salts bath.

❖ Stop smoking and avoid secondary smoke.

❖ REFLEXOLOGY POINT:

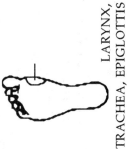

LARYNX, TRACHEA, EPIGLOTTIS

COMMON SYMPTOMS: Sore throat; inability to speak above a whisper because of swollen throat tissues.

COMMON CAUSES: Strep throat; beginnings of a cold or flu; consequence of smoking; lack of sleep; acidic diet; stress.

LEUKEMIA ✧ BONE MARROW CANCER

FOOD THERAPY	VITAMINS/ MINERALS	HERBAL THERAPY	BODYWORK
☙ Start with a macrobiotic diet program (Pg.42) for 3-4 months with no animal protein and lots of alkalizing foods. ◆ Food healing value is lost very quickly in this disease. Make sure the diet is very nutritious to make up for this.	✧ Germanium 150Mg. daily. ✧ Enzymatic Therapy LIVA-TOX and LIQUID LIVER WITH GINSENG 4 daily.	☙ Crystal Star ANEMIGIZE CAPS to rebuild marrow. with DETOX CAPSULES and ANTI-BIO CAPS OR EXTRACT, 4x daily if needed.	✤ OVERHEATING THERAPY is effective. See Airola HOW TO GET WELL. ✤ Avoid pesticides, X-rays, and radiation of all kinds if possible.
☙ High vegetable proteins are the key once initial detoxification is completed.	✤ B Complex 100Mg. with extra Iron, Folic acid, and B6 250Mg. ♀ ✤ Glutathione 50Mg. 2x daily. ♂ with Vitamin E 800IU with selenium and Zinc 50Mg.	☙ Effective red blood cell builders: ◆ Wakasa liquid chlorella ◆ Liquid chlorophyll ◆ Floradix LIQUID IRON ◆ Crystal Star HIGHLY ABSORBABLE IRON EXTRACT	✤ Cortisone and other steroid drugs over a long period of time greatly weaken immunity and bone strength.
☙ To clean vital organs, take a glass of carrot/ beet/cucumber juice every day for the first month of healing; every other day for the second month; once a week the third month.	✤ ENER B INTERNASAL B12 every other day. ✤ Beta Carotene 150,000IU daily for at least 6 weeks. or Sun CHLORELLA 20 tabs daily for 6 weeks. ♂	☙ Mezotrace SEA MINERAL COMPLEX 4 daily. ☙ Effective teas: Yellow Dock Chaparral Pau de Arco Licorice/Sage	✤ See SPLEEN PAGE in this book for additional information. ✤ Avoid all alcohol, junk and chemically processed foods. Omit all refined sugars and red meats.
☙ Take 2-3 glasses of cranberry juice and aloe vera juice daily.			
☙ See CANCER DIET suggestions in this book, and/or "COOKING FOR HEALING" by Linda Rector-Page for a complete healing diet.	✤ Ascorbate vitamin C or Ester C powder, up to 10,000Mg. daily with bioflavonoids and rutin.	☙ Propolis and/or royal jelly capsules, 4x daily. ☙ Garlic/Cayenne caps 8-10 daily.	

COMMON SYMPTOMS: Increase in white blood cells, with no red blood cell production; extreme tiredness; pallor, thinness and weight loss; spleen malfunction or loss; symptoms similar to pernicious anemia.

COMMON CAUSES: Indiscriminate use of X-rays and some drugs, especially in children and pregnant women; poor diet with severe malnutrition; too many refined carbohydrates (especially in children); overfluoridation of the water; thyroid malfunction; deficiencies of vitamin D, iron, B12 and folic acid; hereditary proneness. See Cancer Causes in this book.

LIVER DISEASE
MALFUNCTION ◆ JAUNDICE

FOOD THERAPY	VITAMINS/ MINERALS	HERBAL THERAPY	BODYWORK

BODYWORK

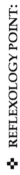 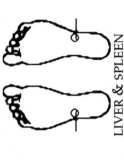

❖ REFLEXOLOGY POINT:

LIVER & SPLEEN

❖ Overheating by raising blood temperature is effective.
See Airola :HOW TO GET WELL"

❖ Eat smaller meals, get adequate rest and sleep, exercise every day with a good brisk aerobic walk.

❖ Take one coffee enema during your cleanse; (1 cup coffee to 1 qt. water.)

❖ Take several saunas if possible during a liver cleanse to induce sweating.

HERBAL THERAPY

🌿 Crystal Star LIV-ALIVE CAPSULES and LIV-FLUSH TEA for intense cleansing.
or
LIV TONIC EXTRACT or MILK THISTLE SEED EXTRACT for gentler longer range cleansing.

🌿 Crystal Star ANEMIGIZE CAPS for rebuilding Liver and Spleen activity. ♂
and/or
HIGHLY ABSORBABLE IRON EXTRACT.

🌿 Royal Jelly 2t. daily with Floradix LIQUID IRON.

🌿 Liver rebuilding tea: Mix 4oz. Hawthorne berries, 2oz. red sage, 1oz. cardamom. Steep 24 hours in 2 qts. of water. Add honey. Take 2 cups daily.

🌿 Other effective teas:
◆ Pau de Arco
◆ Roast Dandelion root
◆ Hibiscus/Burdock
◆ Barberry for jaundice
◆ Oregon Grape/Mullein

VITAMINS/ MINERALS

❖ Take a "spring cleaning inositol cocktail". Lexon B BLEND 1/2t. 3x daily.
and/or
a good lipotropic daily.

❖ Natren LIFE START 2, 1/4t. 3-4x daily.

❖ Liquid chlorophyll 3t. daily, or Sun CHLORELLA 15 daily. ♂

❖ Beta Carotene 100,000IU daily.
with
Ascorbate vitamin C or Ester C 1500Mg. every hour during acute stages, then 3000Mg. daily.

❖ 3% food grade H_2O_2, 1T. in 8oz. water 2x daily for 2 weeks, then 1x daily for 2 weeks.

❖ Alta Health CANGEST W/ Chromium picolinate. ♀

❖ B Complex 100Mg, with extra B₆ 100Mg., Niacin 100Mg., and B₁₂ 2000Mcg

FOOD THERAPY

🐚 If condition is acute, go on a 3 day liquid detoxification diet (see next page) to clean out toxic waste.
Then follow with an alkalizing, rebuilding diet for a month with high quality vegetable protein. (See a brief version on the next page, and a complete diet in "COOKING FOR HEALTHY HEALING" by Linda Rector-Page.)

🐚 Take daily during healing: 2T. each Lecithin granules and brewer's yeast flakes, 2-3 glasses cranberry or cranapple juice and 6-8 glasses of bottled water.

🐚 Avoid red meats, acid-forming foods such as caffeine, alcohol, refined starches and dairy products during all healing phases.

203

COMMON SYMPTOMS: Sluggish system; general depression and melancholy; great tiredness; nausea and shakes; dizziness; dry tongue and mouth; jaundiced skin and/or liver spots; skin itching.

COMMON CAUSES: Too much alcohol and/or drugs; constipation and congestion; too much sugar and refined carbohydrates; stress; hepatitis virus.

LIVER DETOXIFICATION DIET

The liver is a key detoxifying organ. A clean, functioning liver produces natural antihistimines to keep immunity high, metabolizes fats, helps in the formation of red blood cells, and in the control of estrogen production. A cleansing twice a year in the spring and fall is highly recommended, using the extra vitamin D from the sun to help.

ON RISING: take a glass of lemon juice or cider vinegar in water with a little honey, **and 1t. royal jelly** if desired. If an olive oil flush or coffee enema are to be included in the cleanse, now is the time to take them.
BREAKFAST: take a glass of carrot/beet/cucumber juice, or a potassium broth (Pg. 33); **or** a glass of organic apple juice.
MIDMORNING: have a glass of apple or cranberry juice; **or** a cup of Crystal Star LIVA FLUSH TEA.
LUNCH: have a glass of fresh carrot juice.
MIDAFTERNOON: have a cup of peppermint, pau de arco, or roasted danelion root tea; **or** another green drink, or Crystal Star LIVA FLUSH TEA.
DINNER: have an apple, carrot, or celery juice.
BEFORE BED: take another glass of lemon juice or cider vinegar and honey in water. Add 1t. **royal jelly** if desired.

ALKALIZING REBUILDING DIET

This diet is high in alkalizing fresh raw, foods, and vegetable proteins, dairy free, and low in fats. It may be used *after the* above diet, for 1 month, to rebuild healthy liver function, or by itself for a week or more, as a mild "spring cleaning" for the organs at any time.

ON RISING: take a glass of lemon juice and water with a little honey.
BREAKFAST: have a glass of prune, apple or cranberry juice; **then** have some fresh fruits, and a whole grain cereal or muesli with apple juice. Make a mix of lecithin granules, brewer's yeast and flax seed oil, and sprinkle a little on the cereal.
MIDMORNING: take a green drink (Pg. 34) or Crystal Star ENERGY GREEN, or Barley Green or fresh carrot juice;
and/or a cup of Crystal Star LIVER FLUSH TEA.
LUNCH: have a large fresh green salad with lemon/oil dressing, and a cup of miso soup with sea vegetables and crackers; **or** marinated, baked tofu chunks, or fresh fish with brown rice or millet, and a fresh green salad with lemon/oil dressing.
MIDAFTERNOON: have a cup of alkalizing herb tea, such as chamomile, dandelion root, or Crystal Star MEALS END TEA; **and/or** a hard boiled egg with some whole grain crackers and kefir cheese.
DINNER: have a baked potato with kefir cheese or soy cheese dressing, and a large dinner salad;
or a small vegetable omelet with steamed vegetables or tofu;
or a light vegetable stir-fry with a clear oriental noodle soup;
or some steamed vegetables with a whole grain such as bulgar, millet or brown rice and a light italian dressing.
BEFORE BED: have a cup of herb tea, **or** a glass of prune or apple juice, **or** a cup of VEGEX YEAST BROTH.

A continuing diet for liver health should be lacto-vegetarian, low fat, and rich in vegetable proteins and vitamin C foods for good iron absorption.

See "COOKING FOR HEALTHY HEALING" by Linda Rector-Page for a complete liver cleansing and healing diet.

204

LOW BLOOD PRESSURE

FOOD THERAPY

❧ Follow a fresh foods diet for a week, with plenty of green drinks (Pg. 34), potassium broth essence, brewer's yeast, and green salads.
Then follow a modified macrobiotic diet for 1-2 months, stressing vegetable proteins, green salads, miso, onions, garlic and other alkalizing foods, and dried or fresh fruits.

❧ Effective diet liquids:
Grape juice
Celery juice
Pineapple juice
Kukicha/Bancha twig tea
Knudsen's RECHARGE DRINK

❧ Avoid canned and refined foods, animal fats, red meats, and caffeine. Keep cholesterol, starchy and salty foods low.

❧ Complex carbohydrates, such as peas, broccoli, potatoes and whole grains are effective.

VITAMINS/ MINERALS

❖ B Complex 100Mg. daily with extra B_1 500Mg. and Pantothenic acid 1000Mg.

❖ Enzymatic Therapy LIQUID LIVER WITH SIBERIAN GINSENG CAPS.

❖ Twin Lab LIQUID K, up to 6t. daily during healing.

❖ Magnesium 400Mg. 4x daily for extreme cases.

❖ Vitamin E therapy for 8 weeks: work up from 100IU daily the first week, to 800IU daily, adding 100Mg. daily each week. ♂

❖ Vitamin K 100Mg. 2 daily.

❖ Vitamin C with Bioflavs and Rutin 3000Mg. daily.

❖ Avoid phenalalanine and tyrosine amino acids.

❖ Cal/Mag/Zinc 4 daily.♂

HERBAL THERAPY

❧ Crystal Star ANEMIGIZE CAPSULES 2-4 daily for a month, with 6-8 garlic/parsley caps daily. Then, ADRN-ALIVE and POTASSIUM SOURCE CAPSULES 2 daily each for a month.
Then, MASTER BUILDER or ENDOCRINE BALANCE CAPS for a month.

❧ Hawthorne extract 2-3x daily during healing.

❧ Effective capsules:
◆ Siberian Ginseng 4-6 daily
◆ Cayenne/Ginger 4 daily
◆ Garlic 6-8 daily
◆ Kelp 8-10 daily

❧ Effective teas:
◆ Bancha or Kukicha twig
◆ Dandelion Rt.
◆ Prickly Ash

❧ Crystal Star HEMA CLEANSE TEA for prevention and maintenance. ♂

❧ Floradix LIQUID IRON. with Raw Thymus extract

BODYWORK

❖ Acupressure, chiropractic spinal manipulation and shiatzu therapy are all effective in normalizing circulatory function.

❖ Alternating hot and cold hydrotherapy (Pg.31).

❖ Avoid tobacco and secondary smoke.

❖ Consciously try to relax the whole body once a day with short meditation and rest.

❖ Do deep breathing exercises (See Bragg's book) to stimulate circulation and oxygenate the system.

COMMON SYMPTOMS: Malfunction of the circulatory system; thinning of the blood; great fatigue and easy loss of energy; low immunity and susceptibility to allergies and infections.

COMMON CAUSES: Poor diet, causing a "run-down" condition; kidney malfunction causing system toxemia; emotional problems; anemia; over-use of drugs that lower immunity.

205

LUNG DISEASES

SARCOIDOSIS ◆ T.B ◆ CYSTIC FIBROSIS

FOOD THERAPY	VITAMINS/ MINERALS	HERBAL THERAPY	BODYWORK

FOOD THERAPY

🍂 Go on a short mucous cleansing diet (Pg. 25) Then, use the following cleansing diet for at least two weeks:

◆ Lemon juice/water or grapefruit juice each morning.
◆ Fresh Carrot juice or potassium broth daily
◆ 2 fresh green salads daily
◆ Steamed vegetables with brown rice and tofu or seafood for dinner.
◆ Cranberry or celery juice before bed.

🍂 A continuing diet for lung health should be high in vegetable proteins and whole grains, low in refined carbohydrates and starches.

🍂 Include cultured foods such as yogurt and kefir for friendly G.I. flora.

🍂 Pitted fruits, such as apricots, peaches and plums are specifics for the lungs.

🍂 See ASTHMA DIET SUGGESTIONS in this book or "COOKING FOR HEALTHY HEALING" by Linda Rector-Page for a complete healing diet.

VITAMINS/ MINERALS

❖ Beta or Marine carotene 100,000-150,000IU daily. with B Complex 100Mg. with extra B₆ 100Mg, folic acid 400Mcg. and B₁₂ INTERNASAL GEL.

❖ Effective anti-oxidants:
◆ Vit. C 3-5000Mg. daily with bioflavonoids.
◆ Vit. E 400IU with Selenium, 2x daily.
◆ Germanium 100-150Mg. daily.

❖ Food grade H₂O₂ 3% solution, 1 Tbl. to 1 glass, 2x daily for 1 month. Rest for a month, and resume if needed. (see Pg. 45 for instructions).

❖ Enzymatic Therapy AIR POWER as needed.

❖ Enzymatic Therapy RAW LUNG EXTRACT.

❖ Use raw pancreas extract for cystic fibroids. ☺

HERBAL THERAPY

🌿 Crystal Star ANTI-BIO CAPS or EXTRACT 4x daily for 1 week; then 2x daily with RESPIRCAPS 4 daily for 1-2 months. Add RESPIRTEA or DEEP BREATHING TEA 2 cups daily for best results.

🌿 Pau de Arco tea 3 cups daily,
with
Evening Primrose oil capsules 4-6 daily. ♀

🌿 Aloe Vera juice 1 glass daily. ♂
and
Crystal Star HEAVY METAL CAPS if lungs are subject to lots of environmental pollution.

🌿 Effective teas:
◆ Witch Hazel leaf & bark
◆ Licorice ♀
◆ Comfrey/Fenugreek
◆ Mullein/Lobelia
◆ Pleurisy Rt.

🌿 High potency ROYAL JELLY 2t. daily. ♂

BODYWORK

❖ Avoid all chlorofluorocarbons. They are even more harmful to your lungs as they are to the atmosphere and environment.

❖ Avoid tobacco and secondary smoke. Get lots of fresh air and sunshine, away from air pollution.

❖ Scratch the arm lightly, for 5 minutes daily, along the meridian line from the shoulder to the outside of the thumb to clear and heal lungs.

❖ Take a catnip or chlorophyll enema once a week to clear body toxins out faster.

❖ REFLEXOLOGY POINTS:

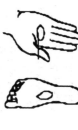

LUNG POINTS

COMMON SYMPTOMS: Constant coughing, inflammation and pain; bloody expectoration; difficult breathing.

COMMON CAUSES: Environmental and heavy metal pollutants, such as chlorofluorocarbons and smoking; malnutrition, and vitamin A deficiency; suppressive over-the-counter cold and congestion remedies that don't allow the lungs to eliminate harmful wastes properly.

LUPUS

FOOD THERAPY

- Follow the ARTHRITIS CLEANSING DIET in this book for three months: The diet should be 60-75% fresh foods during this time.

- Take a potassium broth or essence (Pg. 33) every day for a month, then every other day for a month, then once a week for the 3rd month.

- Then, follow a modified macrobiotic diet (Pg. 42) until blood tests clear, (sometimes 2-3 years, but healing success rate is good).

- Make sure the continuing diet is very low in fat.

- Avoid all red meats, refined sugars and high starch foods.

- See "COOKING FOR HEALTHY HEALING" by Linda Rector-Page for a complete, effective healing diet.

VITAMINS/ MINERALS

❖ Beta Carotene 100,000IU and Vit. D 1000IU daily. (Take Probiologics LIP-ISOL for best Carotene uptake)
with
Twin Lab LIQUID K 3-4t. daily.

❖ Ascorbate vit. C 5000Mg. daily with bioflavs. and/or
Quercitin Plus with Bromelain 2x daily.

❖ Alta Health MANGANESE WITH B₁₂ 2x daily. or
Ener B INTERNASAL B₁₂.

❖ Egg Yolk Lecithin with
High potency ROYAL JELLY (40,000Mg. or more) 2t. daily. ♂

❖ Germanium 100-150Mg. daily, with Sun CHLOR-ELLA 1 packet daily.

❖ Enzymatic Therapy LIQUID LIVER CAPSULES.

HERBAL THERAPY

🌱 Crystal Star LIV-ALIVE CAPS and LIV FLUSH TEA daily for 1 month.
with
BODY REBUILDER, POTASSIUM SOURCE, and ADRN-ALIVE CAPSULES to rebuild energy.

🌱 Pau de Arco tea 3-4 cups daily.

🌱 Black Walnut extract to combat inflammation. ♀

🌱 Crystal Star ANTI-BIO CAPS or EXTRACT or R^TH EASE CAPS as needed.
with
Sun CHLORELLA 15 daily. and
Garlic caps 8 daily.

🌱 Aloe Vera juice 1-2 glasses daily.

BODYWORK, ETC.

❖ Lupus is another immune-deficient disease that is generally not being addressed successfully by the medical community. It responds well to diet and nutritional improvement. It often accompanies arthritis, and many of the same therapies work for lupus.

❖ Our experience over the last 5 years has been that you will feel worse for a month or so til all toxins are released from the body. Then, suddenly, as a rule, you will feel much better. Stick with your program. It is working. A strong immune system is the key.

❖ Over-medication, especially on cortico-steroid drugs is dangerous for this disease, as they weaken the bones and suppress immunity.

❖ Avoid birth control pills, penicillin, and cosmetics with allergens and photoxins.

COMMON SYMPTOMS: Great fatigue; scaly, rough skin patches; chronic fungus infection; nails red at cuticle base; skin pallor; photosensitivity to light; low grade chronic toxemia; rheumatoid arthritis symtoms; kidney problems; anemia; pleurisy; inflammation; low immunity and low leucocyte count.

COMMON CAUSES: Degeneration of the body, often caused by too many anti-biotics or prescription drugs from Hydrazine derivatives; alcoholism; latent diabetes; overgrowth of Candida Albicans yeasts; affects mostly black and hispanic women.

LYME DISEASE

FOOD THERAPY	VITAMINS/ MINERALS	HERBAL THERAPY	BODYWORK, ETC.
❧ A modified macrobiotic diet is recommended for 2-3 months for strengthening the body while cleaning out and overcoming the disease.	❖ Beta or marine carotene 100-150,000IU daily as an anti-infective, with Probiologics LIPISOL AQUEUS solution for optimum uptake.	☙ Crystal Star LIV-ALIVE CAPS or LIV TONIC EXTRACT to enhance liver cleansing activity for a month. Then ANEMI-GIZE CAPS and POTASSIUM SOURCE CAPS to rebuild blood strength.	❖ While anti-biotics are the current medical treatment of choice, and seem to work in the initial phases, symptoms recur after the drugs are withdrawn. Our experience has not been long or extensive with this disease in California, but we have found that holistic alternative treatment _as for a virus_ has been much more successful.
❧ Avoid alcohol, tobacco, all refined and caffeine-containing foods, and sugars. Omit red meat, high gluten and starchy foods.	❖ Vitamin C or Ester C powder, 1/4t. every hour to daily bowel tolerance as an anti-oxidant and toxin neutralizer, especially during acute attacks and recurrences.	☙ Crystal Star ANTI-BIO CAPSULES 4-6 daily for the first week to clean out infection and reduce inflammation, then ANTI-VI EXTRACT in water 2x daily, one week on and one week off to overcome the virus.	❖ This is a serious steadily debilitating and degenerative disease, and difficult to guard against, especially with children. Strong immune enhancement is the best defense.
❧ Take a potassium broth or essence (Pg. 33) twice a week.	❖ Germanium 30Mg. daily, (or dissolve 1 gram powder in 1 qt. water and take 3T. daily.) or	☙ Shark liver oil to enhance leucocytes and overcome virus.	
❧ Take 1 teasp. each daily: ◆ Liquid Whey for orotic acid ◆ Wheat germ oil for body oxygen ◆ Jarrow Egg Yolk Lecithin ◆ Royal jelly	❖ H_2O_2 food grade 3% solution 1T. in 8oz. water.		
	❖ Natren LIFE START ☺ or LIFE START 2, ♂ ♀ to overcome antibiotic effects and restore nutrient assimilation.	☙ Crystal Star RELAX CAPS to rebuild nerve structure with Evening Primrose oil caps 4-6 daily.	❖ Regular exercise for plenty of body oxygen and stress avoidance is a key.
❧ Have a green drink (Pg. 34) or a fresh green salad every day.	❖ Country Life ENERGX VIALS for energy return.	☙ St. John's Wort extract 2-3x daily.	❖ Use Myrrh oil to repel and kill Lyme ticks.

COMMON SYMPTOMS: A large red "bullseye" rash near the site of the bite; initial flu-like symptoms of chills and aches; unusual fatigue, head aches and joint pain, especially in children; later symptoms of heart arrythmia, muscle spasms, chronic bladder problems, arthritis, facial paralysis, and extreme fatigue.

COMMON CAUSES: A spirochete transmitted through the bite of a deer tick; there is no currently known vaccine or anti-dote, but a strong immune system can ward off serious consequences.

FOOD THERAPY	VITAMINS/ MINERALS	HERBAL THERAPY	BODYWORK
❧ Start with a liquid foods diet for at least 24 hours to increase fluid intake as much as possible. Use fresh fruit and vegetable juices, miso soup, bottled water and herb teas such as Catnip, Chamomile or Rosemary, that will mildly induce sweating and clean out toxins faster.	❖ Effervescent EMERGEN-C 2-4x daily in juice, or ascorbate vitamin C 1/4t., 3-4x daily in juice or water.	❧ Crystal Star ANTI-BIO CAPS to curb infection and reduce inflammation, 1 at a time, up to 6 a day. and/or CRISIS CAPS 1-2 daily to break out the fever and rash, and start the healing process.	❖ Use hydrotherapy baths with Comfrey or Calendula flowers to induce sweating, and neutralize body acids.
❧ Then follow with a simple, basic diet featuring vitamin A and C-rich fresh foods. ◆ Give 1t. acidolphilus liquid in citrus juice each morning. ◆ Offer fresh fruits all through the morning, with yogurt if desired. ◆ Have one or two fresh green salads each day. ◆ Have a cup of Miso or clear soup with sea vegies daily. ◆ Have 2-3 cups of therapeutic herb tea during the day, and a cup of VEGEX YEAST BROTH before bed.	❖ Natren LIFE START or Solaray acidolphilus for children 3-4x daily, to replace friendly G.I. flora and rebuild immunity. ☺	❧ St. John's Wort extract, or Mullein/Lobelia tincture for a short period during acute stage. ☺	❖ Take tepid oatmeal baths to relieve skin itch and rash. ☺
	❖ Emulsified vitamin A & D 10,000IU/400IU for children. ☺	❧ Effective body washes to soothe and heal: Elder Flower ☺ Peppermint Chickweed Pleurisy Rt./Ginger Rt. Safflowers	❖ Use marjoram tea internally to sweat out rash; externally to soothe the skin.
	❖ Enzymatic Therapy VIRAPLEX CAPS.		❖ Apply Ginger/Cayenne compresses.
		❧ Catnip, Rosemary, and Chamomile tea, 3-4 cups, to break out the rash; Raspberry or Lobelia tea to heal the skin sores.	❖ Frequent hot baths will often bring out poisons through the rash.
		❧ St. John's Wort capsules.	❖ Take Garlic or Catnip enemas 1-2 times during acute stages to clean out infection fast (Person should be 10 years or older).

COMMON SYMPTOMS: A viral infection with cold-like symptoms. A strong fever is followed by a red rash on the face and upper body which sloughs off when the fever drops. There is coughing, light hurts the eyes, and sometimes hearing is affected permanently.

COMMON CAUSES: Low immunity from a poor diet, or too many immune-depressing anti-biotics or cirtico-steroid drugs. SEE REMEDIES FOR YOUNG CHILDREN ON PAGE 57 & 58 FOR MORE INFORMATION.

FOOD THERAPY	VITAMINS/ MINERALS	HERBAL THERAPY	BODYWORK
Maintain a high level of nutrition to reduce unpleasant menopausal symptoms. Compose the diet of 50% fresh foods, with plenty of vegetable proteins and complex carbohydrates. ◆ Keep the diet low in fats, sugars and mucous-forming foods such as dairy products and carbohydrates.	Stress B Complex 100Mg. with extra B6 100Mg., pantothenic acid 250Mg. and PABA 500Mg.	Crystal Star ESTRAID CAPS 4 daily the first month, 2 daily the 2nd and 3rd month, to control hormone imbalances and bone weakness accompanying estrogen changes. Then take EASY CHANGE CAPS as needed during the year or so of the change; RELAX, ADRN, or FEMALE HARMONY CAPS for a feeling of well-being on a long term basis.	Take a daily brisk walk to keep the system free and flowing. Do deep stretches on rising and each evening before bed.
	Rainbow Light CALCIUM PLUS, or Enzymatic Therapy OSTEOPRIME.		About Estrogen: ◆ Menopause is intended by nature to be a gradual reduction of estrogen by the ovaries with few side effects. In the well-nourished, active woman, the adrenals and other glands pick up the job of estrogen secretion. Most menopausal problems today stem from exhausted adrenals.
Avoid refined foods caffeine, and hard liquor (a little wine is fine).	Effective raw glandulars: ◆ Enzymatic Thyroid/Tyrosine ◆ Enzymatic Mammary ◆ Enzymatic Ovary/Uterus ◆ C. Life Adrenal w/Tyrosine	Evening Primrose oil caps 4 daily for prostaglandin production.	Synthetic Estrogen therapy is often prescribed by the medical community. Be very careful and ask before you agree to this. It can be a lifetime drug. It can destroy Vit. E in the body, making the risk of endometrial or breast cancer, heart and other diseases greater, and is not recommended if there is high blood pressure, fibrocystic breasts, high cholesterol, migraines, or endometriosis. Avoid synthetic estrogen if there is a history of breast cancer, thrombosis, or liver disease.
Avoid chlorinated water. It leaches Vit. E. Drink bottled spring or mineral water.	Nature's Plus VITAMIN E 800IU for several months.	Dong Quai/Damiana caps or extract 2x daily.	
Add to the daily diet 2 t. each: Brewer's yeast Wheat germ oil Lecithin	Ester C with bioflavs. 550Mg. 3-4x daily. and Emulsified A & D 1-2 daily, especially in low solar months.	Effective teas: Dong Quai/False Unicorn Licorice/Rose Hips Black Cohosh/Fennel	
See HYPOGLYCEMIA DIET suggestions in this book, and a complete diet for health during menopause in "COOKING FOR HEALTHY HEALING" by Linda Rector-Page.	For dry vagina: ◆ Vit. B6 500Mg. daily ◆ Apply Vit. E, or A D & E oil ◆ Solaray A D & E CAPS	Kelp tabs 8 daily, or MIODIN or ATOMODINE, or Crystal Star IODINE THERAPY CAPS or EXTRACT for thyroid balance.	◆ Phytoestrogens, or plant estrogens are effective for controlling hot flashes and osteoporosis if the body cannot produce estrogen because of surgical removal or medical directive.
	Enzymatic Therapy NUCLEO-PRO F CAPS, 2 daily. Chew for immediate results.	YS Ginseng tea with honey, 1 cup daily, or Royal Jelly 2t. daily	

COMMON SYMPTOMS: Erratic estrogen and other hormone secretions by the femal glands causing hot flashes, insomnia; lack of sexual interest, irritability, calcium imbalance, unstable behavior and mood swings, and palpitations; disturbance of calcium metabolism causing osteoporosis; skin and vaginal dryness and sometimes atrophy; occasional growth of male characteristics.

COMMON CAUSES: Deficient nutrition and lack of exercise; thyroid imbalance; exhausted adrenals; poor food absorption; B vitamin deficiency; stress;

♀ MENSTRUAL PROBLEMS ♀
EXCESSIVE ◆ SPOTTING

FOOD THERAPY	VITAMINS/ MINERALS	HERBAL THERAPY	BODYWORK
❧ Consciously work on nutrition improvement, with emphasis on vegetable proteins, mineral-rich foods and high fiber foods. ◆ Add plenty of seafood, fish and sea vegetables to regulate metabolism.	❖ Nature's Plus Vit E 800IU with Floradix LIQUID IRON daily. ❖ Enzymatic Therapy RAW MAMMARY CAPS 2-3 daily for almost immediate results; and BIO-CAL if periods are too frequent, or FEM PLUS CAPSULES.	❧ Crystal Star FEMALE HARMONY, 2 daily with 2 bayberry capsules, for 2 months to normalize hormone production. ❧ WOMAN'S BEST FRIEND CAPS or ESTROMONE EXTRACT 2 x daily as a toner and preventive.	❖ ACUPRESSURE: **Press on the insides of the legs about 5" above the knees; 5 minutes each leg to decrease bleeding.** ❖ Apply icepacks to the pelvic area. Get extra sleep during this time.
❧ Avoid caffeine and caffeine-containing foods, hard liquor (A little wine is fine), and red meats (Most are loaded with the hormone DES that has a definite effect on human blood).	❖ Solaray MAGNESIUM ASPOROTATE 4 daily. with Octacosonal 1000Mg. for breakthrough bleeding. ❖ Vitamin K 2 daily with Twin Labs CITRUS BIOFLAVONOIDS AND RUTIN 500Mg/500Mg.	❧ Atomodine, Miodin, or Crystal Star IODINE THERAPY for thyroid balance. ❧ Dong Quai/Damiana caps or extract 4x daily with Shavegrass tea, Crystal Star SILICA SOURCE EXTRACT or Burdock tea.	❖ Get daily regular exercise to keep system and metabolism flowing. ❖ REFLEXOLOGY POINT: 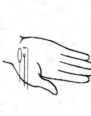 VAGINA, OVARIES, BLADDER
❧ Reduce fried, saturated fatty foods, sugars, and high cholesterol foods.	❖ Rainbow Light CALCIUM PLUS CAPSULES 4 at a time daily.	❧ Effective teas: Shepherds Purse Angelica/Raspberry Bayberry Bk.	❖ Avoid drugs of all kinds, even aspirin and prescription drugs if possible. Many inhibit Vitamin K formation.
❧ Add to the daily diet 2T. each: Brewer's yeast Wheat germ Amaranth Lecithin	❖ Mezotrace SEA MINERAL COMPLEX 4 daily, with raw adrenal glandular.	❧ Sarsaparilla extract daily. ❧ Milk Thistle seed extract as a mild liver cleanse for spotting.	

COMMON SYMPTOMS: Excessive bleeding for 2 or more days, with large dark clots, spotting between periods.

COMMON CAUSES: Nutrition deficient diet with too much caffeine, salt and red meat, causing gladular imbalance; overproduction of estrogen; aspirin; calcium deficiency; underactive, lazy or deficient thyroid; Vit. K deficiency;

♀ MENSTRUAL PROBLEMS ♀
SUPPRESSED ◆ DELAYED

FOOD THERAPY	VITAMINS/ MINERALS	HERBAL THERAPY	BODYWORK
❧ Make sure the diet is very nutritious, with plenty of vegetable proteins and complex carbohydrates. (The body will often not menstruate or conceive if it is malnourished).	❖ B Complex 100Mg. daily with ENER B INTERNASAL GEL VIT. B$_{12}$ every other day. and extra Folic acid 400Mcg.	❧ Crystal Star FLOW ON TEA as directed. and	❖ Horehound compresses on the pelvic area.
	❖ Nature's Plus Vit. E 800IU.	❧ ESTRAID CAPS or ESTROMONE EXTRACT, or WOMAN'S BEST FRIEND CAPS 4 daily.	❖ Alternating hot and cold sitz baths to stimulate pelvic circulation.
❧ Have some brown rice and other B Complex-rich foods every day.	❖ Enzymatic Therapy NUCLEO-PRO F CAPS with ADRENAL COMPLEX and RAW MAMMARY CAPS.	❧ Crystal Star FEMALE HARMONY CAPS AND TEA. or Burdock tea 2 cups daily to balance hormones.	❖ Regular exercise to keep system free and flowing.
❧ Have a green drink (Pg. 34), BARLEY GREEN MAGMA, or Crystal Star ENERGY GREEN DRINK several times a week for healthy blood building.	❖ Cal/Mag/Zinc tabs 4 daily with Kelp tabs 8 daily.	❧ Evening Primrose oil caps 4-6 daily.	❖ Heavy body building and training for marathon or competition sports definitely affects menstruation as the amount of body fat is extremely reduced. The body will not slough off tissue when it feels at risk in forming more.
	❖ Raw female glandular Raw ovary glandular	❧ Dong Quai/Damiana caps or extract 2x daily.	
❧ Take 2T. each daily: Wheat germ Lecithin granules Brewer's yeast		❧ Effective teas: BLack Cohosh Motherwort Ephedra-for delayed menses Pennyroyal	
❧ Avoid caffeine and caffeine-containing foods, such as chocolate and sodas.		❧ Spirulina and Bee Pollen caps 2 each daily for metabolic balance.	

COMMON SYMPTOMS: Absence of menses; irregular menses.

COMMOM CAUSES: Poor health or nutrition;gland and hormone imbalance; too much caffeine; poor organ and abdominal tone; lack of exercise; extreme or very low protein weight loss diet foods; anorexia or excess dieting for weight loss; marathoner's syndrome; hypoglycemia; IUD caused cervical lesions or cysts; venereal disease; stress, emotional shock or depression; adrenal exhaustion; previous birth control pill use causing irregularity.

MENTAL RETARDATION ✧ DOWN'S SYNDROME

FOOD THERAPY	VITAMINS/ MINERALS	HERBAL THERAPY	BODYWORK

🌱 Both Down's Syndrome which represents a glycogen storage problem, and mental retardation can be physically improved and IQ upgraded through nutritional therapy.

❖ Country Life MAXI-B with TAURINE and B_6.
and
B_{15} DMG sublingual 1 daily as an anti-oxidant.
and/or
ENER B INTERNASAL B_{12} GEL every other day.

🌿 Evening Primrose oil caps 4-6 daily for 3-4 months.

🌿 Crystal Star MENTAL CLARITY CAPS 1 daily with YS GINSENG & HONEY TEA 1 cup daily.

❖ Vanguard nutritional work and knowledge is being done and accumulated about this problem. We now know that some retarded disfunction and behavior is <u>learned, not hereditary</u>.

🌱 Eat only fresh foods for 3-4 days to clear the body of toxic waste, and provide a clean working ground for nutritional therapy. Then, insist on a highly nutritious diet of fresh and whole foods, rich in vegetable proteins and magnesium foods.

❖ Mezotrace SEA MINERAL COMPLEX FOR CHILDREN.

❖ Choline 600Mg. 4 daily. with Niacin 100-500Mg and B_6

🌿 Effective teas: 3-4 cups daily for 3-4 months to see noticeable improvement.
◆ Crystal Star CREATIVITEA.
◆ Chamomile ☺
◆ Gotu Kola
◆ European Mistletoe
◆ Sage tea ☺
◆ Siberian Ginseng

❖ Play soothing classical or new age music in the home. It works wonders.

❖ Zinc 50-100Mg daily.

❖ Expose the body to early morning sunshine daily if possible for vitamin D.

🌱 Avoid <u>all</u> refined foods, sugars, pasteurized dairy and alcohol. Reduce high gluten foods.

❖ Glutamine 500Mg. 2 daily. with Ester C 550Mg. with Bioflavs 4 daily.

🌿 Garlic caps 4 daily as brain oxygenators. with Kelp tabs 4 daily for brain potassium.

❖ Avoid pesticides, heavy metals, (cadmium, lead and mercury), and aluminum.

❖ Do deep breathing exercises to oxygenate the brain.

🌱 See HYPOGLYCEMIA DIET suggestions in this book, or "COOKING FOR HEALTHY HEALING" by Linda Rector-Page for an optimal brain nourishment and child's diet.

❖ Country Life RELAXER CAPSULES.

🌿 Crystal Star POTASSIUM SOURCE CAPS or MIN-ZYME-MINOS DRINK for rich herbal minerals. MASTER BUILDER CAPS for pituitary stimulation.

❖ REFLEXOLOGY POINT:

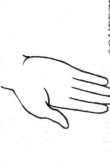

SQUEEZE FOR BRAIN
ALL AROUND FOR BRAIN

❖ CO Q 10, 10Mg. daily with vitamin E 400IU.

🌱 Make a mix and take 2T. daily:
Brewer's yeast
Lecithin
Wheat germ

❖ Tryptophan 500Mg. with Taurine 500Mg. for stress symptoms. ☺

🌿 High potency ROYAL JELLY 2t. daily. ☺

COMMON SYMPTOMS: Slow reactions and motor disfunction; learning disability; withdrawal from and poor behavior with people; gland and hormone deficiencies giving the person a "retarded" appearance.

COMMON CAUSES: Drugs, either given to the childd or taken by the mother when pregnant; excess water fluoridation; too much sugar and refined foods; heavy metal poisoning altering brain chemistry; hypoglycemia; allergies; great emotional shock or stress; birth trauma.

MIGRAINE & VASCULAR HEADACHES

FOOD THERAPY	VITAMINS/ MINERALS	HERBAL THERAPY	BODYWORK
❦ Nutritional awareness is a must for preventing migraines.	❖ Niacin therapy: up to 1000Mg. as needed to open and enhance blood flow. Take with Stress B Complex and extra B₆ for best preventive results.	❦ Crystal Star MIGRAID and RELAX CAPSULES as needed for pain and preventive activity, or HEADACHE DEFENSE EXTRACT WITH FEVERFEW	❖ Biofeedback and chiropractic care have both been successful in controlling migraines.
❦ Trigger foods include: citrus juices, red wine, oxalic acid-forming foods, refined sugars, and cultured foods, such as pickled herring, yogurt and cheeses.	❖ Quercetin Plus with Bioflavonoid and Rutin capsules 4 daily.	❦ HYPO BLUES CAPS or TEA to balance sugar use.	❖ Use ice packs on the neck to draw blood out of the head.
❦ At the first signs of a migraine: take 1-2 cups of strong coffee to prevent vessel dilation; (Avoid caffeine on a regular basis) or a glass of carrot/celery juice if possible.	❖ DLPA for pain control. ♀	❦ Evening Primrose oil caps or royal jelly caps, 4 daily for prevention. ♀	❖ Massage temples for 5 minutes. Breathe deeply. Do 10 neck rolls. Pull earlobes. Pull down and hold each lobe for 5 seconds. Rub back and all around ear shell.
❦ Avoid animal fats, (especially in red meats and dairy products), refined sugars, salt, caffeine,soft drinks (the phosphorus binds up available magnesium), chocolate, smoked meats, avocados, and hard liquor.	❖ Effective preventives: ◆ Germanium 30Mg. ◆ Omega 3 fish or Flax oils ◆ Oral Chelation w/ EDTA ♂ ◆ Alta Health MAGNESIUM CHLORIDE CAPSULES ◆ Mezotrace SEA MINERAL COMPLEX.	❦ Feverfew extract capsules or tea as needed before and during an attack.	❖ Get some fresh air and exercise every day.
	❖ Tryptophan 500Mg.to supplement serotonin deficiency. and	❦ Effective extracts: Valerian/Wild Lettuce Lobelia Passion Flower BioForce MIGRAINE DROPS	❖ AROMATHERAPY: Lavender essence
❦ Make sure you are eating plenty of whole grains, fresh greens, fiber foods and fish for prevention.	❖ Magnesium 400Mg. 2x daily to prevent nerve twitching. ♀	❦ Schiff Garlic/Onion caps on a regular basis as a brain anti-oxidant.	❖ Avoid smoking and secondary smoke. It constricts blood vessels. Avoid pleasure drugs, aspirin, and MSG.
❦ Take 2T. daily lecithin and brewer's yeast as a preventive.	❖ ENER B INTERNASAL B₁₂ GEL. every other day.	❦ Effective teas: Catnip/Peppermint Fenugreek/Thyme Scullcap Rosemary/Sage	❖ Take catnip or coffee enema to stimulate liver.

COMMON SYMPTOMS: A recurrent constriction/dilation of blood vessels in the brain, scalp and face; a preceding aura , light sensitivity, and halos appearing around lights; nausea, made worse by light and movement; intense, long-lasting pain; visual problems.

COMMON CAUSES: Poor diet, with too much caffeine, junk and fast foods, fats and refined sugars; pituitary/hormone imbalance; emotional stress; virus; over-acid system stripping away protective nerve sheathing; food allergies; Vit. B ₆ deficiency and water retention; arthritis; liver toxicity; poor circulation and a lack of blood flow; menstrual dysfunction; over-use of drugs; hereditary weakness.

TO PREVENT AND STRENGTHEN

FOOD THERAPY

❧ A good prevention diet should include plenty of magnesium and potassium-rich foods; leafy greens, brown rice, tofu, sprouts, molasses, etc.
◆ NO soft drinks; they bind up magnesium and make it unavailable.

❧ Take 2T. each daily:
Lecithin
Wheat germ
Brewer's yeast

❧ Be sure to get enough good vegetable protein for the baby's growth: whole grains, sprouts, low fat dairy foods, sea foods, seeds, etc.

❧ Absolutely avoid alcohol, caffeine, and drugs. Reduce sugars and refined foods of all kinds.

❧ Don't smoke. Smokers are twice as likely to miscarry and have low birth weight babies as non-smokers.

VITAMINS/ MINERALS

✢ Take a strengthening prenatal formula such as Rainbow Light PRE-NATAL all through pregnancy for a healthier baby and to help prevent birth defects.

✢ Vitamin C with Rosehips or Ester C with Bioflavs and Rutin to strengthen veins and blood vessels 2-3000Mg. daily.
and/or
Quercitin Plus with Bromelain if problem is severe.

✢ Vitamin E 400IU daily during pregnancy as a miscarriage deterrent.

✢ Rainbow Light CALCIUM PLUS w/high magnesium.

✢ B Complex 50Mg. with Nature's Plus SPIRUTEIN DRINK for protein, and Kal B₁₂ with Folic Acid.

✢ Emulsified A & D. daily.

✢ Solaray ALFAJUICE for chlorophyll and oxygen.

HERBAL THERAPY

🐍 For False Labor:
Take 2 caps each of Cayenne and Bayberry, and get to a hospital or call your midwife.

🐍 Lobelia and cayenne extracts taken together.

🐍 Crystal Star HERBAL PRENATAL CAPSULES for strength and tone during pregnancy.
5 WEEK FORMULA CAPS in the last stages only as directed for an easier birth.

🐍 Effective teas:
Cramp Bark
Wild Yam
False Unicorn

🐍 Red Raspberry and Catnip tea, or Crystal Star MOTHERING TEA all through pregnancy 2-3 cups daily.

🐍 Crystal Star ANTI-SPAZ CAPS or CRAMP CONTROL EXTRACT to help stop bleeding.

BODYWORK

❖ Have the woman lie very still and give a cup of False unicorn tea every 1/2 hour. As hemorrhaging decreases, give the tea every hour, then every 2 hours. Add 5 or 6 Lobelia extract drops as a relaxing agent to the last cup.

❖ Give Comfrey/Wild Yam/Cranesbill tea every hour til bleeding is controlled.

❖ Give Hawthorne extract 1/2 dropperful, and Bee Pollen 2t every hour til bleeding is controlled.

❖ To determine if the fetus is still alive: take body temperature first thing upon waking. Have a thermometer by the bed, already shaken down, move as little as possible, and take the temperature before getting up. The fetus is alive if the body temperature is 98.6 or above. (Unless normal body temperature is low because of abnormally low thyroid metabolism)

COMMON SYMPTOMS: Spotting to profuse bleeding during pregnacy, usually with cramps and severe pain.

COMMON CAUSES: Deficient uterine muscle tone; weak blood vessels and capillaries; lack of protein and sufficient nutrition for both mother and child; improper fixing of the fetus to the womb walls; allergic reaction to drugs.

MONONUCLEOSIS

FOOD THERAPY

🍂 Begin healing with plenty of cleansing/flushing fruit juices and bottled water for 1 week. Do not fast. Strength and nutrition are too low. Particularly use Apple/Sprout, Papaya/Pineapple, and Pineapple/Coconut juices for strength and enzyme enhancement.

🍂 Then, follow with a week of green drinks, potassium broth and vegetable juices to cleanse, strengthen and rebuild liver function.

🍂 Then eat a diet high in vegetable proteins; (brown rice, tofu, nuts, seeds, sprouts,etc.) and cultured foods; (yogurt, kefir, etc.) for building and friendly flora.

🍂 Add vitamin A and vitamin C rich foods.

🍂 See LIVER CLEANSING DIET SUGGESTIONS in this book for more information.

VITAMINS/ MINERALS

❖ Sun CHLORELLA or BARLEY GREEN or Solaray ALFAJUICE during entire healing time.
and

❖ Germanium 100-150Mg.

❖ Beta Carotene 150,000IU daily for 1 month, with
Vitamin C powder, 1/4t. every hour in water to bowel tolerance daily for 1 month. (Reduce dosage on both the 2nd and 3rd months.)

❖ Biotec EXTRA ENERGY ENZYMES 6 daily.
and

❖ ENER B INTERNASAL B12 GEL daily for 1 month, then every other day.

❖ Twin Lab LIQUID K, or WHITE BIRCH MINERAL WATER for potassium. ♂

❖ Natren LIFE START 2, 1/4t. 3-4x daily for 3 months.

HERBAL THERAPY

🍃 Crystal Star ANTI-BIO CAPS or EXTRACT, 4-6x daily for 2 weeks, with
CLEANSING & FASTING or LIV-FLUSH TEA.

🍃 Then, ADRN-ALIVE CAPS with BODY REBUILDER CAPS 2 each daily, or ANEMIGIZE CAPS with POTASSIUM SOURCE CAPS.

🍃 Then, MIN-ZYME-MINOS or ENERGY GREEN DRINK for solid immune building blocks.

🍃 Then, Hawthorne Extract 3-4x daily with FEEL GREAT TEA for last strengthening stages.

🍃 Effective extracts:
Siberian Ginseng ♂
Astragalus
St. John's Wort

🍃 Echinacea and Garlic to clear the Lymph glands of infection.

🍃 Premier 1 or YS ROYAL JELLY 2t. daily. ♀

BODYWORK

❖ Mono is a highly infectious, virulent disease. Its hold is strong; the immune system is usually weak. At least three months of rebuilding are needed to effect real strength.

❖ Liver, Lymph and Spleen systems are the main organs involved in healing. Concentrate your efforts on revitalizing these areas.

❖ Get plenty of rest and early morning sunlight; mild outdoor exercise as soon as possible.

❖ REFLEXOLOGY POINT:

LIVER & SPLEEN

❖ Avoid all pleasure drugs, caffeine and chemical stimulants.

COMMON SYMPTOMS: Severe flu/pneumonia/lung symptoms; extreme fatigue; totally run-down condition; pallor; jaundice as the liver throws off body poisons.

COMMON CAUSES: An opportunistic disease allowed by a weak immune system; overuse and abuse of pleasure drugs and/or alcohol; liver malfunction.

216

MORNING SICKNESS ✧ NAUSEA ✧ VOMITING

FOOD THERAPY

❧ Keep by the bed, and take a few soda crackers before rising to soak up excess acids; eat ice chips to calm spasms; drink a little fresh fruit juice for alkalinity.

❧ For breakfast, have orange juice sweetened with honey; then a little bran or barley cereal.
Take only yogurt in the morning, if friendly flora are needed to settle digestive imbalance.

❧ Take 2T. Brewer's yeast every day for absorbable and non-toxic B vitamins.

❧ Eat plenty of fiber from vegetables and whole grains to keep the system and bowels clean and flowing.
Cucumbers soaked in water and eaten will relieve congestion fast.

VITAMINS/ MINERALS

✤ Acidolphilus powder (1/4t. 2-3x daily), or chewable papaya enzymes to settle stomach imbalance.

✤ Premier 1 or YS ROYAL JELLY 1t. each morning on rising.

✤ Homeopathic NAT. SULPH. or IPECAC as needed.

✤ Stress B Complex 50Mg. daily, with extra B$_6$ 50-100Mg., and magnesium 400Mg., with Rose Hips vitamin C 500Mg. daily.

✤ Comfrey/Pepsin tabs as needed.

✤ Country Life RELAXER CAPSULES as needed.

✤ Cal/Mag/Zinc 2 at a time as needed to settle.

HERBAL THERAPY

❧ Ginger capsules, tea or extract on rising.

❧ Crystal Star FEMALE HARMONY CAPSULES 2 daily.
    and
MOTHERING TEA daily as needed. (Helpful all during pregnancy for balance and fetus health.)

❧ Solaray EUROCALM CAPS and ALFAJUICE CAPS to calm and balance the stomach.

❧ Effective liver decongestants:
 ◆ Dandelion/Yellow Dock
 ◆ Milk Thistle seed

❧ Eucalyptus oil, a small drop on the tongue.

❧ Effective teas:
 ◆ Ginger/Peppermint
 ◆ Red Raspberry
 ◆ Alfalfa/Mint
 ◆ Spearmint/Chamomile
 ◆ Wild Yam

❧ Catnip tea with 1 Golden Seal capsule on rising.

BODYWORK

✤ Deep breathing exercises every morning, and a brisk deep breathing walk every day, for body oxygen.

✤ ACUPRESSURE POINTS:
Press the hollow of each elbow 3x for 10 seconds each.

✤ Both Biofeedback and Hypnotherapy have been effective. See a qualified chirpractor or massage therapist.

✤ Soft classical or new age music in the morning will help calm you and the baby.

COMMON SYMPTOMS: Nausea and heaving in the morning or night during the first stages of pregnancy; gland and hormone upset causing digestive imbalance; sensitivity to food substances.

COMMON CAUSES: Gland and hormone imbalance as the body adjusts to a new biorhythm; congested liver if yellow bile is vomited; low blood sugar.

MOTION SICKNESS

FOOD THERAPY

❧ Before departure, take a cup of Vegex YEAST BROTH with a pinch of cayenne.

　or

❧ Brown rice mixed with 3T. brewer's yeast.

　or

❧ One egg white mixed with Lemon juice.

　or

Suck on a lemon or lime during the trip whenever queasiness strikes.

❧ During the trip, munch soda crackers to soak up excess acids. Take sugar-free, carbonated sodas to neutralize acids. Avoid eating salty, sugary or dairy foods. They can easily cause digestive imbalance.

VITAMINS/ MINERALS

✛ B Complex 100Mg. for several weeks prior to travelling, for better "B" balance.

　and extra

✛ Folic acid and vit. B$_{12}$ 2000Mcg. sublingual.

✛ Glutamine 500Mg. 2-3x before departure.

✛ Vitamin B$_1$, Thiamine. Take 500Mg. like Dramamine before a trip.

✛ Lecithin 1900Gr. 2x

　or

✛ Vitamin E w/ Selenium ♂

HERBAL THERAPY

❧ Take 2-3 ginger caps, or ginger/cayenne caps 1 or 2 hours before traveling.

❧ Ginkgo Biloba extract drops on a regular basis before and during travelling for inner ear balance.

❧ Strong Japanese green tea. ♀

❧ Comfrey/Pepsin tabs, or Comfrey/Fenugreek tea

❧ Crystal Star MEGA MINERAL CAPS for about a month before a trip, and HERBAL ENZYMES for better stomach balance.

❧ Peppermint tea before and during a trip.

BODYWORK

✛ During an attack:
◆ Massage knee caps for 3 minutes.
◆ Massage little finger for 10 minutes.
◆ Massage back of head at base of skull, and behind ears on the mastoids.

✛ Do conscious deep breathing for 1 minute. Get fresh air and oxygen as soon as possible.

✛ REFLEXOLOGY POINT:

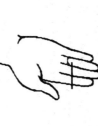

INTERNAL EAR

COMMON SYMPTOMS: Nausea, upset stomach and/or vomiting during a vehicle trip; unsettled stomach; queasiness.

COMMON CAUSES: Inner ear imbalance; mineral deficiency; fear or stress about the trip. Remember that deaf people do not get motion sickness. The inner ear is usually at the root of the problem.

M. S. ✧ MULTIPLE SCLEROSIS

FOOD THERAPY	VITAMINS/ MINERALS	HERBAL THERAPY	BODYWORK

FOOD THERAPY

🐾 Follow a cleansing diet for 1-2 months, similar to a diet for Candida Albicans (Pg. 105). Then follow a modified macrobiotic diet (Pg. 42) for 3-6 months.

🐾 The diet should be 70-80% fresh foods, with plenty of salads and green drinks; 15-20% fresh fruits; and 5-10% vegetable proteins from sprouts, legumes and seeds.

🐾 Take a potassium broth or essence (Pg. 33) at least twice a week.

🐾 Egg Yolk Lecithin 2-3x daily, with high potency ROYAL JELLY 40-50,000Mg. 2t. daily.

🐾 Take 2t. each daily:
Wheat germ oil
Liquid Whey ♂

🐾 Avoid all refined and fried foods, sugars and caffeine-containing foods. Reduce starchy and high gluten foods.

VITAMINS/ MINERALS

✤ Phosphatidyl Choline (PC55) 2-3x daily.

✤ Niacin therapy, 500Mg. 3-4x daily, with B_6 500Mg. for nerves and circulation, and B_1 500Mg.

✤ Beta Carotene 100,000IU (and/or Probiologics LIPISOL), with
Ascorbate vitamin C powder, 1/4t. every hour to bowel tolerance daily for a month; then reduce to 5000Mg. daily.
and
Vit. E 800IU w/ selenium, or Octacosonal 1000Mg.

✤ Country Life ENERGIX VIALS and Threonine as needed for energy.♂

✤ Mezotrace SEA MINERAL COMPLEX daily for nerves.

✤ Omega 3 Flax or fish oils 3 daily,
with
Natren LIFE START #2, 1/2t. 3x daily.

HERBAL THERAPY

🐾 Crystal Star RELAX CAPS to feed and rebuild nerve structure.
and
ANTI-SPAZ CAPS or GINKGO BILOBA EXTRACT for tremor control.
with

🐾 Evening Primrose oil caps 4-6 daily.

🐾 Sun CHLORELLA 2 packets daily.

🐾 Crystal Star LIVER CLEANSE CAPS and LIV-FLUSH TEA to clean out toxins. and ANEMIGIZE CAPS to build blood strength. ♂

🐾 Crystal Star MIN-ZYME-MINOS and ENERGY GREEN DRINKS to rebuild the body.

🐾 Alta Health CANGEST CAPS with meals for food assimilation.

🐾 A catnip enema once a week for several months.

BODYWORK

✤ M.S. must be treated vigorously. A little therapy won't work. Long lasting remission and cure are possible if you catch it in time. Natural therapies take 6 months to a year.

✤ Overheating therapy is effective for M.S. See Airola "How To Get Well" for effective technique.

✤ Avoid smoking and secondary smoke. You need all the oxygen you can retain.

✤ Mild daily exercise, chiropractic adjustment, massage therapy and mineral baths have been useful in controlling M.S.

✤ REFLEXOLOGY POINTS:

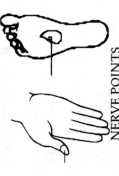

NERVE POINTS

COMMON SYMPTOMS: Numbness; great fatigue and weakness; visual disturbance and loss; slurred speech and mental disturbance; poor motor coordination; tremors; dizziness; nerve degeneration.

COMMON CAUSES: Too many refined carbohydrates and saturated fats, causing poor food assimilation and toxemia from constipation and poor bowel health; lead or heavy metal poisoning; Hypoglycemia; Vitamin B_6 and B_1 deficiency; food allergies; Candida Albicans overgrowth; gland imbalance.

MUSCULAR DYSTROPHY
SPINAL BIFIDA

FOOD THERAPY

🐾 Go on a short 6-10 day cleansing diet to release accumulated toxins. (Pg. 26).
Then follow a macrobiotic diet for degenerative disease for 3 months, and a modified macrobiotic building diet (Pg. 42) for 6 months or more.
See "COOKING FOR HEALTHY HEALING" by Linda Rector-Page for complete details of this diet.

🐾 Avoid all refined foods, caffeine-containing foods, and salty foods.

🐾 Take 2T. each daily:
Lecithin granules
Brewer's yeast
Wheat germ

🐾 Take a potassium broth or essence (Pg. 33) daily for the first 6-8 weeks of healing. Reduce to once a week for the next 6 months. And add at least 1 green drink (Pg. 34) every week.

VITAMINS/ MINERALS

✛ Phosphatidyl Choline (PC55) 4 daily, with Twin Lab LIQUID K 4-6t. daily.
or

✛ Egg Yolk Lecithin 2x daily, with highest potency ROYAL JELLY 50-100Mg. 2t. daily.

✛ Predigested liquid amino acids 1-2t. daily for immediately usable protein building blocks.

✛ Vital Health FORMULA 1 chelation therapy with EDTA for circulation.

✛ Niacin therapy: 500-1000Mg. daily, with Vit E 800IU with Selenium.

✛ Country Life THREONINE and GLYCINE CAPS with CARNITINE 500Mg. 4-6 daily, and ENER B INTERNASAL B₁₂.

✛ Beta Carotene 100,000IU with Ester C, 550Mg. with Bioflavs. & Rutin 6 daily.

HERBAL THERAPY

🐾 Evening Primrose or black currant oil capsules, 4-6 daily.

🐾 Crystal Star RELAX CAPS as needed to rebuild nerve sheath damage.
with
High Omega 3 Flax oil 3x daily.
and
BONZ CAPS and TEA to support muscle atrophy.

🐾 Hawthorne extract 2-4x daily for circulatory tone.

🐾 Crystal Star MIN-ZYME-MINOS DRINK and/or POTASSIUM SOURCE CAPS for rebuilding mineral and enzyme strength.

🐾 3 cups daily, Dandelion, Fennel, Comfrey Root tea.

🐾 Crystal Star MEGA MINERAL CAPS, or HIGHLY ABSORBABLE MINERAL COMPLEX EXTRACT for nerve strength.

BODYWORK

✛ Overheating therapy has been successful in controlling Muscular Dystrophy. See Airola "How To Get Well" for the technique.

✛ Avoid tobacco and alcohol. Question high blood pressure drugs containing sodium.

✛ Use hot and cold hydrotherapy to stimulate circulation. Use mineral and therapeutic baths for cleansing and muscle support. (Pg. 31-32).

✛ REFLEXOLOGY POINT:

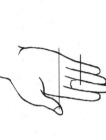

NERVES & MUSCLES

✛ Get early morning sunlight on the body every day possible to rebuild muscle strength.

COMMON SYMPTOMS: Muscle weakness and atrophy; nerve damage and atrophy; tremor and palsy; degeneration in ability to walk; occasional loss of bladder control.

COMMON CAUSES: Poor food assimilation causing deficient minerals; too many refined foods and junk foods; EFA and prostaglandin deficiency.

MUSCLE CRAMPS & SPASMS
LEG CRAMPS ✦ INVOLUNTARY TICS

FOOD THERAPY	VITAMINS/ MINERALS	HERBAL THERAPY	BODYWORK
Eat high vitamin C foods; leafy greens, citrus fruits, brown rice, sprouts, broccoli, tomatoes, green peppers, etc.	Vitamin C or Ester C, up to 5000Mg. daily with bioflavs and rutin.	Crystal Star ANTI-SPAZ CAPSULES 4 at a time, or CRAMP CONTROL EXTRACT with MEGA MINERAL CAPS daily	Take vinegar or epsom salts baths.
	Country Life LIGATEND as needed and MAXI-B COMPLEX w/ TAURINE daily.		Rub Lobelia extract directly on area.
Eat potassium-rich foods; bananas, broccoli, sun seeds, beans and legumes, whole grains and dried fruits.	B Complex 100Mg. daily, with extra B$_6$ 250Mg. and pantothenic acid 250Mg. for nerve repair.	Crystal Star RELAX CAPS daily as needed to rebuild nerve health. with POTASSIUM SOURCE CAPS and/ or IODINE THERAPY CAPS or EXTRACT for deficient minerals. ♀	Massage the legs; elevate the feet, and slap soles and legs hard with open palm to stimulate circulation.
Eat magnesium-rich foods; lettuce, bell pepper, green leafy vegetables, molasses, nuts and seafoods.	For eye tics; CO Q 10, 30Mg. daily.	Alta Health SIL-X silica caps 3-4 daily.	Use alternating hot and cold hydrotherapy, or hot and cold compresses applied to the area to promote circulation.
	Magnesium/potassium/ bromelain 3 daily, with zinc 75Mg. ♂		
Add sea vegetables to the diet for extra iodine and potassium. (or try Crystal Star MIN-ZYME-MINOS DRINK).	Twin Lab LIQUID K 3t. daily, with GABA PLUS.	Evening Primrose oil 4 daily for essential fatty acids.	Shiatzu and massage therapy are effective in releasing and relieving muscle cramps.
Avoid refined sugars, processed and preserved foods. Food sensitivity to these are often the cause.	Solaray CAL/MAG CITRATE 4-6 daily.	Effective teas: ◆ Horsetail/Oatstraw ♀ ◆ Rosehips ♀ ◆ Passion Flower ◆ Alfalfa	
	Mezotrace SEA MINERAL COMPLEX, with Bromelain 500Mg. 3-4x daily.		
Take a good electrolyte drink often for good mineral salts transport.	DLPA or tryptophane for nerve tranquility.	Effective capsules: ◆ Kelp 6 daily ◆ Spitulina 4 daily ◆ Chlorella 15 daily	

COMMON SYMPTOMS: Uncontrollable spasms and twitches of the legs, facial muscles, etc.

COMMON CAUSES: Metabolic insufficiency of calcium, magnesium, potassium, trace minerals, and vitamins D and B$_6$; lack of sufficient HCl in the stomach; Vitamin C and silica deficiency causing poor collagen formation; food allergies to preservatives and colorants; iodine deficiency.

MYASTHENIA GRAVIS
MUSCLE WEAKNESS AND DEBILITATION

FOOD THERAPY

- Recovery from this wasting disease has shown marked success with improved diet. See ARTHRITIS AND HYPOGLYCEMIA DIET SUGGESTIONS in this book for effective diet information.

- Avoid all nightshade plants; tomatoes, eggplant, white potatoes, green peppers, etc.

- Eat potassium and magnesium-rich foods; particularly from whole grains, leafy greens, and green or potassium drinks.(Pg. 33-34)

  ☞ Take EGG YOLK LECITHIN 2-3x daily, with high potency ROYAL JELLY 40-50,000Mg. 2t. daily.

- Take 2t. wheat germ oil daily.

VITAMINS/ MINERALS

✣ Alta Health MANGANESE WITH B_{12} CAPS. with Twin Lab LIQUID K 3-4t. daily.♂

✣ Effective neuro-transmitters:
  ◆ Choline 600Mg. ♂
  ◆ Choline/Inositol ♀
  ◆ Lecithin 3x daily
  ◆ Phosphatidyl Choline (PC 55)

✣ Effective andtioxidants:
  ◆ Octacosonal ♂
  ◆ Vitamin E 800Mg. ♀
  ◆ B_{15} DMG sublingual
  ◆ Solaray TRI O_2 for better oxygen use.

✣ Cal/Mag/Zinc 4 daily, with Vitamin D 1000Mg.

✣ B Complex 100Mg. daily, with extra pantothenic acid 500Mg. and B_6 250Mg. daily.

✣ Glycine 500Mg. and/or Chromium picolinate. ♂

HERBAL THERAPY

❧ Evening Primrose oil caps 4-6 daily for prostaglandin production.

❧ Crystal Star MIN-ZYME-MINOS and ENERGY GREEN DRINKS to build strength.

❧ Crystal Star RELAX CAPS to feed and rebuild nerve strength.

❧ Ginkgo Biloba extract 2-3x daily if there is muscle tremor.♂

❧ White Birch Mineral Water as needed for a high source of potassium.

❧ Siberian Ginseng extract 3-4x daily for circulation increase, and Sun Chlorella for blood building and oxygen.♂

BODYWORK

✣ Avoid smoking, secondary smoke, and oxygen depleting pollutants as much as possible.

✣ Get some outdoor exercise every day for fresh air and aerobic lung and muscle tone.

✣ Massage therapy and shiatzu are both effective in increasing oxygen use and strengthening nerves and muscles.

✣ REFLEXOLOGY POINTS:

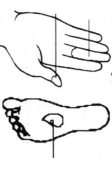

MUSCLES & NERVES

COMMON SYMPTOMS: Severe muscle weakness and fatigue, especially in the upper body; inability to perform even small tasks because of lack of strength; progressive inability, paralysis and exhaustion; double vision; choking; difficult breathing and swallowing; poor articulation and speech.

COMMON CAUSES: Chemistry failure between the nervous system and the muscles; choline and prostaglandin deficiency causing poor neurotransmission.

222

NAILS

FOOD THERAPY	VITAMINS/ MINERALS	HERBAL THERAPY	BODYWORK
Diet and nutrition are the key factors for nail health. ◆ Eat plenty of vegetable protein and calcium foods, such as whole grains, sprouts, leafy greens, molasses, and seafood.	❖ Cal/Mag/Zinc capsules 4 daily with Boron for better uptake. ♀	❧ **If your nail problem is a mineral deficiency; herb and plant minerals are the best choice for supplementation.**	❖ **Do not keep nails constantly polished. Allow them to "breathe" at least 1 day a week.**
To restore color and texture; mix a little honey, avocado oil, egg yolk, and a pinch of salt. Rub onto nails. Leave on 1/2 hour. Rinse off.	❖ **Zinc 50-100Mg. daily for spots or poor growth.**	❧ Horsetail tea or extract 3x daily for a month. or	❖ ACUPRESSURE POINT: Press 3x for 10 seconds each, the moon of each nail, to stimulate circulation.
	❖ Vit. E 400IU daily for ingrown or hang nail infections.	❧ Alta Health SIL-X SILICA CAPSULES 2-4 daily.	
To clear discolored nails; rub fresh lemon juice around the nail base.	❖ **Vit. A&D 25,000/1,000IU for poor growth/ridges.**	❧ Kelp tabs 6-8 daily.	❖ **To tint nails naturally: make a thin paste of red henna powder and water. Paint on and let dry in the sun. Rinse off. Pretty pink nails with no chipping.**
To strengthen weak nails; soak daily for 5 minutes in warm olive oil or cider vinegar.	❖ Betaine HCl for brittleness and white spots. ♂	❧ Crystal Star MEGA-MINERAL CAPSULES, or HIGHLY ABSORBABLE MINERAL COMPLEX EXTRACT for a month.	
	❖ **Raw Thyroid extract for spots or chipping.**	❧ Effective teas: Rosemary/Sage Dulse	❖ Use a green clay poultice to draw out a nail infection; use a wild alum (cranesbill) paste with water to relieve inflammation from ingrown or hang nails.
For hang and splitting nails; take 2T. brewer's yeast daily.	❖ Enzymatic Therapy ACID-A-CAL CAPSULES.	❧ For nail fungus; apply tea tree oil 3-4x daily.	
	❖ Mezotrace SEA MINERAL COMPLEX TABS, 4 daily.		

COMMON SYMPTOMS/ COMMON CAUSES: White spots- zinc, thyroid or HCl deficiency; discolored nails- Vit. B_{12} deficiency, kidney or liver problems; yellow nails- Vit. E deficiency, poor circulation; too white nails- liver malfunction, and general mineral deficiency; blue nails- lung and heart problems, drug reaction, blood toxicity from too much silver or copper; black bands on the nails- chemotherapy or radiation reaction; no half moons or ridged nails- Vit. A or protein deficiency; splitting, brittle or peeling nails- Vit. A & D deficiency, or thyroid problems, or iron, calcium or HCl deficiency; poor growth and shape- iron and zinc deficiency.

Nails can be very useful as an "early warning system" in diagnosing illness and evaluating health. They are one of the last tissues to receive the nutrients carried by the blood, and show signs of trouble before other better-nourished tissues do. Nail trimmings have been chemically analyzed by the medical community for years to determine mineral deficiencies or toxic substances in the body. Reliable analysis may also be done individually (See above). ◆ Give your program at least a month to show improvement. We have found that nothing seems to happen for 3 weeks, and noticeable changes appear in the 4th week.

223

NARCOLEPSY

FOOD THERAPY	VITAMINS/ MINERALS	HERBAL THERAPY	BODYWORK
The diet should be low in fats and clogging foods, such as dairy products and animal proteins; high in light cleansing foods, such as leafy greens and sea vegetables.	B Complex 150Mg. daily, with <u>extra B₆</u> 500Mg. daily.	Ginkgo Biloba extract as needed.	Make sure to take regular daily exercise for circulation and tissue oxygen.
See HYPOGLYCEMIA and THYROID HEALTH pages in this book for more information.	Country Life DMG B₁₅ daily as needed. or Unipro DMG <u>extract</u> under the tongue as needed.	Excel energy formulas, 1 tablet as needed, daily.♂	Biofeedback and chiropractic adjustment have both been effective in correcting the "electrical shorts" involved in brain to motor transmission.
Brewer's yeast and other foods high in B vitamins, such as brown rice, on a regular basis.	Effective neuro-transmitters:	Evening Primrose oil caps 4 daily for prostaglandin formation.	
	Octacosonal 1000Mg.♂ Choline 600Mg. Choline / Inositol	Crystal Star POTASSIUM CAPSULES with ADRN ALIVE CAPS for thyroid and adrenal energy, 2 each daily.♀	
	Enzymatic Therapy THYROID/ TYROSINE CAPSULES, 4 daily, with ADRENAL COMPLEX 2 daily. ♀	Solaray EPHEDRA CAPS 3-4 daily.♀	
	Chromium Picolinate 200Mcg. daily. with Omega 3 fish or flax oils 3-4x daily for sugar and essential fatty acid regulation. and		
	Magnesium 400Mg. 2x daily.		

COMMON SYMPTOMS: A chronic condition of excessive drowsiness, inappropriate and erratic periods of sleep, from which the sleeper is easily awakened; accompanying poor brain and adrenaline function.

COMMON CAUSES: Hypoglycemia; Vit. B₆ deficiency; low thyroid function and metabolism; heredity; poor assimilation and use of body oxygen.

NERVOUS TENSION

HYPERTENSION ♦ ANXIETY

FOOD THERAPY

❦ Diet improvement is a key factor in controlling nervous tension. ♦ Add to the diet regularly: high fiber foods, fresh greens, vegetable proteins, and natural sulfur foods, such as oat bran, lettuce, cucumbers, and celery. B vitamins are a key; eat plenty of brown rice, whole grains and leafy greens.

❦ Effective special foods:
♦ Brewer's yeast for High B vitamins.
♦ Sun seeds and molasses for thiamine and iron.
♦ Carrot/Celery juice for nerve restoration.
♦ Green drinks (Pg. 34) for chlorophyll.
♦ Wheat germ oil 1t. daily

❦ Make sure the diet is low in salt (see pg. 44), and saturated fats.

❦ Avoid acid-forming foods, such as red meats, caffeine, carbonated drinks, (the phophorus binds up magnesium, making it unavailable. Magnesium is a key mineral for controlling hypertension.)

VITAMINS/ MINERALS

✢ Country Life MAXI B COMPLEX w/ TAURINE daily with extra B_1 500Mg

✢ Ascorbate or Ester C 3-5,000Mg. daily with Bioflavonoids and Rutin 500Mg. each.

✢ Alta Health CANGEST with meals, and MAGNESIUM CHLORIDE daily.

✢ Alta Health MANGANESE WITH B_{12} SUBLINGUAL.

✢ Twin Lab TRYPTOPHANE PLUS as needed.

✢ Rainbow Light CALCIUM PLUS with high magnesium, 4 daily.

✢ Nature's Plus MAGNESIUM/POTASSIUM/ BROMELAIN CAPSULES.♂

✢ Mezotrace SEA MINERAL COMPLEX 2-3 daily.

✢ Vitamin E 400IU daily or Phos. Choline 1 daily.

HERBAL THERAPY

❧ Crystal Star RELAX CAPS and TEA as needed.
and
MIN-ZYME-MINOS DRINK and/or HAWTHORNE EXTRACT as a tonic..

❧ Crystal Star HI-PRESSURE CARE CAPS with MEGA MINERAL CAPS 2-4 daily.

❧ Effective capsules:
Ginseng/Gotu Kola ♂
Bee Pollen ♂
Garlic 6 daily
Siberian Ginseng extract

❧ Effective teas:
Chamomile
Peppermint/Hops
Rosemary
Scullcap
Catnip ☺

❧ Deva Flowers ANXIETY DROPS as needed.

❧ Omega 3 Flax oil 3x daily.

BODYWORK

❖ Tobacco and obesity both aggravate nerve disorders and tension. Lose weight and stop smoking.

❖ REFLEXOLOGY POINT:

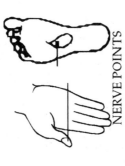

NERVE POINTS

❖ Aromatherapy: Peppermint oil, or Cinnamon oil.

❖ Wear acupressure sandals for a short period every day to clear reflexology meridians.

❖ Take a brisk walk with deep breathing every day.

❖ See HIGH BLOOD PRESSURE DIET SUGGESTIONS for more information.

COMMON SYMPTOMS: Extreme nervousness and irritability; often high blood pressure; lack of energy; chronic headaches; heart disease proneness.

COMMON CAUSES: Too many refined foods, especially sugars; smoking stress; hyperthyroidism and metabolic imbalance; prostaglandin deficiency.

NEURITIS ✧ NEURALGIA

FOOD THERAPY	VITAMINS/ MINERALS	HERBAL THERAPY	BODYWORK

❦ Go on a short 24 hour liquid diet to rebalance body pH,(acid/alkaline). Then, for the rest of the week eat mostly raw fresh foods, with plenty of leafy greens, sprouts, celery sea vegetables, and enzyme foods such as apples and pineapple. **Take a glass of lemon juice and water every morning. Have a potassium broth or essence (Pg. 33) every other day.**

❦ Take 2T. each daily:
Lecithin granules
Sesame Seeds
Brewer's yeast
Wheat germ

❦ **Avoid caffeine, hard liquor and soft drinks, that bind up magnesium.**

❦ Keep salts, saturated fats, and sugars low.

❦ See "COOKING FOR HEALTHY HEALING" by Linda Rector-Page for a complete diet for nerve conditions.

❖ **Niacin Therapy: 500-1500Mg. daily, with Bromelain 500Mg.**
or
Quercitin Plus with Bromelain 3-4 daily
and
Ascorbate or Ester C with bioflavonoids and rutin, 5000Mg. daily, to rebuild connective tissue.

❖ **Stress B Complex 150Mg. with extra B$_6$ 250Mg. and pantothenic acid 500Mg.**
and
Phosphatidyl Choline.

❖ Ener B$_{12}$ INTERNASAL GEL every other day.

❖ **Hylands NERVE TONIC.**

❖ **Country Life LIGATEND CAPS as needed.**

❖ **Chromium Picolinate 200Mcg. 2-3 daily.**

❖ **DLPA 750Mg. as needed for pain.**

❧ **Crystal Star RELAX CAPS as needed for rebuilding the nerve sheath 2-4 daily.**

❧ **Evening Primrose oil caps 4 daily, with the following tea daily to rebuild nerves.**
Equal parts: St. John's Wort, Peppermint, Lavender, Valerian, Lemon Balm, Blessed Thistle.

❧ Effective extract:
Lobelia
valerian
Passion Flower
Scullcap
Ginkgo Biloba

❧ Crystal Star BONZ CAPS to relieve inflammation, 4 daily.
PANEX or ANTI-SPAZ CAPS as needed for pain.

❧ **Crystal Star POTASSIUM SOURCE CAPSULES 4 daily as an effective source of sea vegetables.**

❖ Get some regular mild exercise every day for body oxygen and circulation.

❖ Use hot and cold hydrotherapy to stimulate circulation (Pg.31-32).

❖ Do 10 neck rolls as needed at a time to relieve nerve trauma.

❖ Chiropractic adjustment, shiatzu, and massage therapy are all effective in controlling these nerve disorders.

❖ REFLEXOLOGY POINT:

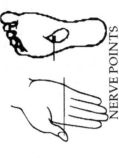

NERVE POINTS

❖ Apply B&T TRI-FLORA ANALGESIC GEL.

COMMON SYMPTOMS: Muscle weakness and degeneration; burning, tingling, numbness in the muscles; motor and reflex weakness; nerve inflammation.

COMMON CAUSES: Spinal pinch or lesions; excess alcohol or prescription drugs; prostaglandin deficiency; diabetic reaction; herpes; poor circulation; multiple sclerosis type weakness and numbness; kidney and gallbladder malfunction; arthritis; lupus; migraines; heavy metal poisoning.

NUMBNESS ✧ NERVE PARALYSIS

FOOD THERAPY	VITAMINS/ MINERALS	HERBAL THERAPY	BODYWORK
❦ Go on a short 24 hour liquid diet (Pg.27) to lighten the circulatory load and clean out waste.	✤ Rainbow Light CALCIUM PLUS CAPS with high magnesium, 4 daily.	❧ Crystal Star RELAX CAPS to rebuild nerve sheathing, with HEMA-CLEANSE TEA daily.	✤ Apply Cayenne/Ginger compresses to the area.
❦ Then, eat only fresh foods for 3-4 days to alkalize and clean the bloodstream. Follow with a modified macrobiotic diet (Pg. 42) for 3-4 weeks, emphasizing whole grains and vegetable proteins, til condition clears.	✤ Barley GREEN MAGMA, 2 packets daily for nerve restoration. or Sun CHLORELLA TABS, 15 daily.	❧ Kukicha twig tea, 2 cups daily with Cayenne/Ginger caps 3 daily for 1-2 months.	✤ Apply B&T TRIFLORA ANALGESIC GEL.
	✤ B Complex 100Mg. daily with extra B₆ 500Mg. if the extremeties are periodically numb. or B₆ 250Mg. 6-8x daily, if numbness is from nerve interference or a stroke.	❧ Ginkgo Biloba extract as needed to balance circulation.	✤ Use alternating hot and cold hydrotherapy (Pg. 31-32).
		❧ Butcher's Broom capsules, 2-4 daily.	✤ Acupuncture, massage therapy, shiatzu, and chiropractic adjustment have all shown excellent results with these conditions.
❦ Take 2T. each daily: Brewer's yeast Unsulphured molasses	✤ Niacin Therapy: 500Mg. or more daily. with Vitamin C up to 5000Mg. daily with bioflavonoids and rutin for nerve connective tissue.	❧ Effective teas: best taken at night. Ginger/Oatstraw Scullcap	✤ REFLEXOLOGY POINT:
	✤ Enzymatic Therapy THYROID/TYROSINE CAPS, 4 daily.	❧ Crystal Star CIRCU-EXTRA EXTRACT as needed to increase circulation.	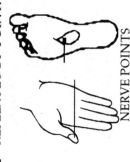 NERVE POINTS

B Complex 100Mg. daily with extra B_6 500Mg.
B_6 250Mg. 6-8x daily

COMMON SYMPTOMS: Lack of feeling in various parts of the body; "going to sleep" in the extremeties.

COMMON CAUSES: Poor circulation; thyroid deficiency; pinched nerve or spinal lesions; stroke and brain dysfunction; multiple sclerosis type nerve damage; poor diet with too many mucous-forming foods.

OSTEOPOROSIS

FOOD THERAPY

❧ **Vegetarians have denser, stronger bones. Avoid red meats. Have a fresh green salad every day.** Take a high protein drink several times a week.

❧ **Eat plenty of calcium and potassium foods;** broccoli, sea vegetables, fish and seafood, eggs, yogurt, kefir, sprouts, miso, beans, leafy greens, tofu, bananas, dry fruits, molasses.

❧ Avoid sugar, caffeine and caffeine-containing foods, hard liquor, tobacco, and nightshade plants that interfere with calcium absorption.

❧ **Contrary to popular belief, pasteurized milk is not a very good source of absorbable calcium. It actually interferes with mineral assimilation.**

❧ See "COOKING FOR HEALTHY HEALING" by Linda Rector-Page for a complete bone-building diet.

VITAMINS/ MINERALS

❖ Vitamin C or Ester C with Bioflavs. and rutin, up to 5000Mg. daily for connective tissue health.
with
Vit. D 1000IU, Marine Carotene 50,000IU, and Zinc 30Mg. daily.

❖ Alta Health SIL-X SILICA, 10 daily for 15 days, then 5 daily for 15 days, then 2 daily for 3-4 months.
with
Manganese with B_{12}.

❖ **Calcium Citrate 1500Mg. and Magnesium 1000Mg. with Boron for absorption and metabolism.**

❖ Solaray TRI O_2 CAPS for germanium and CO Q 10,
with
Ener B INTERNASAL B_{12} GEL every other day.

❖ **Enzymatic Therapy OSTEOPRIME CAPSULES.**

❖ Mezotrace SEA MINERAL COMPLEX, **with** Betaine HCl for absorption.

HERBAL THERAPY

❧ Crystal Star BONZ CAPS and/or TEA 2X daily, with other estrogen-forming herbs, such as SUPER LICORICE or DONG QUAI/ DAMIANA EXTRACT, or ESTR-AID or **Black Cohosh caps for marrow development.**

❧ Other Crystal Star mineral formulas for bone health:
◆ MEGA-MINERAL CAPS
◆ POTASSIUM SOURCE CAPS
◆ CALCIUM SOURCE CAPS AND EXTRACT
◆ SILICA SOURCE EXTRACT (dietary Silica biologically engenders calcium production in the body).

❧ Solaray ALFAJUICE CAPS

❧ Evening primrose oil caps 6 daily, with Crystal Star MIN-ZYME-MINOS DRINK.

❧ Effective teas: Horsetail/Comfrey Rt. Dandelion/Nettles Sarsaparilla

BODYWORK

❖ **Exercise is one of the best ways to build bone and prevent bone loss. It is a prime nutrient in itself.**

❖ Avoid fluorescent lighting, electric blankets, aluminum cookware, non-filtered computor screens, etc..All tend to leach calcium from the body.

❖ **Get some early morning sunlight on the body every day possible for Vitamin D.**

❖ Cortico-steroid drugs over a long period of time leach potassium from the system and weaken the bones.

❖ REFLEXOLOGY POINT:

SPINE

COMMOMSYMPTOMS: Decrease in bone mass and density; porous and open spaces in the bones where supporting structure is lost; weight and height loss; easy bone breaks; thin, brittle bones.

COMMON CAUSES: Menopause and estrogen deficiency; poor use of synthetic estrogen; mineral, (calcium and magnesium) protein and collagen deficiency; poor Vitamin C use and assimilation; prostaglandin deficiency; too much cortisone and antibiotics; smoking; excess sugar and hard liquor consumption; heavy metal and environmental pollutants,(especially cadmium); stress.

IMPORTANT FACTS TO HELP YOU ARREST & AVOID OSTEOPOROSIS & POST-MENOPAUSAL BONE LOSS

Osteoporosis is an extremely complex problem with multiple facets, and multiple factors contributing to its onset. These primarily include 1)a drop in estrogen levels; 2) thyroid and parathyroid malfunction; 3) low intake of dietary calcium and minerals; 4) poor collagen/protein development; 5) general poor nourishment.

Osteoporosis can be treated nutritionally. It can be arrested and current bone mass maintained. But the program must be continued, or bone loss will continue.

Bone and cartilege are an ever-changing infrastructure of the body. They need mineral-rich nutrition for strength and health. Minerals and trace minerals are the building blocks of the body, the most basic elements needed for growth. Healthy bones act as reservoirs for the body's mineral needs. They are also the bonding agents between you and your food. Without them the body is not able to absorb nutrients or utilize food. **Minerals and trace minerals** cannot be made by the body, and must be taken in regularly through food and drink. Dietary calcium from food, herbs and food source supplements, is far superior in absorption and benefits, because it occurs naturally with estrogen-forming, and other substances to insure assimilation. Dietary silica for instance, biologically engenders to calcium production in the body. **Minerals are of prime importance to bone health.** Organically grown foods and herbs are the best way to get them.
Vitamin D deficiency, not older age, is a more usual cause of poor calcium absorption. Get some early morning sunlight on the body every day possible, preferably while taking a brisk daily walk.

Life style, heredity, and body type all play significant parts in an osteoporosis risk profile. Here are the higher risk factors:
- ❖ Female, small-boned, white or asian, with a family history of osteoporosis.
- ❖ Lifelong low calcium and vitamin D intake.
- ❖ Removal of ovaries before menopause, or early menopause, before 45 years old.
- ❖ No child-bearing.
- ❖ Irregular or no menstrual periods.
- ❖ Consistently high consumption of hard alcohol, cigarettes, caffeine and animal proteins.
- ❖ Regular and consistent use of certain medications, such as corticosteroids.
- ❖ Have reached an advanced age.

Remember that poor hormone production greatly increases the risk of osteoporosis regardless of age. Hormone and calcium deficiencies appear regularly in women with irregular menstrual cycles because of excessive running or exercise, or who are bulemic or anorexic. Over 50% of American women suffer from calcium deficiency alone. (Taking a calcium citrate **supplement before a period can let you know if this is your problem.** Calcium deficiencies show up premenstrually as back pain, tooth pain, and cramping. **Calcium supplementation should help these symptoms disappear).**

You can test yourself for probable osteoporosis. Use pH paper (sold in most health food stores), and test your urine. A habitual reading below pH 7 (acid) usually leads to calcium and bone loss. Above pH 7 (alkaline) indicates a low risk system.

◆NOTE: Since few men experience osteoporosis because of their increased testosterone supply, new research is centering on natural testosterone sources such as Smilx for supplementation in arresting bone loss. Herbal extracts of Sarsaparilla are now being used experimentally with some hope for success.

♀ OVARIAN & UTERINE CYSTS & FIBROIDS ♀

FOOD THERAPY

❧ Follow a low fat, fresh foods vegetarian diet. High fats mean high estrogen production. (too much estrogen is a common cause of cysts and fibroids)
◆ Get adequate high quality protein daily (about 60-70 grams from largely vegetable sources, to avoid saturated fats): whole grains, sprouts, tofu, sea foods, low fat dairy, etc.
◆ Increase intake of B vitamin foods, such as brown rice, wheat germ and brewer's yeast.
◆ Avoid red meat, caffeine and refined sugars that can cause iodine deficiency.
◆ Add miso, sea vegetables, and leafy greens to alkalize the system.
◆ Avoid fried and salty foods, especially during menses.
◆ Avoid concentrated starches, full fat dairy products, and hard liquor on a continuing basis.

❧ Keep the diet high in fresh foods (about 50-60%). Drink only bottled water

❧ Take 4t. wheat germ oil daily for tissue oxygen.

❧ Have some fresh apple or carrot juice every day.

VITAMINS/ MINERALS

❖ Nature's Plus Vitamin E 800IU during healing. with Twin Lab MARINE CAROTENE 100,000IU daily.

❖ High Omega 3 oils or Shark Liver oil as an anti-infective.

❖ Ascorbate Vitamin C, Ester C with Bioflavonoids, or Quercitin Plus, 5000Mg. daily. with Alta Health SIL-X SILICA for collagen regrowth.

❖ Food grade H₂O₂ PEROXY GEL rubbed on the fibroids. Noticeable reduction in 3-6 weeks.

❖ Sun CHLORELLA 20 daily and Germanium 100Mg. daily as antioxidants.

❖ Enzymatic Therapy RAW MAMMARY CAPS or RAW OVARY CAPS, or NucleoPro F CAPS.

HERBAL THERAPY

❧ Crystal Star WOMAN'S BEST FRIEND CAPSULES, 4 daily for 3 months. with Evening Primrose oil caps 4-6 daily for 3 months. then

❧ Crystal Star FEMALE HARMONY CAPSULES 2 daily as a hormone balancer to prevent return.

❧ Iodine Therapy: (often effective in 3-4 months.) ATOMODINE or MIODIN DROPS 2-3X daily. and/or Crystal Star IODINE THERAPY CAPS/ EXTRACT. (Take with vit.E for best results)

❧ Effective extracts: Echinacea Sarsaparilla (as a source of progesterone) Dong Quai/Damiana C.Star.SILICA SOURCE

❧ Crystal Star ANTI-SPAZ CAPS or CRAMP CONTROL EXTRACT for cramping.

BODYWORK

❖ Be careful of jumping into surgery. Many of these cysts/fibroids disappear by themselves.

❖ Avoid IUDs and X-rays as causes of fibroid tumors.
Remember that synthetic estrogen increases the risk of uterine, ovarian and breast cancer.

❖ REFLEXOLOGY POINT:

UTERUS & OVARIES

❖ Pain in the heels, and swollen breasts at times other than menses, indicate ovarian cysts.

❖ See ENDOMETRIOSIS and BREAST FIBROIDS pages in this book for more information.

COMMON SYMPTOMS: Acute or chronic pain in the fallopian tubes or ovaries; disturbance in the normal menstrual cycle, with unfamialiar pain and discomfort in the lower abdomen; painful intercourse; infertility;unusual abdominal swelling gas and pain; fever and coated tongue.

COMMON CAUSES: IUDs and/or radiation and X-rays that change cell function and structure; prostaglandin and EFA deficiency; too much caffeine and saturated fats in the diet; high dose birth control pills and synthetic estrogen; obesity; hypertension; diabetes; high stress lifestyle and over-acid diet producing acid wastes in the body that are poorly eliminated because of chronic constipation.

FOOD THERAPY	VITAMINS/ MINERALS	HERBAL THERAPY	BODYWORK
Diet can be a key factor in preventing PMS. A mild LIVER CLEANSING DIET, or a modified HYPOGLY-CEMIA DIET are both effective. (See those pages in this book).	Enzymatic Therapy RAW OVARY and RAW MAMMARY CAPS daily. or NUCLEOPRO F CAPS. (May also be chewed for almost immediate results.) or PMX CAPSULES.	Evening Primrose oil 4-6 daily the 1st month, then 2-4 daily the 2nd month. with Crystal Star FEMALE HARMONY CAPSULES 2 daily each month. Add 2 CRISIS CAPS, or 2 Bayberry capsules daily if flow is excessively heavy.	Treat yourself to a good massage or shatzu session before your period to loosen and release clogging mucous and fatty formations and to cleanse the system.
Get plenty of low fat protein from vegetable sources, such as whole grains, legumes, soy foods, sprouts, or sea foods. Or take a protein drink such as Nature's Plus SPIRUTEIN each morning.	Nature's Plus vitamin E 800IU. with Alta Health MAGNESIUM, & sublingual B_{12} 2500Mg.	Crystal Star WOMAN'S BEST FRIEND CAPS on a regular basis to prevent cramping and pain. During the period, use ANTI-SPAZ CAPS, 4 at a time, FLOW EASE TEA, or CRAMP CONTROL EXTRACT as needed.	Stop smoking and avoid secondary smoke, Nicotine inhibits good hormone function.
Keep the diet low in fats salt and sugar, high in greens and whole grains. Eat plenty of cultured foods, such as yogurt and kefir for friendly flora.	Effective brand products: ◆ Schiff PMS FORMULA 1 & 2 ◆ Natrol SAF capsules ◆ Country Life RELAXER CAPS ◆ Rainbow Light PMS CAPS	Crystal Star RELAX CAPS for stress and tension.	Get plenty of fresh air and sunshine during your period. Take a brisk walk every day.
Avoid caffeine, caffeine-containing foods, red meat, and saturated fat animal products.	Vitamin B_6 250Mg. 2x daily.	Woman's Health RELEAF FORMULA 3-4 daily.	Apply ice packs to the pelvic area.
	MIODIN or ATOMODINE DROPS, or Source Naturals FRAC to relieve breast swelling and soreness.	Effective extracts: ◆ Dong Quai/Damiana ◆ Sarsaparilla ◆ Nature's Way ANTSP ◆ Cramp Bark	For facial blemishes at period time, apply liquid chlorophyll as needed.
Take 2T. each daily: Brewer's yeast Lecithin granules	For daily prevention: B Complex 100Mg. with extra B_6, vitamin C with bioflavonoids and rutin, and emulsified A&D 25,000IU/1,000IU.		REFLEXOLOGY POINT:
Drink only bottled water.	High omega 3 oils 3 daily.	Effective teas: ◆ Hops/Blue Cohosh ◆ Burdock Rt. ◆ Licorice/Sarsaparilla	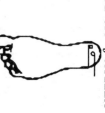 UTERUS & OVARIES

MORE INFORMATION ABOUT P.M.S.

The intricacies of a woman's body are very delicately tuned, and can become unbalanced or obstructed easily, causing pain, poor function, and lack of "oneness" that often results in physiological and emotional problems, especially during the menstrual cycle. Drugs, chemicals and synthetic medicines, standing as they do outside this natural cycle, often do not bring positive results for women. These substances usually try to add something to the woman's body, or act directly on a specific problem area. A highly nutritious diet, herbs as concentrated foods, and naturally-derived vitamin compounds are identified and used by the woman's own individual enzyme action. These nutrients encourage the body to do its own work, providing balance and relief that is much more gratifying.

The suggestions outlined above usually take 2 months to effect complete relief, as the body works through both ovary cycles. The first month, there is noticeable decrease in P.M.S. symptoms; the second month finds them virtually gone. Since the problem is so frequently a hormone imbalance (too much estrogen, too little progesterone), continuing with the diet recommendations, and lower doses of the herb and/or vitamin choices, make sense toward preventing P.M.S. return.

Prostaglandin formation is a key to controlling P.M.S. Prostaglandins are vital hormone-type compounds that act as transient hormones, regulating all body functions electrically. Supplementing the body's essential fatty acid supply through dietary means, such as ocean fish, sea foods and olive, safflower, or sunflower oils, or herbs, such as Evening Primrose and flax oils, can have the strong benefit of controlling P.M.S. Conversely, excess saturated fats in the body, especially from fatty animal foods, inhibit both prostaglandin production and flow.

COMMON SYMPTOMS: Mood swings, tension, irritability, and depression; argumentative, aggressive behavior; water retention, bloating, and constipation; headaches and lower back pain; sore and swollen breasts; nausea; heavy cramping and excessive menstrual flow; low biorhythm and low energy; food cravings for salt and sweets with extreme thirst; alcohol craving; nerve pain; acne and skin eruptions; light-headedness.

COMMON CAUSES: Prostaglandin malfunction and/or deficiency; estrogen excess or imbalance because of liver malfunction; glandular insufficiency (especially the thyroid); lack of regular exercise; poor diet with lack of B vitamins, and magnesium, calcium and protein deficiencies; poor circulation; too much salt, red meat, sugar and caffeine; stress and emotional tension

232

PAIN

CHRONIC ◆ LOWER BACK ◆ JOINT & NERVE

FOOD THERAPY	VITAMINS/ MINERALS	HERBAL THERAPY	BODYWORK
❧ Make sure the diet is rich in complex carbohydrates and vegetable proteins for strength: plenty of whole grains, broccoli, peas, brown rice, legumes, sea foods, etc.	✥ DLPA 500-750Mg. as needed daily, ♀ with CO Q 10 30Mg. 2x daily and/or Quercitin Plus with Bromelain 500Mg. ♂	❧ Crystal Star PANEX CAPS or ANTI-SPAZ CAPS , 4 at a time, and/or CRAMP CONTROL EXTRACT, or RELAX CAPS as needed.	❖ Chiropractic adjustment, shiatzu massage, bio-feedback, acupuncture, and massage therapy are all effective in controlling pain.
❧ Have a green drink(pg. 34), and/or a green leafy salad every day.	✥ Solaray Calcium Citrate 1000Mg. daily, with Ascorbate vitamin C with bioflavonoids and rutin 5000Mg. daily for connective tissue formation.	❧ Crystal Star BONZ CAPS 4-6 daily, with MIN-ZYME-MINOS DRINK or MEGA MINERAL CAPS to alkalize and rebuild body and muscle strength.	❖ Effective compresses: Plantain/Marshmallow Comfrey Lobelia
❧ Take 2 T. each daily: ◆ Brewer's yeast ◆ Cider Vinegar and honey in water.		❧ Apply B&T TRI-FLORA ANALGESIC GEL.	❖ Effective oil rubs: Mullein Tea Tree Tiger Balm Wintergreen/Cajeput
❧ Avoid caffeine, salty foods and refined sugars.	✥ Country Life LIGATEND CAPSULES as needed daily with RELAXER CAPSULES .	❧ Effective extracts: ◆ Valerian/Wild Lettuce ◆ Crystal Star HIGHLY ABSORBABLE CALCIUM ♀	❖ Acupressure: pinch and massage webs between the thumb and index finger to reduce pain.
❧ Add high mineral foods to the diet for strength. Emphasize magnesium and calcium foods for bone and muscle health. (See "COOKING FOR HEALTHY HEALING" by Linda Rector-Page for an effective high mineral diet.)	✥ Enzymatic Therapy MYOTONE CAPSULES.		❖ REFLEXOLOGY POINT: 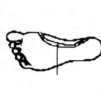 SPINE
	✥ Twin Lab GABA PLUS CAPS with Tryptophane 1000Mg daily.		
	✥ B Complex 100Mg. with ENER B INTERNASAL B_{12} .		

COMMON SYMPTOMS: Pain is a mechanism to draw attention to a problem that the autonomic system cannot handle by itself. Pain signals to consciously address the underlying cause. Muscle wasting; poor reflexes; numbness; sorenesss in the sensory nerves.

COMMON CAUSES: Poor posture; poor nutrition with lack of green vegetables and calcium-rich foods; poor muscle development; adrenal and pituitary gland exhaustion; flat feet; obesity; internal or external tumors or growths.

PARASITES ✧ INTESTINAL WORMS

FOOD THERAPY

🍃 **Go on an apple juice fast and mono diet for 4 days.** (One day for a child) ☺

◆ Take 6-8 garlic capsules daily during this time, and chew fresh papaya seeds mixed with honey frequently.

◆ On the 3ʳᵈ day, add papaya juice with 1 T. wormwood tea, and 1 T. molasses.

◆ On the 4ᵗʰ day, add 2 cups senna/peppermint tea with 1 T. castor oil, and eat a handful of raw pumpkin seeds every 4 hours.

🍃 **After worms are gone, eat a high vegetable protein diet and lots of culture foods, such as yogurt, to rebuild intesinal tract.**

🍃 **Then, a high resistance diet must be followed to prevent recurrence. Eat lots of onions and garlic. Avoid sweets, pasteurized milk and refined foods. Eat a leafy green salad every day.**

🍃 **No junk foods!**

VITAMINS/ MINERALS

✤ **Take garlic oil capsules in the morning. Refrain from eating or drinking til bowels have moved. Repeat for 3 days.**

✤ Solaray GARLIC/BLACK WALNUT CAPSULES. ♀

✤ Nature's Way HERBAL PUMPKIN FORMULA. ♂

✤ Floradix HERBAL IRON LIQUID for strength during healing.
with
✤ B Complex 50Mg. daily. ♀

✤ Beta Carotene 50,000IU daily as an anti-infective.

✤ Aloe Vera juice 2-3 glasses daily.

HERBAL THERAPY

🐛 Take psyllium husk in water 3x daily, and 2 cups daily senna tea to purge.

🐛 **Black Walnut extract 4-6x daily.**
with
Barberry tea as an anti-infective.

🐛 Crystal Star VERMEX CAPSULES, 4 daily <u>with</u> 2 garlic capsules, after every meal for 2 weeks.
<u>and</u>
4 cups fennel tea daily.
and/or
Crystal Star ANTI-BIO CAPS 4 daily.

🐛 For crabs and lice; apply Thyme oil
Tea Tree oil

🐛 Effective teas:
Valerian
Chaparral
Wormwood/Tansy
Chamomile
Pau de Arco

BODYWORK

❖ Dietary and nutritional therapy is a good choice for thread and pin worms, but is very slow in cases of heavy infestation. Short term allopathic means can be more beneficial for masses of hook and tape worms.

❖ **Garlic enemas daily as needed during healing.**

❖ **Apply Zinc oxide to opening of anus. Then take a warm sitz bath using 1 1/2 cups epsom salts per gallon of water. Repeat for 3 days. Worms will often expel into the sitz bath.**

COMMON SYMPTOMS: Diarrhea and other abnormal bowel conditions; stomach pains and chronic indigestion; appetite and weight loss; colic and weakness in children; irritability; fatigue; anal inflammation and irritation.

COMMON CAUSES: Lowered immune defenses allowing infestation; poor diet with too much sugar and refined carbohydrates(junk foods); too much red meat; poor hygiene; fungal and yeast overgrowth conditions; infested, uncooked, poorly cooked, or spoiled meat.

PARKINSONS DISEASE

FOOD THERAPY

❧ Go on a completely fresh foods diet for 3 days to cleanse and alkalize the body. **Use organically grown foods wherever possible.**
Then, follow a modified macrobiotic diet (Pg. 42) for 3-6 months til condition improves.
Use short 24 hr. juice fasts (Pg.27) once every two weeks during healing.

❧ Take green drinks (Pg. 34) frequently, at least once a week.

❧ Drink only bottled water.

❧ Take 2T. each daily:
Lecithin granules
Brewer's yeast

❧ Eat smaller meals more frequently. No large, heavy meals.

❧ See ANEMIA and M.S. DIET SUGGESTIONS in this book for more information.

VITAMINS/ MINERALS

✤ Twin Lab GABA PLUS, or Country Life RELAXER CAPS as needed.
or
DLPA 500-750Mg. as needed for depression.

✤ Tyrosine 500Mg. 2x daily for L-Dopa production.
with
Tryptophane 500Mg. to aid serutonin formation.

✤ High Omega 3 flax or fish oils 3x daily.

✤ Niacin Therapy: 500Mg. 2x daily.
with
B Complex 100Mg. with extra B₆ 500Mg.daily.
and
Ener B INTERNASAL GEL

✤ Phosphatidyl Choline (PC 55) 2 daily.

✤ Nature's Plus Vitamin E 800Mg. with Dyna Mins Magnesium 500Mg. ♀

✤ Enzymatic Therapy Raw Brain & Adrenal complex.

HERBAL THERAPY

❧ Evening Primrose oil caps 4-6 daily for GLA.
with
Crystal Star RELAX CAPS to rebuild nerve sheath.
and
MENTAL CLARITY CAPS or GINKGO BILOBA EXTRACT for brain and tremor.
then
ADRN CAPS with MIN-ZYME-MINOS DRINK to restore strength.

❧ Ginseng/Royal Jelly vials, 1 daily. ♂

❧ Solaray Ginseng/Damiana and Cayenne/Ginseng.

❧ Sun CHLORELLA or BARLEY GREEN MAGMA 1 packet daily.

❧ Effective teas:
Pau de Arco
Crystal Star FEEL GREAT
Sun SIBERIAN GINSENG

❧ Aloe Vera juice daily, with
❧ Unsprayed bee pollen 2t. daily. ♂

BODYWORK

✤ Chiropractic treatment, shiatzu, acupuncture and acupressure have had some success in reversing early Parkinsons.

✤ REFLEXOLOGY POINT:

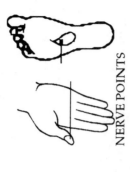

NERVE POINTS

✤ Take long warm baths. Crystal Star LOVE BATH FOR MEN has had some success.

✤ Use catnip enemas once a week to encourage Liver/Kidney function.

✤ **Avoid aluminum** (cookware, deodorants with aluminum chloride, condiments with alum, etc.)and heavy metals that lodge in the brain and nerve centers.

COMMON SYMPTOMS: Central nervous system dysfunction affecting normal posture and movement; clear brain abnormality; muscle rigidity and lethargic movement speech difficulty; vision problems; depression (which can show dramatic improvement with supplementation); tremor.

COMMON CAUSES: Aluminum and heavy metal toxicity; over-use of some drugs; allergy reaction; nerve malfunction; poor diet allowing degeneration.

PHLEBITIS ♦ EMBOLISM ♦ THROMBOSIS

BLOOD CLOTS

FOODS THERAPY	VITAMINS/ MINERALS	HERBAL THERAPY	BODYWORK
❧ Have a leafy green salad every day. Have one glass of each every other day: ◆ Black Cherry juice ◆ Fresh carrot juice ◆ Crystal Star ENERGY GREEN DRINK or other green drink (Pg.34)	❖ Nature's Plus vitamin E 800IU to keep body oxygen in good compound form. ❖ Bromelain 500Mg. 2 daily. and/or Quercitin Plus as an anti-inflammatory for fragile veins.	❧ Crystal Star HEMA-CLEANSE TEA with CARDI-STRENGTH CAPS and HAWTHORNE EXTRACT 2-4x daily. ❧ Butcher's Broom capsules and/or Kukicha Twig tea ♀	❖ Deep vein thrombosis is life-threatening. Get medical help immediately! ❖ Elevate legs whenever possible. No prolonged sitting. Consciously stretch and walk frequently during the day. Take a brisk half hour walk daily.
❧ Drink 6-8 glasses of bottled water daily. ❧ Take 2T. each daily: Lecithin granules Brewer's yeast	❖ Kal Pycnogenol caps with Ascorbate vitamin C crystals with bioflavs and rutin, 1/4t. daily to bowel tolerance. and High Omega 3 flax or fish oils 3 daily. ♂	❧ Evening Primrose oil caps 4-6 daily. with Crystal Star ANEMIGIZE CAPS 3 daily to stimulate spleen activity.	❖ Avoid smoking and secondary smoke. It constricts blood vessels and restricts oxygen use.
❧ Avoid all starchy, fried and fatty foods. Avoid refined sugars, caffeine and hard liquor.	❖ Niacin Therapy: 500Mg. 3x daily, with Chromium picolinate 200Mcg. daily. or Solaray CHROMIACIN ♀	❧ Effective extracts: ◆ Bilberry ◆ Echinacea ◆ Enzymatic Therapy HERBAL FLAVONOIDS ♀	❖ Avoid chemical anti-coagulants and oral contraceptives unless absolutely necessary.
❧ Eat plenty of onions, garlic and other high sulphur foods. Have an ONION/GARLIC BROTH at least 2-3x a week (Pg. 36).	❖ Biotec EXTRA ENERGY ENZYMES 6 daily for free radical scavenging.	❧ Effective compresses: ◆ Plantain ◆ Witch Hazel ◆ Fresh Comfrey leaf	❖ Take alternating hot and cold sitz baths, and/or apply alternating hot and cold ginger/cayenne compresses to stimulate leg blood circulation.
❧ See HEALTHY HEART DIET in this book for more information.	❖ Enzymatic Therapy SPLEEN & LYMPH COMPLEX	❧ Apply B&T CALIFLORA GEL	❖ Keep weight down to relieve pressure on weak circulatory system.

COMMON SYMPTOMS: Swelling, inflammation; redness and aching in the legs; fever with blood clots in the legs.

COMMON CAUSES: Clogged and toxic bloodstream from excess saturated fats, especially from too much red meat and fried food; inactivity, lack of daily exercise, and sedentary life style; poor circulation from constipation, obesity or weak heart; oral contraceptive side-effect; prolonged emotional stress.

PITUITARY & PINEAL GLANDS

MASTER GLAND HEALTH TO RETARD AGING, RELEASE ENERGY, AND INCREASE BODY BUILDING

FOOD THERAPY	VITAMINS/ MINERALS	HERBAL THERAPY	BODYWORK
❧ Eat plenty of green leafy vegetables every day. Have a green drink (Pg. 34) once a week.	✤ Mezotrace SEA MINERAL COMPLEX 3-4 daily.	❧ Crystal Star MASTER BUILDER CAPSULES 2 daily. with	✤ ACUPRESSURE POINTS: Press for 10 seconds, 3x each over the left eyebrow for pituitary stimulation; on the forehead where the eyebrows meet for pineal stimulation.
❧ Eat plenty of complex carbohydrates; broccoli, potatoes, sprouts, peas, dried fruits, whole grains and brown rice, etc.	✤ Vitamin C or Ester C with Bioflavonoids and Rutin, 550 Mg. 4x daily. with Choline or Phosphatidyl choline.	❧ IODINE THERAPY CAPS or EXTRACT for brain potassium and iodine, and ENERGY GREEN DRINK for blood & oxygen building.	
❧ Have plenty of fresh fruit juices.	✤ Alta Health Sɪʟ-X SILICA CAPSULES 2 daily and MANGANESE w/ B₁₂.	❧ WHITE BIRCH MINERAL WATER daily.	✤ REFLEXOLOGY POINTS: 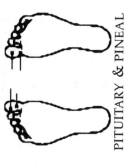 PITUITARY & PINEAL
❧ Drink only bottled water.		❧ Sun CHLORELLA 15 daily.	
❧ Avoid beer, sweet wines, refined flour, sugar, heavy pastries, and canned foods. Avoid all MSG-containing foods and preserved foods.	✤ B Complex 100Mg. daily with extra B6 250Mg. and PABA 1000Mg. daily.	❧ Effective teas: Alfalfa Burdock Saw Palmetto ♂ Prickly Ash	
	✤ Argenine/Ornithine caps 500/500Mg. daily. ♂		✤ AROMATHERAPY: Bergamot oil
	✤ Enzymatic Therapy RAW PITUITARY CAPS 4 daily. ♀	❧ Crystal Star ENDOCRINE BALANCE for overall gland activity.	
	✤ Ener B₁₂ INTERNASAL GEL every other day.	❧ Solaray ALFAJUICE CAPS.	
		❧ SOLARAY Gotu Kola/ Damiana caps 4 daily.♂	

Pituitary secretions affect all physical body growth and weight distribution functions. Pineal development affects metaphysical understanding, and higher consciousness thinking.

COMMON SYMPTOMS: Fatigue; mental stress; lack of growth and/or poor growth; inability to understand metaphysical or higher consciousness concepts; gastritis and ulcers; obesity and water retention; recurrent diarrhea.

COMMON CAUSES: Heavy metal toxicity (the pituitary is particularly vulnerable, and is affected first of all the glands); hypoglycemia; diabetic, pancreatic, and sugar regulation abnormalities; poor nutrition, especially protein deficiency; stress; emotional pressure and adrenal exhaustion.

237

PNEUMONIA ✧ PLEURISY

FOOD THERAPY	VITAMINS/ MINERALS	HERBAL THERAPY	BODYWORK
☙ Go on a mucous cleansing liquid diet for 1-3 days during the first and acute stages. (Pg. 25). ◆ Take a hot lemon and honey drink with water each morning. ◆ Have a fresh carrot juice, and a strong potassium broth or essence (Pg. 33) each day. ◆ Drink plenty of fruit juices, herb teas and bottled water. Avoid alcohol.	✤ Ascorbate vitamin C crystals with bioflavonoids and rutin, 1/4t. every half hour to bowel tolerance, daily for 2 weeks; then every 2 hours for 2 weeks; then 3000Mg. daily for another month. with Beta Carotene 150,000IU daily for the first 2 weeks.	✿ Crystal Star ANTI-BIO CAPSULES or EXTRACT 6X daily to clean out toxins, with CRISIS CAPS to sweat out mucous.	✤ Apply a cayenne poultice: Mix 1/2t. cayenne, 1T. Lobelia, 3T. Slippery Elm and enough water to make a paste. Leave on 1 hour.
		✿ Crystal Star RESPIRCAPS and TEA after crisis has passed to heal lungs and encourage more oxygen uptake.	✤ Apply a mustard plaster to chest to stimulate lungs and draw out poisons: Mix 1T. mustard powder, 1 egg, 3T. flour and enough water to make a paste. Apply and leave on til skin turns pink.
☙ Then follow a largely fresh foods, cleansing diet for 1-2 weeks.	✤ Food Grade H$_2$O$_2$ PEROXY GEL rubbed on the chest daily, and/or taken internally, 1/2t. in a glass of water 2x daily for a week.	✿ Take fresh grated Horseradish root in a spoon with lemon juice. Hang over a sink immediately to expel quantities of mucous.	✤ Take an oxygen bath. Use 1-2 cups food grade H$_2$O$_2$ to a tub of water. Soak 20 minutes.
☙ Then eat a diet high in vegetable proteins, low in meat, dairy and animal fats, to allow lungs to heal easily.	✤ Effective extracts: Liquid DMG 2x daily ♂ Raw Lung	✿ Cayenne/Ginger/Golden Seal caps 4 daily. ♂	✤ Take hot and cold showers to stimulate lung circulation.(Pg. 31-32) REFLEXOLOGY POINT: 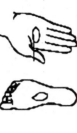 LUNG POINTS
	✤ Vitamin E 400IU 2x daily.	✿ Effective extracts: Echinacea / Golden Seal Mullein/Lobelia ☺	
☙ Add cultured foods, such as yogurt and kefir.	✤ Garlic capsules 6-8 daily.	✿ Effective teas: Ephedra Comfrey Root Comfrey / Fenugreek Slippery Elm Pleurisy Root	✤ Get plenty of rest.
☙ See LUNG DISEASE PAGE in this book for more suggestions.			

COMMON SYMPTOMS: Inflamed lungs and chest area; aggravated flu and cold symptoms; swollen lymph glands; difficult breathing; heavy coughing and expectoration; back, muscle and body aches; chills and fever; sore throat; inability to "get over it"; lung infection and inflammation; great fatigue.

COMMON CAUSES: Low immunity; respiratory infection; clogged lymph nodes; allergies; stress and fatigue.

POISONING FROM FOOD

ARSENIC ✦ SALMONELLA ✦ BOTULISM

FOOD THERAPY

🐍 Take 1/2 cup olive oil very slowly through a straw to remove poison from the stomach area. OR, take warm water with 1t. baking soda in it. Take no milk, fruit juice, alcohol or vinegar until poison has moved out of the stomach.

🐍 Effective neutralizers:
◆ 1-2 heads of iceberg lettuce
◆ bamboo shoots
◆ strong black tea
◆ burnt toast
◆ 2 raw eggs
◆ milk of magnesia
◆ onions and garlic

🐍 Effective protectors against pesticides and poisons in food: ◆ high soluble fiber foods, citrus fruits, wheat germ, whole grains, dark green and yellow vegetables.

🐍 Take a glass of aloe vera juice morning and evening for a week after poisoning to cleanse the digestive tract.

🐍 Eat largely fresh foods for a week after poisoning to realkalize the system.

VITAMINS/ MINERALS

❖ Activated charcoal tabs to absorb poison; 3-5 every 15 minutes.
    and/or
❖ Ascorbate vitamin C powder, 1/2t. every 1/2 hour to bowel tolerance to flush and alkalize the tissues.

❖ Niacin therapy to sweat out poisons; 250-500Mg. every hour until improvement is felt. (about 3-4 capsules) ♂

❖ Enzymatic Therapy LIV-ATOX CAPSULES 3 daily.

❖ Protector supplements against food poisons:
◆ Vit. E with Selenium 400IU
◆ Vit. C with bioflavs and rutin
◆ Beta Carotene 25-50,000IU
◆ Biotec EXTRA ENERGY ENZYMES-SOD W/ CATALASE
◆ Glutathione 50Mg.

❖ Natures Life CAL-MAG LIQUID, PHOS. FREE..

❖ Rainbow Light FOOD SENSITIVITY SYSTEM if there are allergies.

HERBAL THERAPY

🐦 Crystal Star CLEANSING & FASTING TEA as needed, several times daily.
    and/or
ENERGY GREEN DRINK for potassium and iodine.

🐦 Apple Pectin caps. ♂

🐦 Sun CHLORELLA TABS 10 every 4 hours to neutralize and then rebalance the system.

🐦 Effective teas:
Plantain
Scullcap
Elecampane
Wormwood

🐦 Solaray MONTMORILLITE CAPS to absorb and pass poisons.

🐦 For arsenic poisoning: Yellow Dock/Nettles tea

🐦 Kelp tabs 8-12 daily. ♀

BODYWORK

❖ Use an emetic of strong Lobelia tea with 1/4-1/2t. cayenne to throw up poisons and empty the stomach.
Follow with White Oak tincture to neutralize and normalize the stomach.

❖ Sweat out pesticides and poisons in a long, low heat sauna.

❖ Overheating therapy is effective. See P. Airola "How To Get Well" for correct technique.

COMMON SYMPTOMS: Nausea and vomiting; cold sweats after eating severe indigestion; hot flushes; chills; diarrhea; red, rashed skin.

COMMON CAUSES: Pesticides and fungicides; food additives and preservatives; sulfites; food allergy reaction; MSG; breathing noxious fumes.

POISONING FROM HEAVY METALS

LEAD ◆ CADMIUM ◆ MERCURY ◆ RADIATION

FOOD THERAPY	VITAMINS/ MINERALS	HERBAL THERAPY	BODYWORK
✿ Go on a short 3-7 day liquid diet (Pg. 26) to start poisons releasing from the body. Have one each of the following daily: ◆ a glass of fresh carrot juice ◆ a potassium broth (Pg. 33) ◆ 2 cups Miso soup	✤ Glutathione 50Mg. 3 daily with Enzymatic Therapy CHEMEX CAPS.	☙ Evening Primrose oil caps 4 daily with 2 cysteine caps each time.	✤ For chemical burns; apply a green clay poultice.
✿ Take 2T. each daily: Brewer's yeast Wheat germ Lecithin granules	✤ Ascorbate vitamin C powder, 1/2t. every hour to bowel tolerance daily as a tissue flush. with Solaray Calcium citrate 6 daily, or Nature's Life CAL-MAG PHOS. FREE LIQUID.	☙ Aloe Vera juice, 1 glass every 4 hours. ☙ Liquid chlorophyll 1t. every 4 hours. ☙ Pau de Arco tea every 4 hours, or Crystal Star LIV-FLUSH TEA.	✤ Avoid antacids; they interfere with enzyme production, and the ability of the body to carry off heavy metals. ❖ See pages 43 and 47 on neutralizing the effects of chemotherapy and radiation.
✿ Drink only bottled water. ✿ Eat organically grown foods as much as possible. Avoid canned foods.	✤ Biotec EXTRA ENERGY ENZYMES S.O.D. W/ CATALASE, 6 daily.	☙ Crystal Star HEAVY METAL or DETOX CAPS for 2-3 months, with CLEANSING & FASTING TEA.	❖ Avoid smoking and secondary smoke, pesticides and fungicides, phosphorus fertilizers, fluorescent lights, aluminum cookware and deodorants, electric blankets; microwave ovens, and non-filtered computor screens.
✿ Avoid caffeine; it inhibits liver filtering function.	✤ Twin Lab LIQUID K PLUS.	☙ Effective capsules: ◆ Astragalus ♂ ◆ Kelp 8-10 ◆ Garlic 6-8 ◆ Siberian Ginseng extract caps	
✿ Crystal Star ENERGY GREEN and MIN-ZYME-MINOS DRINKS are both good detoxifiers and blood builders.	✤ Vital Health FORMULA 1 ORAL CHELATION/EDTA. 2 packets daily. ♂ ✤ Protection nutrients: ◆ Beta Carotene 150,000Iu ◆ Vit. E 400Iu w/ Selenium ◆ Solaray SELENOMETHIONINE ◆ Alta Health SELENIUM PLUS	☙ Sun CHLORELLA or BARLEY GREEN MAGMA 20 daily. (especially to overcome radiation and chemotherapy)	
✿ To excrete lead; eat beans and sea vegetables	✤ Zinc 50-100Mg daily.	☙ Crystal Star LIV-ALIVE and IODINE THERAPY CAPS 2-6 daily. ♀	

COMMON SYMPTOMS: Seizures; Schizophrenic -like, uncontrolled psychotic behavior as poisons react in the system; memory loss and senility; infertility and impotency; insomnia; bad breath and body odor as the body tries to throw off the alien substances.

COMMON CAUSES: Industrial pollution and exposure to toxic chemicals; nicotine; insecticides; dental fillings; over-treated water; copper paints and pipes; hair dyes; aluminum cookware and deodorants; smoke and smog; zinc depletion.

POISON OAK

FOOD THERAPY

❧ Apply cider vinegar, denatured alcohol, or a cornstarch paste to blisters to control itching and neutralize acid poisons.

❧ Follow a fresh foods diet during acute blistering to cleanse systemic poisons out of the bloodstream.

❧ Take several green drinks during acute phase.(Pg. 34).

VITAMINS/ MINERALS

✣ Effective topicals:
   ◆ Liquid chlorophyll
   ◆ H₂O₂ PEROXY GEL.
   ◆ Vitamin E oil
   ◆ Nature's Life CAL-MAG LIQUID

✣ Enzymatic Therapy CORTOTONE CAPS, with DERMAZYME OINTMENT.

✣ Ascorbate vitamin C crystals, 1/4t. every hour to bowel tolerance, til itching lessens, then reduce to 1/4t. 4x daily til clear.

✣ Hylands homeopathic POISON OAK TABS to build immunity against poison oak.

HERBAL THERAPY

❧ Effective topicals:
   ◆ Comfrey/Aloe salve
   ◆ Tea Tree Oil ☺
   ◆ B & T CALIFLORA GEL
   ◆ Calendula ointment
   ◆ Witch Hazel
   ◆ Echinacea cream

❧ Crystal Star P.O. #1 AND P.O. # 2 CAPSULES ☺ alternately as directed.

❧ Crystal Star ANTI-HST CAPSULES 4-6 daily til clear, to help the liver produce natural anti-histimines.

❧ Crystal Star ADRN EXTRACT or ADRN-ALIVE CAPS 2 x daily to strengthen the adrenal glands as a protection factor.

❧ Black Walnut tincture. Apply locally. Take internally.

❧ Jewelweed tea. Apply locally. Take internally.

❧ Apply Dusty Miller tea.

BODYWORK

❖ Take epsom salts baths.

❖ Swim in the ocean if possible, as effective neutralizing therapy.

❖ Apply ALOE ICE GEL. ♂

❖ Apply Chinese WHITE FLOWER OIL.

❖ Apply Aloe Vera gel.

COMMON SYMPTOMS: Itching, burning blisters on the skin that ooze, erupt and spread the systemic plant poisons.

241

FOOD THERAPY

❧ Take lemon juice and water every morning to cleanse sediment; then cider vinegar and honey in water daily to prevent.

❧ Follow a fresh foods diet the first week of healing, with lots of leafy green salads, sea vegetables, fresh fruits, juices and steamed vegetables. Then, add simply cooked whole grains, and sea foods for 3 weeks. Keep the diet very low in fats.

❧ Make a mix and take 4T. daily:
Lecithin granules, wheat germ, pumpkin seeds, oat bran, brewer's yeast flakes, sesame seeds.

❧ Avoid caffeine, hard liquor, tobacco, carbonated drinks, and tomato juice during healing.

❧ Avoid all fried, fatty and refined foods.

VITAMINS/ MINERALS

✢ Zinc 100Mg. daily for 1 month, then 50Mg. daily for 1 month.
with
Marine Carotene 100,000IU to control infection.
and
Nature's Plus vitamin E 800IU daily.

✢ Ascorbate vitamin C crystals, 1/2t. every hour to bowel tolerance daily for 2 weeks, then 1/2t. 4x daily for 2 weeks, then 3000Mg. daily for 1 month.

✢ High Omega 3 fish or flax oils 3x daily.

✢ Enzymatic Therapy NUCLEO-PRO M CAPS.

✢ Solaray PROSTAGEUM.

✢ Biotec EXTRA ENERGY ENZYMES 6 daily.

✢ Sun CHLORELLA 20 tabs daily for prevention.

HERBAL THERAPY

❧ Crystal Star PROSCAPS 4-6 daily as needed for 1 month, then 2-4 daily for 1 month.
take with
Evening Primrose oil caps 4-6 daily for 1 month, then 2-4 daily for 1 month.
and
ANTI-BIO CAPS or EXT-RACT 6x daily to reduce inflammation and infection.
then
MALE CAPS for area regeneration; IODINE THERAPY CAPS / EXTRACT for prevention. (Take with vitamin E for best results).

❧ Effective extracts:
◆ Echinacea
◆ White Oak

❧ Effective capsules:
◆ Kelp 6-8 daily
◆ Bee Pollen 2-4 daily

❧ Effective teas:
◆ Pau de Arco
◆ Saw Palmetto
◆ Damiana

BODYWORK

✜ Use chamomile tea enemas (pg. 32) once a week during healing to cleanse the body of harmful acids.
Or take warm chamomile sitz baths for 20 minutes at a time morning and evening.

✜ Apply ice packs to the area to reduce pain.

✜ Avoid chemical antihistimines. Overuse impairs liver function, that then results in prostate trouble.

✜ Sex life should be normal in frequency and desire with a natural climax. Avoid prolonged sex and interrupted climax.

✜ REFLEXOLOGY POINT:

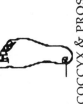

COCCYX & PROSTATE

COMMON SYMPTOMS: Inflamed, swollen, infected prostate gland; frequent, painful desire to urinate with not much urine passed; incontinence in severe cases; fever; lower back and leg pains; impotence, and/or paiful orgasm; loss of libido; unusual fatigue.

COMMON CAUSES: Poor diet with too little fiber, and too many over-acid foods; too much alcohol and caffeine; EFA and prostaglandin depletion; exhausted lymph system from from too many over-the-counter antihistimines; internal congestion and poor circulation; lack of exercise; zinc deficiency; venereal disease.

RHEUMATIC FEVER
A STREP INFECTION

FOOD THERAPY	VITAMINS/ MINERALS	HERBAL THERAPY	BODYWORK
❧ Adhere to a fresh juice and liquid diet for the acute stages of healing to reduce body work and strain. ◆ Take potassium broth or essence, and apple/alfalfa sprout juice daily during acute period. ◆ Take VEGEX YEAST PASTE BROTH and Miso soup daily for B vitamins and strength.	✤ Ascorbate vitamin C crystals with bioflavonoids. 1/4t. every hour in juice, to bowel tolerance during acute periods, then reduce dosage to 3-5000Mg. daily. ☺ with Beta Carotene 50-100,000IU daily as an anti-infective.	ꙮ Evening Primrose oil caps 4 daily. ꙮ Crystal Star ANTI-BIO CAPS 4 daily for at least a month to totally overcome virus. Then CARDI-STRENGTH or BODY REBUILDER and ADRN-ALIVE CAPS to strengthen the system against recurrence.	✤ Get lots of bed rest. Yoga and mild muscle-toning exercises, and/or massage therapy during confinement (which can last for several weeks) will prevent loss and atrophy of body strength.
❧ Then eat fresh and steamed foods, adding plenty of vegetable protein from whole grains, tofu, sprouts, etc.	✤ Shark oil caps 2 daily to overcome the virus.	ꙮ Garlic tabs 6 daily.	✤ Catnip enemas once a week to reduce fever.
❧ Take only small meals.	✤ Effective anti-oxidants: Vitamin E 4-800IU daily.♀ B15 DMG Germanium 25-30Mg. CO Q 10 30Mg. daily	ꙮ Sun CHLORELLA or BARLEY GREEN MAGMA GRANULES 1 packet daily.	✤ Avoid aspirin as an anti-inflammatory in the case.
❧ Drink only bottled water.	✤ Ener B12 INTERNASAL GEL	ꙮ Lobelia tincture. ☺	
❧ Avoid all sugars, salty and refined foods during healing. Keep fats low. No fried foods. No caffeine or carbonated drinks during healing.	✤ High potency ROYAL JELLY 2t. daily. ♂	ꙮ Apply Wintergreen oil compresses to chest. Take wintergreen/White Willow tea internally.	
	✤ Raw Thymus extract ☺		

Rheumatic fever can be prevented if the strep virus is killed within 10-12 days of infection. The body's own immune defenses can overcome the disease within that time. Homeopathic medicines are very effective in this case, and may be taken even if chemical anti-biotics are already being used. ◆ Remember to reduce doses for children.☺

COMMON SYMPTOMS: Extreme weakness; heart weakness affecting joints and skin; shortness of breath; poor circulation and lack of blood flow.

COMMON CAUSES: Holes in the heart ventricles; inflammation of the main circulatory system; allergic reaction; low immunity, especially in children; often accompanied by acute viral disease; toxic exposure to harmful chemicals, environmental pollutants, or radiation.

RHEUMATISM

FOOD THERAPY

🍂 Avoid all acid-forming foods, such as red meats, cooked spinach and rhubarb, caffeine, sodas and caffeine-containing foods; and nightshade family plants, such as tobacco, tomatoes, eggplant, etc.

🍂 Avoid pasteurized dairy products, refined, fatty, and fried foods.

🍂 Take a glass of lemon juice and water each morning.
   ◆ Take a glass of pineapple or grapefruit juice at mid-morning.
   ◆ Take a glass of fresh celery juice at night to put inorganic sediments into solution so they may be flushed in the morning.

🍂 Take 2T. each daily:
   Brewer's yeast
   Lecithin
   Wheat germ

🍂 See ARTHRITIS and GOUT PAGES in this book for more dietary information.

VITAMINS/ MINERALS

✤ Quercitin Plus with Bromelain 500Mg. 3 or more times daily to bring down inflammation.

✤ Enzymatic Therapy ACID-A-CAL and HERBAL FLAVONOIDS CAPS.♀

✤ BioForce RHEUMATISM FORMULA DROPS.

✤ Twin Lab LIQUID K PLUS 2-3t. daily.

✤ Ascorbate vitamin C or Ester C powder with bioflavonoids and rutin, 1/2t. every 4 hours to bowel tolerance daily for a month, to neutralize acid wastes and rebuild connective tissue.

✤ Source Naturals Germanium 100Mg. daily.

✤ DLPA 750Mg. for pain.

✤ High Omega flax oil 3 x daily, with Sun CHLORELLA granules 1 packet daily.

HERBAL THERAPY

🍃 Crystal Star R^TH EASE CAPSULES and TEA for 2-3 months.
   with
🍃 Crystal Star PANEX CAPS with POTASSIUM SOURCE CAPS or SILICA SOURCE EXTRACT 2x daily.

🍃 Take 2 glass aloe vera juice daily.♂

🍃 Effective extracts:
   ◆ Valerian/Wild Lettuce
   ◆ Mullein/Lobelia
   ◆ Hawthorne
   ◆ Bilberry

🍃 Effective capsules:
   ◆ Solaray Yucca 4 daily
   ◆ Solaray Devils Claw extr. caps
   ◆ Alfalfa 8 daily
   ◆ Solaray ALFAJUICE CAPS
   ◆ Cayenne/Ginger 6 daily
   ◆ Cayenne/Garlic 8 daily

🍃 Effective teas:
   ◆ White Willow
   ◆ Horsetail/Rosemary
   ◆ Slippery Elm
   ◆ Nettles/Burdock

🍃 Alta Health SIL-X SILICA CAPS 4 daily.♀

BODYWORK

✤ Use an occasional catnip enema in the morning to alkalize and cleanse. (Take a cup of senna tea the night before for best results).

✤ Apply hot Comfrey compresses to draw out acid waste.

✤ Effective topicals:
   ◆ **CamoCare cream**
   ◆ **Cajeput/Wintergreen oil**
   ◆ **White Flower oil**
   ◆ **B & T TRiFLORA ANALGESIC GEL**

✤ Crystal Star ALKALIZING ENZYME BODY WRAP to change body pH.

✤ REFLEXOLOGY POINT:

COMMON SYMPTOMS: Painful, swollen and often deformed joints; painful muscle activity; acidosis; stiffness and body aches; fatigue; often affects women in young adulthood; worsening symptoms in cold weather.

COMMON CAUSES: Lowered immunity; environmental/chemical pollutants; inflammation in the muscles; poor diet with too many acid-forming foods.

SCARS ✧ STRETCH MARKS

FOOD THERAPY

🌿 Wheat germ oil. Apply locally. Take 2t. daily internally.

🌿 Have a green drink at least three times a week during first healing stages. (Pg. 34).

🌿 Apply sesame oil.

🌿 Apply avocado oil. Eat avocados for skin elasticity.

🌿 Eat a high vegetable protein diet for faster healing. Include plenty of whole grains, sprouts, tofu, and a protein drink every morning, such as Nature's Plus SPIRUTEIN.

VITAMINS/ MINERALS

❖ Apply vitamin E oil. Take E 400IU internally daily.

❖ Vitamin C therapy, for collagen production and connective tissue growth: ascorbate C powder; take up to 500Mg. daily, and mix with water into a solution and apply directly.

❖ Enzymatic Therapy DERMAZYME OINTMENT and HERBAL FLAVONOIDS CAPS.

❖ Germanium 25-30Mg. for wound healing, for at least a month.

❖ A & D oil capsules. Take 25-50,000IU internally daily. Puncture a capsule and apply directly 2-3x daily.

❖ UNIPRO BCAAs to accelerate healing tissue.

HERBAL THERAPY

🌿 Home Health SCAR-GO.

🌿 Crystal Star ENERGY GREEN DRINK for blood and tissue building.

🌿 Effective applications:
◆ Aloe Vera gel
◆ C.S. CALENDULA GEL
◆ Tea Tree oil
◆ B&T CALIFLORA GEL
◆ Comfrey/Aloe salve
◆ Golden Seal salve
◆ BioForce ECHINACEA CREAM

🌿 Highest potency YS or Premier 1 ROYAL JELLY 2t. daily.

🌿 Superior GINSENG/ BEE SECRETION.♀

🌿 Sun CHLORELLA or BARLEY GREEN MAGMA GRANULES 1 packet daily.

🌿 Alta Health SIL-X SILICA CAPS, 4 daily. (Organic Silica biologically engenders organic calcium formation, and is identified by the body as collagen for healing)

BODYWORK

❖ Get regular exercise daily for muscle and skin tone, and body oxygen.

❖ Massage the scar thoroughly when rubbing your choice of topical application, to bring up healthy circulation and skin tone.

❖ Apply Collagen and Elastin ampule concentrates.

COMMON SYMPTOMS: Non-healing or slow healing skin wounds, often with continuing redness, roughness, and irregular weals.

COMMON CAUSES: Protein deficiency; vitamin A & D deficiency; zinc deficiency; poor overall nutrition.

245

SCHIZOPHRENIA ✧ PSYCHOSIS ✧ MENTAL ILLNESS

FOOD THERAPY	VITAMINS/ MINERALS	HERBAL THERAPY	BODYWORK

FOOD THERAPY

❧ Start with a short liquid, juice and cleansing diet to normalize blood levels. (Pg.26)

❧ Minimize fruit juices if hypoglycemia is involved.

Then, eat largely fresh foods for the remainder of the week.

Then, gradually add vegetable proteins, gluten-free grains (especially brown rice), sea foods, fish, nuts and seeds.

❧ Take 2T. each daily:
Brewer's yeast
Lecithin granules

❧ Avoid all refined sugars, red meats and preserved foods.

❧ See HYPOGLYCEMIA DIET SUGGESTIONS in this book for more information.

VITAMINS/ MINERALS

✤ Ascorbate vitamin C powder with bioflavonoids and rutin, 1/2t. every hour to bowel tolerance daily for the first month of healing. (Remember that vitamin C is a natural tranquilizer. It will help in withdrawal from chemical tranquilizers and drugs)

✤ Niacin Therapy: 1-3000Mg. daily. (Take a baby aspirin before taking to remove niacin flush).♂

or

✤ Solaray CHROMIACIN.♂

✤ Glutamine 1000Mg. and Tyrosine 1000Mg daily.

✤ B Complex 150Mg. with extra B₆ 500Mg. and B₁₂ 2500Mcg.♀

✤ Phosphatidyl Choline (PC55) 2-3x daily. with

✤ Zinc 50Mg. 2x daily. and

✤ Tryptophane 1000Mg.♂

HERBAL THERAPY

❧ Evening Primrose oil caps 4-6 daily for prostaglandin production.

❧ Crystal Star RELAX CAPS as needed.

with

IODINE THERAPY CAPS or EXTRACT, or MEGA-MINERAL CAPS 6-8 daily.

and

ADRN-ALIVE CAPS or FEEL GREAT CAPS or TEA for balance.♀

❧ Miodin or Atomodine drops 2-3x daily.

❧ Kelp tabs 6-8 daily.

❧ Effective teas:
Sage ♂
Gotu Kola
Prickly Ash

❧ Country Life MOOD FACTORS as needed.♂

BODYWORK

✤ Get some exercise every day, especially running, walking or jogging. The oxygen will do wonders for your head.

✤ Massage therapy and spinal adjustment have had some success.

✤ Ocean walks for sea minerals, or a visit to a mineral-rich spring and spa are effective.

✤ Avoid all pleasure drugs, and as many prescription drugs as possible. For many people, permanent brain change and psychosis can result.

COMMON SYMPTOMS: Severe mental depression; lethargy; emotional swings, often to violent actions; delusions and hallucinations; detachment from reality.

COMMON CAUSES: Hypoglycemia; diabetes; gluten and/or dairy allergies; heavy metal toxicity; general poor nutrition with too many junk foods, and refined sugars causing constipation and auto-toxemia; prescription and/or pleasure drug abuse; vitamin B₁₂ deficiency; iodine deficiency; elevated histimine levels; hypothyroidism; glandular imbalance.

SCIATICA

FOOD THERAPY

- Take a potassium broth or essence (Pg. 33) every other day for a month to rebuild nerve health.

- Have a leafy green salad every day. Take a little white wine with dinner to relieve tension and nerve trauma.

- Eat calcium and magnesium rich foods, such as green vegetables, sea vegetables, shellfish, tofu, whole grains, molasses, nuts and seeds.

- Drink bottled mineral water, 6-8 glasses daily.

VITAMINS/ MINERALS

- Cal/Mag/Zinc 4 daily with vitamin D 400IU.

- Country Life LIGATEND CAPSULES as needed. with Vitamin E 400IU daily.

- Quercitin Plus 3-4 daily with Bromelain 500Mg.

- Ascorbate vitamin C or Ester C with bioflavonoids and rutin, 3-5000Mg. daily for connective tissue development.

- DLPA 500-750Mg. 2x daily as needed for pain.

- B Complex 100Mg. with extra B_1 100Mg., B_6 250Mg. and Niacin 250Mg. ♀

HERBAL THERAPY

- Crystal Star RELAX CAPS as needed for rebuilding the nerve sheath. and CALCIUM SOURCE CAPS or HIGHLY ABSORBABLE CALCIUM EXTRACT. ♀

- Apply MINERAL ICE GEL, or apply ALOE ICE GEL.

- Mix wintergreen, Cajeput, Rosemary oils. Massage into area.

- Liquid chlorophyll 3t. daily with meals. or BARLEY GREEN MAGMA 1 packet daily, for nerve rebuilding.

- Mezotrace SEA MINERAL COMPLEX 4 daily.

- Garlic/Parsley caps 4-6 daily.

BODYWORK

- REFLEXOLOGY POINT:

SCIATIC

- Massage therapy and chiropractic adjustment are both effective.
- Apply ice packs to relieve pain.

- Gentle morning and evening stretches, and daily Yoga exercises are effective.

- Take hot epsom salts baths.

- Apply alternating hot and cold, or Hops/Lobelia compresses to stimulate circulation

- Effective topicals: Olive oil Tiger Balm White Flower oil B & T TRIFLORA GEL.

COMMON SYMPTOMS: Neuritis of the sciatic nerve; lower back pain and aching; muscle weakness and wasting; uncomfortable sensation in the legs and thighs; reduced reflex activity.

COMMON CAUSES: Poor posture and muscle tone; poor bone and cartilege development; exhausted pituitary and adrenal glands; menopause symptoms; obesity; lack of exercise; high heels; protein and calcium depletion; not enough green vegetabes; flat feet; spinal imbalance.

247

♂ SEXUALITY ✧ LIBIDO ♀

FOOD THERAPY	VITAMINS/ MINERALS	HERBAL THERAPY	BODYWORK
⚘ Lack of normal libido can often be overcome simply by improving a poor diet. Junk foods, chemical and processed foods are a key factor in the body's not feeling "up to it".	MALE: ✤ B₁₅ DMG liquid or sublingual tablets. ✤ Country Life ENERGIX VIALS 1 daily. ✤ Carnitine 500Mg. with Raw Orchic glandular and Arginine. ✤ Zinc 50Mg. 2x daily.	MALE: ☙ Yohimbe casules 500-1000Mg. for testosterone production. ☙ Crystal Star LOVING MOOD EXTRACT FOR MEN and/or LOVE CAPS MALE (2-4 daily as needed.) ☙ BioForce GINSAVENA EXTRACT as needed. ☙ Highest potency YS ROYAL JELLY 60,000-120,000MG. daily.	✤ Crystal Star LOVE BATHS FOR MEN & WOMEN. ✤ Get regular exercise such as dancing, walking, and swimming to stimulate circulation and increase body oxygen.
⚘ Add mineral-rich foods to the diet; from shellfish, leafy greens, sea vegetables, whole grains, nuts, legumes, and molasses.			✤ Hypnotherapy has been effective when the problem is psychologically based.
⚘ Avoid red meats; keep saturated fats, salt and sugar low. (All inhibit the free-flowing quality of the system.)	FEMALE: ✤ Vitamin E 800IU daily. ✤ B₁₅ DMG liquid or sublingual tablets.	FEMALE: ☙ Crystal Star LOVE CAPS FEMALE (2 for several days before a weekend as needed.)	✤ Remember that Ginseng is a re-generative herb. It does not make the normal body "supernormal".
⚘ While there are no real "aphrodisiac foods", there are some superfoods that have a lot of the nutrients for healthy sex and desire: broccoli, whole grains, brewer's yeast, spinach, peas, oysters, salmon and other sea foods, eggs, cantaloupe, carrots, and soybeans.	✤ Tyrosine 500-1000Mg. and/or Phenalalanine 500Mg. or Nature's Plus PIZZAZZ (Liquid phenalalanine) ✤ Highest potency YS ROYAL JELLY 60,000-120,000MG. daily.	☙ Crystal Star DONG QUAI/ DAMIANA EXTRACT ☙ Yohimbe 500Mg. capsules	✤ Many drugs, both pleasure and prescription, can have the side effect of impaired sex drive. Take a good look at any you may be using.
⚘ A whole and fresh foods diet definitely encourages more zest for life.	BOTH: ✤ Country Life ADRENAL W / TYROSINE CAPS.	BOTH: ☙ Ginseng/Damiana capsules 4 as needed. ☙ Crystal Star CUPID'S FLAME TEA.	

COMMON SYMPTOMS: Impotence; frigidity; lack of normal sexual interest.

COMMON CAUSES: Emotional stress and tension from job, relationship unhappiness or life style; poor diet resulting in physical malfunction; childhood abuse and trauma; prescription and/or pleasure drug reaction.

FOOD THERAPY

❧ Go on a short 3 day cleansing diet to eliminate acid wastes and alkalize the blood (Pg. 26).
◆ Take a Carrot/Beet/Cucumber juice, and a cranberry juice each day. Take an apple juice or celery juice each night.
◆ Then, eat only fresh foods for 1-2 weeks, with lots of alkalizing salads and fruits.

❧ Keep the diet consciously alkaline, with plenty of miso soup, brown rice, vegetables and leafy greens.

❧ Include cultured foods, such as yogurt and kefir for friendly GI flora.

❧ Avoid food with preservatives, additives and colorings. Avoid refined foods, sugars, aspirin, tetracyclenes, nitrates and nitrites.

❧ Avoid acid-forming foods, such as red meats, caffeine, fried foods, and carbonated drinks.

VITAMINS/ MINERALS

✢ Stress B Complex 150Mg. with extra B_6 250Mg. and B_{12} 2500Mcg.
with
Lysine 1000Mg, and apply LYSINE PLUS cream locally to blisters.

✢ Quercitin Plus with Bromelain for instant action against inflammation. with Phosphatidyl choline (PC 55)

✢ Ascorbate vitamin C or Ester C powder with bioflavs., 1/4t. every hour in water up to 10,000Mg or bowel tolerance daily during an attack.

✢ Emulsified A & D 50,000/ 1,000IU daily.
with
Vit. E 400IU 3x daily. Apply E oil directly.♂

✢ Enzymatic Therapy HERPILYN CAPSULES. ♀

✢ DLPA 750Mg for pain.

HERBAL THERAPY

❧ Crystal Star THERADERM or HERPEACE CAPSULES.
and
THERADERM TEA, internally, and topically, patted on blisters to neutralize acids coming out through the skin.
with
RELAX CAPS to rebuild strong nerve structure.

❧ Crystal Star ANTI-VI CAPSULES 2-4 daily. with High Omega 3 Flax oil 3t. daily.

❧ Effective teas:
Alfalfa
St. John's Wort extract
Red Clover/Nettles
Burdock Rt.

❧ Kelp tabs 6-8 daily.

❧ Effective topicals:
◆ BioForce Echinacea cream
◆ Aloe Vera/Golden Seal solution or ointment.
◆ B & T CALIFLORA GEL
◆ calendula gel
◆ B&T SSSTING STOP GEL

BODYWORK

✤ Effective topical applications to relieve pain:
◆ petroleum jelly
◆ B & T TRiFLORA ANALGESIC GEL.

✤ Take epsom salt or oatmeal baths to neutralize acids.

✤ Get early morning sunlight on the body for healing vitamin D.

✤ Remember that corticosteroid drugs taken over a long period of time for shingles greatly weakens the immune system, allowing future attacks.

✤ Relaxation and tension control techniques are effective. Stress creates an acid body condition, and erodes protective nerve sheathing.

✤ See HERPES PAGE in this book for more information.

COMMON SYMPTOS: Swollen red skin blisters, usually around the upper part of the body; pain radiating along one or several nerves preceding outbreaks; attacks last from 2 days to 2 weeks, leaving irritated nerves even after blisters are gone; accompanied by fever, weakness, chills and nausea.

COMMON CAUSES: Food allergies, particularly to shellfish, wheat, MSG, food additives and preservatives, milk products; over-chlorined drinking water; stress; adrenal and/or liver exhaustion; histimine reaction; acidosis and HCl depletion; poor circulation and constipation; too many prescription drugs; caffeine, or hard liquor; proneness if had chicken pox as a child.

SHOCK ✧ TRAUMA

SHOCK is the condition that develops when blood flow is reduced below the levels needed to maintain vital body functions. Obviously, shock and trauma can happen during serious injuries or illnesses where a great deal of blood and other body fluids are lost. But it can also occur during severe infections, allergic reactions (such as anaphylactic shock), and malfunction of the nervous system (as a severe reaction to a poisonous insect or snake bite).

Every significant injury is accompanied by some degree of shock, because the autonomic nervous system responds to the trauma of injury by altering blood flow. It is usually wise to treat any severely injured person for shock in addition to treating them specifically for the injury. If there is lots of bleeding, major burns, or a head wound, treatment for shock should be very high priority.

Have the person lie down with the legs elevated slightly above the head. Don't bend the legs. Loosen clothing at the neck, waist and chest. Protect the person from extremes of warmth and cold. If there is the chance of serious or life-threatening injury, do not move the person. Give small sips of fluids only if fully conscious; no solid food.

GET MEDICAL CARE IMMEDIATLY!

The following emergency measures are beneficial until medical help arrives:

1) Deva Flowers FIRST AID REMEDY, or Bach Flowers RESCUE REMEDY; 2-4 drops on the tongue every 5 minutes til breathing normalizes.

2) Cayenne solution in water (1-3 teasp. or 2-4 capsules); give with an eyedropper on the back of the tongue if necessary every 10 minutes to restore normal heart rate.

3) Gingko Biloba extract; a few drops in water, given on the tongue can help with stroke, and allergic reactions such as dizziness, loss of balance, memory loss or ringing in the ears.

4) Arnica drops are usually the first homeopathic remedy to give for injury; every 1/2 hour to 1 hour on the tongue

5) Bromelain 500Mg., or Quercitin Plus with Bromelain to control body trauma; open 1-2 capsules in water and give in small sips. Acts like aspirin, an anti-inflammatory without the stomach upset.

6) Hops/Valerian tincture; 5-6 drops in water. Give in small sips every 10-15 minutes for calmness.

COMMON SYMPTOMS: General weakness; cold, pale skin; rapid weak heartbeat; heart attack or stroke; reduced alertness and consciousness; shallow, irregular breathing; confusion.

COMMON CAUSES: Major burns; heat prostration; major accident and injury; loss of blood; head injury; poisonous insect or snake bite; bone breaks, sprains, and falls.

Thanks and credit to "Everybody's Guide to Homepoathic Medicines" for this page. It is needed for a family reference, and our experience has not included emergency shock trauma.

SINUS PROBLEMS ✧ SINUSITIS

FOOD THERAPY

🐚 Go on a short 3 day mucous cleansing liquid diet.(Pg. 25) ◆ Take a glass of lemon juice and water each morning. ◆ Add an extra glass of fresh carrot juice the 1st day. ◆ Add a pineapple/ papaya juice the 2nd day. ◆ Add a glass of apple juice the 3rd day.

🐚 Then, eat fresh foods only for the rest of the week to cleanse encrusted mucous deposits.

🐚 Take an ONION/GARLIC, or MUCOUS CLEANSING BROTH (pg. 36) each day.

🐚 Slowly add back whole grains, vegetable protein, and cultured foods to your own tolerance.

🐚 Avoid heavy starches, red meats, pasteurized dairy products, caffeine and refined sugars.

🐚 See "COOKING FOR HEALTHY HEALING" by Linda Rector-Page for a complete diet for respiratory health.

VITAMINS/MINERALS

❖ Vitamin C therapy: Use ascorbate or Ester C powder, 1/4t. every hour to bowel tolerance daily during acute phase. Also, dissolve crystals in water and drip into nose with an eyedropper.

❖ Beta Carotene 100,000IU.

❖ Enzymatic Therapy AIR POWER CAPSULES, LIQUID LIVER CAPS, and RAW ADRENAL COMPLEX.♂

❖ Nutrition Resource NUTRIBIOTIC LIQUID CONCENTRATE diluted as directed, as an anti-biotic nasal rinse.

❖ Propolis tincture drops ♂ and/or

❖ High potency ROYAL JELLY 2t. daily.♀

❖ B Complex 100Mg. with extra B₆ 250Mg., pantothenic acid 500Mg., and B₁₂ 2500Mcg. sublingual.

HERBAL THERAPY

🐚 Crystal Star ALRG CAPSULES and TEA. or ANTI-HST EXTRACT and OPEN UP TEA.

🐚 BioForce SINUSAN DROPS or TABLETS.

🐚 Apply Tiger Balm or Chinese WHITE FLOWER OIL to sinuses.

🐚 Unsprayed Bee Pollen 2t. daily.

🐚 Effective teas: Comfrey/Fenugreek Fenugreek/Thyme Ephedra

🐚 Mix fresh grated horseradish root with lemon juice in a spoon. Take and hang over a sink to expel lots of mucous all at once.

🐚 Steam face and head with Eucalyptus/Mullein steam.

BODYWORK

❖ Take a hot sauna for 20 minutes daily during acute phases.

❖ ACUPRESSURE POINTS: Massage under the big toes for 1 minute every day. Squeeze ends of each finger and thumb hard for 20 seconds every day.

❖ REFLEXOLOGY POINTS:

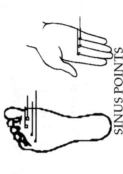

SINUS POINTS

❖ Mix 1t. food grade H₂O₂, or several drops of Tea Tree oil in a vaporizer. Use at night for clear morning sinuses.

COMMON SYMPTOMS: Headaches; runny nose and inflamed nasal passages; post-nasal drip; a mucous-clogged head; sore throat; indigestion because of mucous overload; pain behind the eyes; loss of smell and taste; swollen, tender face; bad breath from low grade infection.

COMMON CAUSES: Too many mucous-forming foods, such as pasteurized dairy products and refined carbohydrates; too many salty, fatty and overly-spiced foods; poor food combining; lack of green vegetables; constipation and poor circulation; lack of exercise and deep breathing; suppressive over-the-counter sinus drugs.

SKIN
BEAUTY & HEALTH

FOOD THERAPY

❧ **Great skin starts with a good diet:** ◆ Eat plenty of mineral-rich foods, such as leafy greens, bell peppers, broccoli sesame and sunflower seeds, fish and sea vegetables. ◆ Eat plenty of cultured foods, such as yogurt, tofu and kefir. ◆ Eat plenty of flushing and cleansing foods, such as fresh fruit and cucumbers. ◆ Eat vitamin C-rich foods such as citrus fruits and fresh vegetables.

❧ **Drink watermelon juice whenever it is available. It is rich in skin nourishing natural silica, and keeps the systemflushed and alkaline.**

❧ Make a mix and take 2 Tblsp. daily:
◆ Sesame seeds
◆ Wheat germ
◆ Molasses
◆ Brewer's yeast

❧ **Drink 6 glasses of bottled water every day.**

❧ **Avoid red meats, caffeine, fried, fatty and fast foods. Reduce dairy foods and heavy starches**

VITAMINS/ MINERALS

❖ **Alta Health** SIL-X SILICA TABS 4 daily. Organic Silica is biologically engenders organic calcium formation, and is identified by the body as collagen.

❖ **Ascorbate vitamin C or Ester C with bioflavonoids, 3000Mg. daily for connective tissue growth.** with DDS (dairy free) acidolphilus caps at meals.

❖ Super-natural facial: Prick open and squeeze out 1 vitamin A&D 25,000IU, and 1 vitamin E 400IU capsule. Grind up 1 zinc 30Mg. tablet and 1 PABA 100Mg. tablet. Mix with 1-2t. wheat germ oil and smear on face. Let dry and rinse off.

❖ **Zinc picolinate 50-100Mg. daily, with B$_6$ 250-500Mg.**

❖ **High Omega 3 Flax oil** internally for dry flaking skin.

❖ **Enzyme Therapy HAIR & SKIN NUTRITION, and HERBAL FLAVONOIDS.**

❖ Collagen tabs or powder.

HERBAL THERAPY

❧ **Evening Primrose oil caps 4 daily.**

❧ **Crystal Star** BEAUTIFUL SKIN TEA. **Use internally & pat on problem spots.**

❧ Other Crystal Star effective skin blends:
◆ MEGA-MINERAL CAPS 2 daily
◆ MIN-ZYME-MINOS DRINK for elasticity.
◆ ADRN-ALIVE CAPS for spots and freckling.
◆ SKIN THERAPY # 1 for internal cleansing.
◆ SKIN THERAPY #2 for smoothing.
◆ IODINE THERAPY for thyroid stimulation and minerals.

❧ **High potency YS or Premier 1 ROYAL JELLY, and/or Superior GINSENG/ BEE SECRETION.**

❧ Effective teas to hydrate:
◆ Calendula
◆ Chamomile
◆ Witch Hazel
◆ Rose Hips / Lemon juice
◆ Peppermint / Eucalytus for a freshening scrub.

❧ **CamoCare concentrate**

BODYWORK

❖ Use a gentle, balancing mask once a week, such as Crystal Star HERBAL TONING MASK, or Zia SUPER HYDRATING MASK.
◆ Follow with a blend of Aloe Vera gel and vitamin E oil.

❖ Good softening agents:
◆ Jojoba oil
◆ Sesame oil
◆ Crystal Star SOFT TONE OIL
◆ Wheat germ oil

❖ Effective exfoliant/cleansers for glowing skin:
◆ Loofa sponges
◆ Cucumber/Papaya skins
◆ Oatmeal baths
◆ Crystal Star MINERAL SALT GLOW
◆ Honey / Almond / Oatmeal scrub

❖ Get 20 minutes of early morning sunlight on the skin every day possible for Vitamin D.

❖ Effective soaps/cleansers:
◆ Zia SEA TONIC WITH ALOE
◆ Aubrey JOJOBA CLEANSER
◆ Olive oil soap
◆ Tea Tree oil soap

COMMON SYMPTOMS: Unbalanced skin and acid mantle, with sores, spots, cracks, oiliness or dryness, scaling, itching, chapping, redness and rashes.

COMMON CAUSES: Emotional stress; poor diet of excess refined foods and sugars; too many saturated fats; caffeine overload; food allergies; too high copper levels causing blotching; poor digestion and assimilation; PMS; irritating cosmetics; essential fatty acid depletion; liver malfunction.

MORE NATURAL THERAPY FOR SKIN PROBLEMS:

Remember that all great skin starts from the inside with a diet high in minerals and fresh foods. Natural cosmetic and food supplements can help stimulate healthy cell growth, smoothness, elasticity, tone and color.

* **FOR WHITE HARD BUMPS ON THE UPPER ARMS AND CHEST:** Emulsified vitamin A 25,000IU 2 daily, zinc picolinate 50Mg. daily, and Ester C 550Mg. with bioflavonoids and rutin 2-3 daily.

* **NATURAL SUPPLEMENTS WITH RETIN A EFFECTS:** Aloe juice 1 glass daily, 1 teasp. aloe gel mixed with 1 pricked vitamin E 400IU capsule, Reviva LIGHT SKIN PEEL, and NIGHTCREAM/DAYCREAM, Zia PAPAYA PEEL. Apply high potency Royal Jelly.

* **FOR VITILIGO** (DEPLETION AND LACK OF SKIN PIGMENTATION): Some effectiveness has been shown when treated as for radiation poisoning (see that page in this book). Also, Solaray Turmeric capsules 4 daily; PABA 1000Mg. with 2T. unsulphured molasses daily as an iron source, and Pantothenic acid 1000Mg., and Betaine HCl tabs with meals; Alta Health SIL-X SILICA CAPS; Smart COLLAGEN TABS OR POWDER; Sun CHLORELLA 1 packet daily, with Egg Yolk Lecithin and Ginkgo Biloba extract. Calendula gel is an effective topical. Always wear UV poisoning sunscreen defense creams because of this probable reaction to ozone depletion.

* **FOR LIVER SPOTS/ AGE SPOTS:** High potency Premier one or YS ROYAL JELLY 2t. daily, Biotec AGELESS BEAUTY to release rancid fats, Reviva BROWN SPOT REMOVER, PABA 100Mg. with Pantothenic acid 1000Mg., high Omega 3 flax oil 3t. daily.

* **FOR DRY AND DAMAGED SKIN:** Apply Aloe gel mixed with vitamin E oil, or ALOE ICE GEL; rub face with papaya peels, take high omega 3 flax oil 3t. daily, Evening Primrose oil capsules 4 daily.

* **FACIAL BLOTCHING AND EXCESS PIGMENTATION:** Reduce too high copper levels by adding more zinc and iron-rich foods. Keep the body free of clogging waste with a herbal laxative.

* **FOR POOR SKIN TONE AND COLOR:** Crystal Star MINERAL SALT GLOW, ALOE ICE GEL, jojoba oil.

* **FOR FREE RADICAL SCAVENGING AND PROTECTION FROM ENVIRONMENTAL POLLUTANTS:** Twin Lab SUPER GERMANIUM WITH SUMA CAPSULES 3-4 daily, Biotec AGELESS BEAUTY CAPSULES 6 daily, Vitamin E with Selenium 400IU, Egg Yolk Lecithin capsules, Ginkgo Biloba extract, cosmetics and skin care products with azuline.

* **TO BALANCE SKIN pH:** Twin Lab GERMANIUM WITH SUMA CAPSULES, Jason SUMA MOISTURIZER, Crystal Star BEAUTIFUL SKIN TEA, lemon juice to restore acid mantle.

* **FOR WRINKLING AND DRY CRACKS:** Zia PAPAYA PEEL, Revivia LIGHT SKIN PEEL, 1 teasp. aloe gel mixed with 1 pricked vitamin E 400IU capsule. Rub face with papaya skins, and add apples, papaya and citrus fruits to the diet.

* **NATURAL MAKE-UP REMOVERS:** Make a mix of apricot, avocado, almond and sesame oils; good for all skin types - makes your skin feel wonderful.

FOOD THERAPY	VITAMINS/ MINERALS	HERBAL THERAPY	BODYWORK
Keep the diet simple and alkaline during healing. Add more fresh fruits and vegetables. Consciously add vegetable protein sources for faster healing; whole grains, soy foods, sea foods and cultured foods.	**BASAL CELL CARCINOMAS:** Open sores, chronic reddish patches, small mole growths, shiny bumps; usually in areas exposed regularly to the sun. ◆ H$_2$O$_2$ PEROXY GEL ◆ Calendula gel ◆ PABA 500-1000Mg. **STRAWBERRYS/BROWN PIGMENT MARKS.** ◆ B&T Califlora ointment ◆ Pantothenic acid 1000Mg. ◆ B6 500Mg.	Highest potency YS or Premier 1 ROYAL JELLY 2t. daily.	Get early morning sunlight on the skin every day for 15 minutes. Use an SPF sun screen of 15 or higher.
Take 1t. each in a glass of aloe vera juice 2x daily: Wheat germ oil, Brewer's yeast	**SQUAMOUS CELL CARCINOMAS:** Pink, opaque nodules or patches anywhere on the body. ◆ Beta Carotene 100,000IU ◆ Vit. E 400IU w/ Selenium ◆ Tea Tree oil	Solaray Turmeric capsules 4 daily with Burdock tea 2 cups daily.	Effective applications: ◆ Hot comfrey compresses ◆ Dry mustard plaster ◆ Green clay poultice
Drink 6-8 glasses of bottled water daily to keep acid wastes flushed.	**MALIGNANT MELANOMAS:** Small or large brown-black patches, or multi-colored patches, or irregular nodules. ◆ Calendula gel ◆ Vitamin C solution ◆ H$_2$O$_2$ PEROXY GEL	Evening Primrose oil caps 4-6 daily, with Pau de Arco or Burdock tea 2 cups daily.	Apply H$_2$O$_2$ peroxy gel directly to affected area, and on to soles of feet. Usual noticeable change in 3 weeks.
Avoid saturated fats, sugars, caffeine and caffeine-containing foods.	Ascorbate or Ester C powder, 1/2t. hourly to bowel tolerance during healing for collagen production and connective tissue growth.	Crystal Star THERADERM CAPS 4-6 daily, and THERADERM TEA. Take internally and pat on with cotton externally.♀	Avoid all pleasure drugs, especially cocaine. Most constrict the blood vessels and leave the skin without nutrients. It shrivels and dies quickly.
Eat Vitamin C and A rich foods for collagen and interstitial tissue health.	Bromelain 500Mg. with Omega 3 Flax oil 3x daily.	Effective applications: ◆ BioForce Echinacea cream ◆ Tea Tree oil ◆ Propolis tincture ◆ Golden Seal/Myrrh solution ◆ Enzymatic Therapy DERMAZYME OINTMENT ♀ ◆ Calendula gel ◆ B & T CALIFLORA GEL ALOE ICE GEL for 24 hour renewal.	Remember that corticosteroid drugs over a long period of time for skin problems, can greatly weaken the immune defenses and allow cancers to take hold.

COMMON SYMPTOMS: Festering, non-healing skin sores and lesions that appear in different forms: hard, sub-cutaneous nodes; chronic scaling and itching patches, growing warts and moles, shiny bumps, pink nodules, multicolored or brown patches; old skin patches that won't come off, etc.

COMMON CAUSES: UV radiation from the sun because of ozone depletion; too many antibiotics, especially in children; malfunctioning sebaceous glands; allergies to sugars, wheat or pasteurized dairy; too much saturated fat and red meat, causing over-acid system; B vitamin depletion; fungus infection; Candida Albicans; inherited thin sensitive skin.

SMOKING & TOBACCO
HOW TO STOP

FOOD THERAPY

- There must be a lifestyle and diet change for there to be permanent success. **Start with a 3 day liquid fast (Pg. 25) with fresh fruit and vegetable juices and miso soup to neutralize and clear the blood of nicotinic acid and fortify blood sugar.** Then, follow a fresh foods only diet for the rest of the week, with carrot juices, plenty of carrots and celery, leafy green salads, and lots of citrus fruits to promote body alkalinity. pH 7 and above readings definitely show decreased desire for tobacco.

- **Include lots of vegetable proteins. Eat smaller meals more frequently.**

- **Avoid junk foods and sugar that aggravate cravings.**

- See HYPOGLYCEMIA DIET suggestions in this book for more information.

VITAMINS/ MINERALS

✤ **Enzymatic Therapy NICOTABS for 2 months.**

✤ **Ascorbate vitamin C powder, 1/2t. in water every hour** (about 10,000Mg. or to bowel tolerance) **while trying to quit**

✤ For nicotine toxicity, take twice daily each:
  1 Cysteine capsule
  1 Glutamine capsule
  2 Vitamin C 1000Mg. tablets
  2 Evening Primrose capsules

✤ Vitamin E w/ Selenium as an anti-oxidant, with Mezotrace SEA MINERAL COMPLEX 4 daily.

✤ **Niacin Therapy: 500-1000Mg. daily. ♂**

✤ **Brain stimulants to replace nicotine stimulation:**
  ◆ Phosphatidyl Choline
  ◆ Choline/Inositol ♂

✤ **Folic Acid 800Mcg. with B₁₂ 2000Mcg. to prevent cell/lung tissue damage.**

HERBAL THERAPY

☙ **Crystal Star NICOSTOP TEA, 2 cups taken over the day in sips to keep the tissues flooded with elements that discourage the taste for nicotine.**
  and
  RELAX CAPS as needed to rebuild nervous system and calm withdrawal tension.
  with
  DEEP BREATHING TEA to keep lungs clear.

☙ Chew Licorice root sticks, calamus root or cloves for oral gratification that curbs the craving.

☙ **Effective extracts:**
  ◆ **Crystal Star SUPER LICORICE EXTRACT ♀**
  ◆ **Echinacea**
  ◆ **Valeriana/Wild lettuce**
  ◆ **Lobelia extract**

☙ Effective teas:
  ● Sassafras Bark ♂
  ● Peppermint
  ◆ Scullcap ♀

☙ Sun Chlorella 15 tabs or 1 packet daily.

BODYWORK

✤ Each cigarette takes 8 minutes off your life; a pack a day takes 1 month off your life each year; 2 packs a day, takes 12-15 years off your life. Cigarettes have over 4000 known poisons, any of which can kill in high enough doses. ONE DROP of Nicotinic Acid can kill a man. Depending on the age that you quit, your life expectancy can increase from 2-5 years.

✤ Even secondary or passive smoke has been shown to increase the instance of cervical, uterine and lung cancer.

✤ **Do deep breathing exercises for more body oxygen whenever you feel the urge for tobacco til the desire decreases.**

✤ **Don't be discouraged. Quitting is hard work, but it gets easier every day, as your body loses the dependence on nicotine.**

COMMON SYMPTOMS: Chronic bronchitis; constant hacking cough; difficult and shortness of breath; lung and respiratory depletion and infection; emphysema and dry lungs; often eventual lung cancer and other degenerative diseases; adrenal exhaustion and fatigue; poor circulation affecting vision; high blood pressure; premature aging and wrinkled, dehydrated skin with no color or elasticity; stomach ulcers; osteoporosis; low immunity; etc., etc., etc.

COMMON CAUSES: System stress and disease from nicotine poisoning; emotional insecurity; hypoglycemia; dietary deficiencies; nicotine addiction.

SNAKE BITE ✧ POISONOUS SPIDER BITE

Get emergency medical help immediately! The methods below are to be used only until this help arrives.

SEE SHOCK & TRAUMA PAGE IN THIS BOOK FOR MORE EMERGENCY INFORMATION. (Pg. 250)

FOOD THERAPY	VITAMINS/ MINERALS	HERBAL THERAPY	BODYWORK
❥ **Wash bite with soap and water. No ice compresses. No alcoholic drinks. (The poison will spread faster).**	✛ **Niacin therapy: up to 500Mg. after poison is out of the body, to dilate and tone blood vessels.**	❧ **Cayenne, 2 capsules or 8-10 drops of Cayenne extract in warm water as a shock preventive to strengthen the heart.**	❖ **Put a constricting band 2-4" above the wound. Do not cut off circulation. (Move band up if swelling reaches it.)**
❥ Give the victim only small sips of water.	✛ **Calcium ascorbate vitamin C powder, 1/4t. every 1/2 hour to bowel tolerance during acute reaction phase.**	❧ Apply Aloe/Comfrey Salve or Aloe Vera gel or Comfrey extract.	❖ Use suction by mouth or suction cup <u>as soon as possible after the bite.</u> Make a small cut <u>up and down, not across,</u> through each fang mark. Suction with mouth or cup for at least 30 seconds. Do not swallow. Rinse immediately.
❥ Plant onions and garlic around the house to keep snakes away.	✛ Vitamin E 400IU. Take internally; prick capsule and apply locally.	❧ **Yellow Dock tea every hour til swelling goes down.**	
❥ Make a tobacco and saliva poultice and apply to bite.	✛ Vitamin A & D 25,000IU; take internally; prick capsule and apply locally.	❧ Plantain or Rue compresses.	❖ Keep victim still and calm. Immobilize the bite area and keep it lower than the heart.
		❧ Apply Chinese WHITE FLOWER OIL.	
		❧ Apply Calendula gel or lotion.	

COMMON SYMPTOMS: Slow upward spreading red lines as poison moves toward the heart; swelling, pain and nausea; sweating; dizziness and fainting; breathing difficulty.

SORE THROAT ✧ STREP THROAT ✧ SWOLLEN GLANDS

FOOD THERAPY

❧ Go on a short 24Hr. liquid cleansing diet (Pg. 27), or a 3 day mucous cleansing diet (Pg.25).

◆ Take lemon juice and honey in water, and a potassium broth (Pg. 33) each morning. Take citrus juices throughout the day.

◆ Then eat mainly fresh foods during healing. Have plenty of leafy greens.

❧ Follow a cleansing diet for at least another week to overcome low grade infection; eat some steamed vegetables, tofu, fresh fruits, and brown rice every day.

❧ Avoid all dairy foods, sugars and fried fatty foods during healing.

❧ Effective gargles:
Lemon juice and brandy
Black tea
Sea salt water
Cider vinegar and water

❧ Apply hot parsley compresses to the throat.

VITAMINS/ MINERALS

❖ Zinc gluconate or propolis lozenges every few hours as needed. ☺

❖ Alacer EFFERVESCENT C. every few hours. Hold in the mouth as long as possible for best absorption.
and/or
Vitamin C chewable 500Mg. with Rose Hips or Acerola cherries, every hour during acute stages.

❖ N.F. Factors HERBAL SEPTIC as needed. ⬡

❖ BioForce SANTASAPINA THROAT DROPS, or SANTASAPINA or DROSINULA SYRUPS. ☺

❖ Solaray MULTIDOLPHILUS or Nature's Plus JUNIOR DOLHILUS CHEWABLES.☺

❖ Hylands HYLAVIR TABS.

❖ ENZYMATIC THERAPY VIRAPLEX CAPS and/or ORAL-ZYME LOZENGES.

HERBAL THERAPY

❧ Crystal Star ANTI-BIO or ANTI-VI CAPSULES, 6 daily (depending on the cause)
with
COFEX TEA as needed for a soothing throat coat.

❧ Shark Liver oil caps as a strong anti-infective.

❧ Garlic capsules 6 daily.

❧ Effective gargles:
◆ Golden Seal/Myrrh
◆ Fenugreek/Honey
◆ Liquid chlorophyll

❧ Effective tinctures:
◆ Zand HERBAL INSURE
◆ Crystal Star SUPER LICORICE
◆ Licorice Root ♂
◆ Wild Cherry
◆ Myrrh Gum

❧ Effective teas:
◆ Horehound
◆ Slippery Elm
◆ Barberry Bark

❧ Effective herbal lozenges:
◆ Zand HERBAL INSURE
◆ Olbas

BODYWORK

❖ Apply hot ginger compresses to the throat.

❖ Use Eucalyptus steams.

❖ Take hot 20 minute saunas daily if possible.

❖ Stick tongue out as far as it will go. Hold for 30 seconds. Release and relax. Repeat 3 times to increase blood supply to the area.

COMMON SYMPTOMS: Sore, aching, inflamed, throat and tonsils; swollen throat tissues; difficult talking; laryngitis.

COMMON CAUSES: Viral infection; low immunity; tonsilitis; too many mucous-forming foods; adrenal exhaustion.

SPINAL MENINGITIS ✧ ENCEPHALITIS

FOOD THERAPY	VITAMINS/ MINERALS	HERBAL THERAPY	BODYWORK
❥ There must be diet and life-style change for there to be effective, permanent improvement. ☺	✛ Niacin Therapy: 100-500Mg. daily. (If a child, give a baby aspirin first to avoid niacin flush). ☺	❦ Comfrey tea 5 cups daily as an anti-flammatory.	❖ Immerse back of the head in warm epsom salts solution to draw out inflammation, several times daily. ☺
❥ No sugar, refined, or junk foods at all. ☺	✛ Beta Carotene 50,000IU as an anti-infective.	❦ Evening Primrose oil caps 4-6 daily.	❖ Alternate hot and cold packs on the neck and back of the head to stimulate circulation to the area.
❥ The diet should be 50-75% fresh foods and vegetable juices, with a fresh carrot juice and a potassium broth (Pg.33) or green drink (Pg.34) 2-3x a week.	✛ Quercitin Plus with Bromelain to control inflammation.	❦ Kelp tabs 6-8 daily.	
	✛ Phosphatidyl Choline (PC 55), to nourish brain tissue. ♂	❦ Scullcap tea for nerve support. ♀	❖ Use catnip enemas during acute phase to clear body quickly of infection. ☺
❥ A 24 hour liquid diet should be used one day each week to keep the body flushed and alkaline. (Pg. 27).	✛ Ascorbate vitamin C or Ester C powder with bioflavonoids, 1/4t. every hour during acute phases. Reduce dosage by 1/2 for maintenance til remission.	❦ Enzymatic Therapy VIRAPLEX CAPS, 4 daily.	❖ Avoid aluminum cookware, deodorants, and other alum containing products.
		❦ Crystal Star ANTI-VI EXTRACT one week on, one week off to control infection. with MIN-ZYME-MINOS DRINK to strengthen a weakened system.	❖ Get some fresh air and early morning sunshine every day.
❥ Add cultured foods, such as yogurt and kefir, for friendly G.I. flora establishment. ☺	✛ Vital Health Formula ONE ORAL CHELATION with EDTA to increase blood flow to the brain.♂	❦ High Omega 3 flax oil 3t. daily.	❖ Remember that cortico-steroid drugs taken for this problem over a long period of time weaken both bone structure and immunity.
❥ Drink only bottled water, 6-8 glasses daily.	✛ B Complex 50Mg., with extra B6 100Mg. and B12 sublingual lozenges 2500Mcg. daily.	❦ Sun CHLORELLA for inflammation and healthy tissue growth.	

COMMON SYMPTOMS: Inflammation and damage to the brain because of nerve/spinal inflammation; consequent deficient blood supply and oxygen to the brain; lethargy, and slowness of thought and movement; brain retardation; constant chronic colds and respiratory conditions.

COMMON CAUSES: Nutritional depletion, especially in children; too many mucous-forming foods; heavy metal or chemical poisoning; cerebro-vascular disease; psychological trauma.

258

SPLEEN & LYMPHATIC SYSTEM HEALTH

FOOD THERAPY

☙ To revitalize through diet:
◆ Take carrot/Beet/Cucumber juice every day for 1 week, then every other day for another week to "spring clean" these glands of stored toxins.
◆ Then, build up red blood cells with a potassium broth (pg.33), green drink (pg.34), (or Crystal Star ENERGY GREEN DRINK), and a leafy green salad every day. Include brown rice and alfalfa sprouts frequently.

☙ Take a glass of lemon juice and water regularly in the morning, and a glass of papaya juice in the evening.

☙ Include plenty of potassium-rich foods regularly, such as sea vegetables, broccoli, bananas and seafood.

☙ See LIVER CLEANSING & DIET SUGGESTIONS in this book for more details.

☙ Avoid caffeine, sugar and alcohol during healing.

VITAMINS/ MINERALS

✤ Marine Carotene 50-100,000IU daily. with
Liquid chlorophyll 3t. daily with meals.

✤ Enzymatic Therapy LIQUID LIVER WITH GINSENG, and RAW SPLEEN COMPLEX ♂

✤ Shark Liver oil for leucocyte production.

✤ Alta Health CANGEST daily with
Evening Primrose oil caps 4 daily. ♀

✤ Raw spleen glandular Raw Thymus glandular

✤ Vitamin E 400IU daily for red blood enhancement.

✤ Zinc picolinate 30Mg. or Solaray BIO-ZINC. ♂ and

✤ Natren LIFE START #2.

HERBAL THERAPY

❧ Crystal Star ANTI-BIO CAPS for white blood cell enhancement; and ANEMI-GIZE CAPS with HAWTHORNE EXTRACT for blood building and tone.

❧ Effective extracts:
◆ Crystal Star SUPER LICORICE
◆ Hawthorne Lf. and Bry.
◆ Siberian Ginseng
◆ Floradix HERBAL IRON

❧ Effective capsules:
◆ Golden Seal
◆ Chaparral/Dandelion
◆ Garlic/Cayenne
◆ Solaray ALFAJUICE

❧ Effective oxygen teas:
◆ Barberry
◆ Chaparral
◆ Yellow Dock/Sage
◆ Burdock Rt.

❧ Spleen enhancing tea: 4oz. Hawthorne, 1oz. Cardamom, 1oz. Safflowers, 1oz. Lemon Balm, 1oz. Red Sage; take 2 cups daily.

❧ Sun CHLORELLA GRANULES 1 packet daily.

BODYWORK

✤ No aluminum cookware, food additives, or aluminum-containing foods.

✤ Regular exercise is a key to the health of this system.

✤ REFLEXOLOGY POINT:

LYMPH & SPLEEN

COMMON SYMPTOMS: The spleen destroys worn out and ineffective red blood cells, and stores and renews healthy cells, providing oxygen for the bloodstream and brain. It can be an absolute necessity in times of hemorrhage or shock trauma. Depletion symptoms include anemia, pallor, extreme slimness; lack of energy and memory; sluggishness.
◆ The Lymphatic system flushes waste from the body, and filters through microphages, that can engulf foreign and harmful particles and render them harmless.

COMMON CAUSES: Too many saturated fats and refined carbohydrates reduce activity of these glands; liver exhaustion and stress; protein and B$_{12}$ deficiency all affect efficiency.

SPORTS INJURIES ✦ SPRAINS ✦ MUSCLE PULLS

FOOD THERAPY

❦ A basic diet should consist of about 65-70% complex carbohydrates, (from vegetables, fruits, whole grains and legumes); 20-25% protein, (from nuts, seeds, soy foods, poultry, seafood, and low fat dairy products); and 10-15% fats from quality sources, (unsaturated vegetable oils, nuts, seeds, low fat dairy, butter, and fish).

❦ Athletes nutritional needs are considerably greater than those of the average person, (about 2000-6000 calories and 4-6 meals a day) since they need to reach peak performance and avoid easily occuring injuries.

❦ Eat chromium-rich foods: Lobster, low fat cheeses, brewer's yeast, and organ meats.

❦ Drink plenty of mineral water every day.

❦ Effective foods for massaging into injury:
  ◆ Cider vinegar/sea salt paste
  ◆ Hot linseed or flax oil
  ◆ Cayenne/Vinegar solution
  ◆ Wheat germ oil

TORN LIGAMENTS

VITAMINS/ MINERALS

✣ Quercitin Plus with Bromelain 500-750Mg. 2-4 caps daily as an anti-inflammatory.
  or

✣ Country Life LIGATEND CAPS 4 daily. ♀

✣ Vitamin C crystals, 1/2t., or Alacer Emergen-C every hour during acute stress for collagen and connective tissue healing.

✣ Enzymatic Therapy ACID-A-CAL CAPS 4 daily. ♀

✣ Dyna-Mins Cal/Mag 500/500Mg. 6 daily.
  with
  Zinc 75Mg. daily. ♀

✣ Vitamin E 800IU daily with methionine 500Mg. for torn cartilege.

✣ Chromium picolinate 200Mcg., or Nutrition 21 CHROMAX 2, or Solaray CHROMIACIN CAPS

✣ DLPA 500-750Mg. as needed with CO Q 10 30Mg. for pain relief.

HERBAL THERAPY

❧ Alta Health SIL-X SILICA CAPS 4-6 daily, for new collagen and interstitial tissue regrowth. ♀

❧ Crystal Star HIGH PERFORMANCE CAPS 2-4 daily to provide long range energy and prevent lactic acid buildup.
  and
  ADRN-ALIVE with BODY REBUILDER CAPS ♀, or MASTER BUILDER CAPS. ♂

❧ Biotec EXTRA ENERGY ENZYMES 6 daily for arthritis-like symptoms.

❧ Siberian Ginseng extract for lactic acid build-up, increased oxygen use and glycogen storage. ♂

❧ Country Life ENERGIX VIALS 1 daily. ♂

❧ Mezotrace SEA MINERAL COMPLEX 6 daily for preventive strength.
  and
  White Birch mineral water to replace lost potassium.

BODYWORK

✣ *Elevate the area.*
  1) Apply ice packs immediately. Leave on for 30 minutes. Remove 15 minutes. Repeat for up to 3 hours. This decreases bleeding from injured vessels by causing them to constrict.
  2) Wrap the strain or sprain snugly with an elastic bandage (over the ice if desired) to limit swelling.
  3) Apply alternating hot and cold packs the next day to stimulate circulation/relax muscle cramps.

✣ Effective applications:
  ◆ Ginger/Thyme compresses
  ◆ B & T ARNIFLORA CREAM
  ◆ MINERAL ICE
  ◆ Tiger Balm
  ◆ B & T ANALGESIC RUB
  ◆ Chinese White Flower oil
  ◆ Cajeput/Wintergreen oil
  ◆ Tea Tree oil
  ◆ DMSO solution.

✣ Crystal Star DRAWING & SWEATING WRAP as a steam room treatment.

✣ Make a healing paste: mix 2t. Aloe vera gel, 1t. each golden seal, comfrey and slippery elm powders; apply.

260

COMMON SYMPTOMS: Wrenched knees; twisted ankles; sprained wrists; shin splints; tennis elbows; torn ligaments; muscle pulls; arthritis-like symptoms; bruises; tendon inflammation; Achilles heel; shooting pains in the ankles, feet and knees.

MORE SPECIFICS ABOUT NATURAL SUPPLEMENTS FOR SPORTS MEDICINE

Athletes cannot get by any longer just adding anabolic steroids to gain body mass. (See page 51 for more on the hazards of chemical steroid use). Over and above the well-known debilitating hormone changes brought on by these drugs, they also greatly effect immune system balance, preventing the body from healing easily after injury. In addition, after all the expense and body trauma, the muscles "deflate" quickly when the steroids are stopped. The only effective alternative for mature muscle growth is optimum nutrition and/or food-source supplementation.

❖ NATURAL ANABOLIC STEROID REPLACEMENTS ❖

❖ **CHROMIUM PICOLINATE:** This trace mineral form acts as a safe alternative to anabolic steroids. It promotes a noticeable difference in free-form amino acid uptake by the cells from the bloodstream. It boosts muscle structure (particularly in bicep and calf circumference) by decreasing body fat without decreasing muscle, and helps build leaner body mass without sugar or cholesterol problems. Refined sugars rob the body of chromium. The most effective products include complexes with Niacin for Chromium uptake: Nutrition 21 CHROMAX 2, Solaray CHROMIACIN, Weider, CHROMATE.
❖ **HERBS WITH ANABOLIC EFFECT:** Smilax (Sarsaparilla), Siberian Ginseng (Eleuthero), Brazilian Ginseng (Suma), Korean Ginseng, Chinese Red Ginseng (Panax), Astragalus, Fo-Ti-Tieng, Saw Palmetto, Damiana, Gotu Kola, Ma Huang, Licorice and Alfalfa, BioForce GINSAVENA DROPS.
❖ **INOSINE:** A nucleotide precursor and breakdown product for ATP (Adenosine Tri-phosphate) production, and short-range, intense energy bursts.
❖ **BCAAS (BRANCHED CHAIN AMINO ACIDS):** for muscle work effeciency, energy, and new tissue development after injury.
❖ **DIBENCOZIDE:** The most active form of vitamin B_{12} for cellular development; a safe, effective steroid alternative. Use with Carnitine or CO Q 10 for best effects.
❖ **FREE FORM AMINO ACIDS:** Many have anabolic properties without the side effects; Argenine and Ornithine as GH producers, and Carnitine for heart health and circulation.
❖ **OTHER NATURAL ALTERNATIVES TO STEROIDS:** Bee Pollens and Royal Jelly, Germanium for utilization of oxygen, and heart and artery fitness, Country Life ENERGIX VIALS, Enzymatic Therapy LIQUID LIVER WITH SIBERIAN GINSENG, Octacosonal, and Source Naturals FRAC and GAMMA ORYZONOL (GO) CAPSULES.
❖ **HERBS FOR FOUNDATION MINERALS:** The most concentrated, absorbable mineral sources in the world today are herbs. Particular effectiveness comes from herbal iron, calcium and potassium sources. Effective products include Crystal Star HIGHLY ABSORBABLE IRON and CALCIUM EXTRACTS, POTASSIUM SOURCE and MEGA-MINERAL CAPSULES, and MIN-ZYME-MINOS DRINK; FLORADIX HERBAL IRON, Enzymatic Therapy BIO-K, and Vital Health WHITE BIRCH MINERAL WATER, for highly available potassium.
❖ **PROTEIN & PROTEIN POWDERS:** Champion METABOLOL 2, Nature's Plus SPIRUTEIN, NUTRI-TECH ALL 1 POWDER, RichLife PRO-MUSCLE.
❖ **ELECTROLYTE REPLACEMENTS:** Take electrolyte replacements to rebuild lost mineral strength. Knudsens RECHARGE CARBO COOLERS, Twin Lab ULTRA FUEL.
❖ **NATURAL ANTI-INFLAMMATORIES:** Crystal Star BONZ CAPS 4-6 daily as an anti-inflammatory. (Also effective made into a paste with water and applied), B & T Califlora gel, Enzymatic Therapy CORTOTONE CAPSULES and SIMI-CORT CREAM.

See NUTRITION & BODYWORK COMPONENTS OF THE NEW PHYSICAL FITNESS in this book for more information, pp 48.

261

STOMACH & DUODENAL ULCERS

FOOD THERAPY

❧ **Go on a short 3 day liquid diet to cleanse and alkalize the G.I. tract.**
  ◆ Take 2-3 glasses of your choice of juices daily: Potassium broth or essence (pg. 33), Green drinks (pg. 34), Cabbage/Carrot/Parsley juice, Carrot/Spinach juice, Apple/Alfalfa sprout juice with 1t. Spirulina powder added.

❧ Then, add easily digestible, fresh alkaline foods, such as leafy greens, vegetables, whole grains and fruits.

❧ Eat lots of cultured foods for friendly G.I. flora.

❧ Drink 2-3 glasses mineral water daily.

❧ **Chew all food slowly and well.**

❧ Avoid sugars, pasteurized dairy products, red meats, fatty, fried and refined foods. Reduce alcohol (a little white wine is ok), and heavy spices during healing.

VITAMINS/ MINERALS

❖ **Enzymatic Therapy DGL CHEWABLE TABS with Sun CHLORELLA TABS 15 daily**, or liquid chlorophyll 3t. daily with meals.

❖ **High potency YS or Premier One ROYAL JELLY 2t. daily.** ♀

❖ Ascorbate vitamin C or Ester C, 3000Mg. daily with **Vitamin E 400IU 2x daily** and Emulsified A 100,000IU, for 3 months.

❖ Stress B Complex 100Mg. with extra pantothenic acid 500Mg. ♀

❖ Natren LIFE START #2, 1/2t. before meals.

❖ Enzymatic Therapy RAW ADRENAL COMPLEX CAPS.

❖ Propolis tincture as needed. ♂

HERBAL THERAPY

❧ Crystal Star ULCR CAPSULES or EXTRACT, **with meals as needed.** and RELAX CAPS or ANTI-SPAZ CAPS as needed to calm and rebuild nerve structure.
  ◆ ANTI-BIO CAPS 4-6 daily if there is infection.

❧ Yerba Prima Aloe Vera juice with herbs daily.

❧ Effective extracts:
  ◆ Nature's Way ANTSP ♂
  ◆ Golden Seal/Myrrh
  ◆ Ginkgo Biloba
  ◆ Licorice ♂

❧ Effective teas:
  ◆ Comfrey/Mint
  ◆ Slippery Elm
  ◆ Comfrey/Fenugreek
  ◆ Chamomile/Red Sage

❧ Effective capsules:
  ◆ Solaray "COOL CAYENNE"
  ◆ Golden Seal/Cayenne
  ◆ GREEN MAGMA TABS
  ◆ Garlic/Parsley

❧ High omega 3 flax oil 3t. daily. ♀

BODYWORK

❖ Remember that Tagamet and Zantac drugs for ulcers (1 billion dollars in sales yearly) suppress HCl formation in the stomach, inhibit bone formation, and cause eventual liver damage. DGL (De-glycyrrhizinated Licorice), can normalize after these drugs.

❖ Remember that herbal remedies and vegetable juices are excellent and gentle for ulcerated tissue.

❖ **Avoid smoking and caffeine, two of the key culprits in aggravating ulcers.**

❖ Take a catnip or garlic enema once a week during healing to detoxify the G.I. tract.

❖ For duodenal ulcers: take a mild olive oil flush with 2T. of oil through a straw before going to bed, for a week.

COMMON SYMPTOMS: Open sores or lesions in the stomach/duodenum walls, causing burning, nausea and diarrhea; happens especially after eating.

COMMON CAUSES: Prolonged stress and nervous tension creating an acid system; poor food combining and too many acid-forming foods; eating too fast; commercial antacids; food allergies; too many sugary foods; too much caffeine and alcohol; tobacco; anemia; Candida Albicans; Hypoglycemia.

STRESS ◆ ANXIETY

NERVOUS TENSION

FOOD THERAPY	VITAMINS/ MINERALS	HERBAL THERAPY	BODYWORK
☙ Good nutrition is often the answer to stress and tension. As stress increases, protein needs go up. Add vegetable proteins from whole grains, sea vegetables, seafoods, soy foods and sprouts.	✢ DLPA 500-750Mg. as needed daily. with Tyrosine 500Mg. 2 daily, or Glycine 500Mg.	☙ Feed your nerves. Crystal Star RELAX CAPS 2-4 daily as needed, or STRESS RELIEF EXTRACT. and if desired CALCIUM SOURCE CAPS or MEGA MINERAL CAPSULES.	✤ You have to unwind before you can unleash. Deep breathing aerobic exercise every day is one of the best things you can do for stress.
☙ Take 2T. each daily: Brewer's yeast Wheat germ Lecithin	✢ Stress B Complex 100Mg. 2-3x daily, with extra B₆ 250Mg. (Take with Fennel tea if appetite increases).♀	☙ Feed your adrenals; Crystal Star ADRN ALIVE CAPS or ADRN EXTRACT.	✤ Consciously take a rest and relaxation period every day. Listen to soft music. Meditate. Do 3 minutes of neck rolls.
☙ Have fresh carrot juice and fresh fish or seafood at least once a week.	✢ Ascorbate vitamin C with bioflavonoids, 500Mg. every 4 hours during acute periods. with Magnesium/Potassium/ Bromelain capsules.♂	☙ Effective extracts: ◆ Valerian/Wild Lettuce ◆ Hops/Valerian ◆ Scullcap ◆ Astragalus ◆ Passion Flower ♀	✤ Hypnotherapy, aromatherapy, (Chamomile oil), massage therapy and shiatzu have all shown effective results against stress.
☙ Add other magnesium-rich foods, such as green vegetables, whole grains and molasses.	✢ Alta Health MANGANESE WITH B₁₂ LOZENGES.	☙ Effective teas: ◆ Crystal Star RELAX TEA ◆ Chamomile ◆ Wood Betony ◆ Fennel seed	✤ Go on a short vacation. Take a long weekend. It will do wonders for your head.
☙ Observe good food combining to relieve digestion. Take a small glass of wine before dinner. No liquids with meals.	✢ Dyno-Mins Calcium 500Mg./Magnesium 500Mg. 4 daily. with Tryptophane 500Mg. ♀	☙ Evening Primrose oil caps 2-4 daily.	✤ Have a good laugh every day.
☙ Drink only bottled water.	✢ COQ 10 15-30Mg. daily.♂	☙ High potency ROYAL JELLY 2t. daily for effective pantothenic acid.	✤ Don't smoke. Nicotine constricts the blood vessels, causing increased body stress.

COMMON SYMPTOMS: Chronic indigestion; high blood pressure; weight loss or gain from anxiety eating; depression; P.M.S. and menstrual disorders; bad breath and body odor; poor skin; heart attack.

COMMON CAUSES: Emotional and/or psycholgical problems; overuse of drugs or prescription medicines; nerve damage; fatigue and lack of rest; too much tobacco, caffeine or alcohol; allergy reaction; hypoglycemia; gland imbalance; mineral depletion; niacin deficiency; noise, air and environmental pollutants; overcrowding; unemployment; poverty; marital and social problems.

SUNBURN ✧ HEATSTROKE

FOOD THERAPY	VITAMINS/ MINERALS	HERBAL THERAPY	BODYWORK
❧ Effective natural electrolyte replacements: Celery juice Lemonade Mineral water Suck on Limes Potassium broth (pg.33)	✤ Ascorbate vitamin C with bioflavonoids and rutin, 1/4t. in water every hour during acute stage; also pat solution on burned areas frequently.	❧ Apply Aloe Vera gel. Drink 1-2 glasses aloe juice daily.	❖ For heat stroke: apply ice packs and wrap in a cold wet sheet. Get medical help immediately. Treat for shock (pg. 250).
❧ Add plenty of complex carbohydrates and vegetable proteins to the diet for good skin repair and renewal.	✤ Canthaxanthin caps, 4-6 daily for prevention and better tanning. ♀	❧ High potency ROYAL JELLY 2t. daily for heathy skin regrowth. ♀	❖ If burns are severe, see BURNS PAGE in this book. Apply cold compresses, or take a cool bath immediately (do not use soap or hot water).
❧ Apply yogurt, honey or cider vinegar to burned areas. Apply grated apple to burned eyelids for immediate relief.	✤ B Complex 100Mg. daily with extra PABA caps 1000Mg. and Raw Adrenal extract. ♀	❧ Effective applications: ◆ Comfrey/Aloe salve ◆ Jojoba oil ♀ ◆ Green clay poultice ◆ B&T CALIFLORA GEL ☺ ◆ Plantain compresses ◆ Crystal Star CALENDULA GEL	◆ Take an electrolyte drink, or a little salty water. No alcoholic beverages (they dehydrate).
❧ Take 2T. each daily for faster healing: Brewer's yeast Lemon juice Wheat germ Lecithin	✤ Vitamin E 400IU daily internally. Prick a capsule and apply externally with an A & D capsule.	❧ Crystal Star MEGA-MINERAL CAPS, 2 daily, or MIN-ZYME-MINOS DRINK for electrolyte minerals.	❖ Mix 1 teasp. vinegar and 1/2 cup sunflower oil and pat on burns.
	✤ Effervescent C 1-2 packets daily as a drink for lost electrolytes. ♂	❧ Mezotrace SEA MINERAL COMPLEX 2-3 daily.	❖ Pat on Tea Tree oil.
	✤ PABA caps and cream with Zinc oxide cream for protection. ♂	❧ Apply a wheat germ oil, vitamin E oil, comfrey leaf, and honey poultice.	❖ Regularly use SPF 15 or more sunburn prevention cream or oil.

COMMON SYMPTOMS: Sunburn and dehydration; over-reaction to heat and sun exposure; headache; numbness; high blood pressure; often confusion and delerium; rapid pulse and shock condition, if serious, which can lead to brain damage.

Remember to take sunburn prevention supplements, and use sunburn cream SPF 15 or above, regularly. If the tissues are loaded with carotene A, vitamin C, E w/ Selenium and B complex, whether from food or a good food source supplement, it will be difficult for your skin to even get a sunburn, let alone be damaged.

TASTE & SMELL LOSS

FOOD THERAPY

- Make sure the diet is low in salt and refined sugars.

- Use herbal salt-free seasonings.

- Keep the diet free of mucous-clogging foods, such as heavy starches, red meats and pasteurized dairy foods.

- Have some brown rice, miso soup, and sea vegetables every day for 3 months to boost minerals and B vitamins.

- See THE LOW SALT DIET(pg.44) for more information.

VITAMINS/ MINERALS

❖ Zinc, up to 100Mg. daily.

❖ ENER B₁₂ INTERNASAL GEL every other day.♀

❖ B Complex 100Mg. daily, with extra B₆ 100Mg. with

❖ Ester C 550Mg. with bioflavonoids 4-6 daily.♀

❖ Marine Carotene up to 100,000IU daily, with
   Cal/Mag Citrate capsules 4-6 daily.♀

❖ Glutamine 500Mg. 2 daily, with
   Mezotrace SEA MINERAL COMPLEX TABS 3 daily.♂

❖ Enzymatic Therapy LIQUID LIVER WITH GINSENG CAPSULES 3-4 daily.♂

HERBAL THERAPY

🌿 Crystal Star MEGA MINERAL CAPSULES 4 daily, or MIN-ZYME-MINOS DRINK daily, or POTASSIUM SOURCE CAPSULES 4 daily for at least 3 months to increase natural foundation minerals in the body.

🌿 Kelp tabs 6 daily.

🌿 Ginkgo Biloba extract 3-4x daily.

🌿 Twin Lab Propolis extract 3-4x daily.♂

🌿 Siberian Ginseng extract capsules 2 daily,
   or
   Superior GINSENG/ROYAL JELLY VIALS 1 daily.♂

BODYWORK

❖ Use a catnip or chlorophyll enema to cleanse clogging mucous.

❖ REFLEXOLOGY POINT:

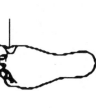

NOSE & TONGUE POINTS

❖ Regular exercise with deep breathing to keep passages clear.

COMMON CAUSES: Zinc deficiency; too many anti-biotics, causing zinc excretion; deviated septum; chronic low grade throat and sinus infection; poor circulation and mucous clogged system; atrophied nerve endings; high blood pressure medicine; over-the-counter cold medicines; chemical diuretics; gland imbalance and poor hormone secretions; hereditary proneness.

265

FOOD THERAPY

❧ Effective applications:
  ◆ Garlic oil if there is infection.
  ◆ Sea salt and honey mix.
  ◆ Wine or brandy if there is swelling.
  ◆ Clove oil if there is redness and swelling.

❧ Feed plenty of chilled foods; fresh fruits, yogurt, etc. to relieve discomfort.

❧ Give lots of cool water daily.

VITAMINS/ MINERALS

✤ Natra-Bio TEETHING DROPS.

✤ Hylands TEETHING TABLETS.

✤ Ascorbate vitamin C powder with bioflavonoids, make a weak solution in water. Give internally and apply to gums every few hours.

✤ Chewable Mezotrace childrens SEA MINERAL COMPLEX.

✤ RichLife CHEWABLE CALCIUM TABS.

✤ Apply Aloe Vera gel to gums as needed.

HERBAL THERAPY

❧ Rub on Lobelia extract.

❧ Rub on Peppermint oil.

❧ Rub on Myrrh extract.

❧ Rub on Bilbery extract drops as an anti-inflammatory.

❧ Make a weak Golden Seal solution in water. Give internally with an eye dropper on the back of the tongue. Rub on gums.

❧ Effective weak teas:
  ◆ Slippery Elm
  ◆ Chamomile
  ◆ Raspberry
  ◆ Catnip
  ◆ Peppermint
  ◆ Fennel

❧ Soak Yarrow flowers in bran and water for 3 days. Strain and rub on gums as needed.

❧ Let the child chew on natural Licorice sticks.

BODYWORK

✤ Make a weak Tea Tree oil solution with water, and rub on gums if there is swelling and infection.

✤ REFLEXOLOGY POINTS:

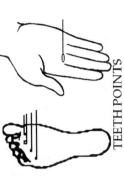

TEETH POINTS

COMMON SYMPTOMS: Sore, inflamed gums where teeth are pushing through the skin; often slight fever and infection; crying and discomfort.

See CHILDREN'S REMEDIES PAGE in this book for more information, pp.57-58.

FOOD THERAPY	VITAMINS/ MINERALS	HERBAL THERAPY	BODYWORK
Concentrate on fresh foods (at least 50% of the diet) during healing. Include plenty of vegetable proteins for faster healing, and magnesium-rich foods for muscle tension. Add a weekly potassium broth (Pg. 33) for needed electrolytes.	DLPA 500-750Mg. for pain relief.	Crystal Star RELAX CAPS to rebuild nerve sheath, with ANTI-SPAZ CAPS or CRAMP CONTROL EXTRACT as needed for pain. ♂	Apply ice packs immediately. Elevate legs and slap them hard with open palms to stimulate circulation.
	Quercitin Plus with Bromelain 500Mg. 2-4x daily as an efficient anti-inflammatory. with Magnesium/Potassium/ Bromelain caps 2 daily.	Crystal Star BONZ CAPS and/or ADRN-ALIVE CAPS or EXTRACT to rebuild adrenal cortex.	Effective applications: ◆ DMSO liquid ◆ B&T TriFlora analgesic gel ◆ TIGER BALM ◆ Chinese White Flower oil
Eat high vitamin C foods, particularly lemon juice, honey and water at night, and grapefruit or pineapple juice in the morning.	Enzymatic Therapy ACID-A-CAL, MYOTONE, or CORTOTONE CAPS. ♂	Liquid Chlorophyll 3t. daily with meals, or Crystal Star ENERGY GREEN DRINK, or Sun CHLORELLA 15 tabs daily.	Effective compresses: ◆ B&T ARNIFLORA GEL ◆ Calendula gel ◆ Comfrey ◆ Hot Burdock tea
	Twin Lab LIQUID K		Massage affected areas well and frequently. Massage therapy and shiatzu are both effective treatments.
	Country Life LIGATEND.	Lobelia extract drops. ☺	
Take 2T. each daily: Brewer's yeast Wheat germ Lecithin	Mezotrace SEA MINERAL COMPLEX 4 daily.	Rub on H_2O_2 PEROXY GEL or Aloe Vera gel.	Use alternating hot and cold compresses on affected areas to increase circulation, and take down swelling.
Avoid acid-forming foods, such as red meats, caffeine and carbonated drinks.	Alta Health SIL-X SILICA CAPS 4 daily, with Manganese and B12 lozenges 2 daily.	Crystal Star HIGH PERFORMANCE CAPSULES 2-4 before stressing the muscles to prevent lactic and uric acid buildup. SILICA SOURCE EXTRACT for collagen formation.	See SPORTS INJURIES PAGE in this book for more information.
See the ARTHRITIS DIET in this book for more suggestions.	Dyno-Mins Calcium 500Mg., Magnesium 500Mg. 4 daily. ♀		

COMMON SYMPTOMS: Cramping and soreness during and after muscle exertion; painful joints and nerve endings; leg cramps at night.

COMMON CAUSES: Calcium, Magnesium, and general mineral deficiency; poor diet, high in acid-forming foods, low in green vegetables and whole grains; too much saturated fat and sugar; HCl depletion; poor circulation.

THYROID HEALTH

FOOD THERAPY

🐍 Follow a 50% fresh foods diet for a month to rebalance the system for better metabolism.

🐍 Eat Iodine-rich foods: Sea vegetables, sea foods and greens.

🐍 Eat vitamin A-rich foods: yellow vegetables, eggs, carrots, dark green vegetables, raw dairy.

🐍 Take 2T. Brewer's Yeast and 2t. Wheat Germ oil daily.

🐍 Avoid refined foods, saturated fats, sugars, white flour and red meats.

🐍 Avoid cabbages, brussels sprouts, etc . They have anti-thyroid substances.

VITAMINS/ MINERALS

✢ Emulsified A 25,000IU 3x daily, or Beta carotene 100,000IU daily.
   with
   Vitamin E 400IU daily.

✢ Magnesium/Potassium Bromelain caps 2 daily, with Zinc 75Mg. daily. ♂

✢ Taurine 500Mg. with Lysine 500Mg. 2x daily.

✢ Enzymatic Therapy THYROID/ TYROSINE ♀

✢ Ester C with Bioflavonoids 3000Mg. daily.

✢ B Complex 100Mg. with extra B_2 100Mg., B_1 500Mg., and B_6 250Mg.

✢ CO Q 10 30Mg. daily.

✢ Raw Thyroid
   Raw Pituitary
   Raw Adrenal substance

HERBAL THERAPY

🐍 Crystal Star IODINE THERAPY CAPS and EXTRACT 3x daily.
   or
   THY-METABS 2x daily.
   and
   ADRN EXTRACT 2x daily.
   Crystal Star MIN-ZYME-MINOS DRINK.

🐍 N.F. MIODIN DROPS or Heritage ATOMODINE. ♀
   with
   Nature's Plus Vit.E 800IU.

🐍 Evening Primrose oil caps 4 daily.

🐍 Kelp tabs 6-8 daily
   with
   Cayenne caps 3 daily.

🐍 Sun CHLORELLA, or Wakasa Gold drink daily.

🐍 Siberian Ginseng extract under the tongue. 2x daily. ♂

BODYWORK

✤ Take a half hour brisk walk daily to oxygenate and stimulate circulation.

✤ Sun bathe in the morning. Sea bathe and wade whenever possible.

✤ ACUPRESSURE POINT: Press hollow at the base of the throat to stimulate thyroid, 3x for 10 seconds each.

✤ REFLEXOLOGY POINT:

THYROID / THYMUS

✤ Avoid fluorescent lights as much as possible. They deplete calcium and vitamin A in the body.

The Thyroid is the thermostat of the body. TO DETERMINE YOUR THYROID CONDITION: Take your basal temperature for 10 minutes on rising in the morning. It should be between 97.8 and 98.2 for health. Below this, and a sluggish thyroid still exists. Temperature will return to normal as nutritional therapies become effective.

COMMON SYMPTOMS: Thyroid hormone is the body's carburetor. If it is depleted or deficient, the rest of the body functions poorly. *Weak, sluggish system; dry, cold skin; slow thinking; chronic fatigue; weight gain because of poor metabolism.*

COMMON CAUSES: Iodine depletion, often from X-rays or low dose radiation tests, such as mammograms; pituitary and thyroid malfunction; air and environmental pollutants that deplete vitamin A in the body; over-use of diet pills and other drugs; vitamin A, E and Zinc deficiency.

FOOD THERAPY

🌱 Go on a short 3 day mucous cleansing diet (Pg. 25). Then eat largely fresh foods for the rest of the week. Have plenty of salads and citrus fruits.

🌱 Then, for a month, eat a mildly cleansing diet. Avoid all clogging, saturated fat foods. Reduce dairy products. Add plenty of soluble fiber foods from vegetables and whole grains.

🌱 Have a glass of lemon juice and water each morning.

🌱 Drink only bottled water.

🌱 Keep the diet very low in sugars, salt, and dairy foods on a regular basis.

🌱 See HYPOGLYCEMIA DIET PAGES in this book for more suggestions.

VITAMINS/ MINERALS

❖ Oral chelation (such as Vital Health FORMULA ONE WITH EDTA) to open clogged arteries and blood flow to the brain. and extra

❖ Beta Carotene 100,000-150,000IU daily.

❖ Niacin Therapy: 500-1000Mg. daily.♂

❖ Vitamin C with bioflavonoids, 3000-5000Mg. daily for 3 months.

   with

Alta Health MANGANESE AND B$_{12}$ LOZENGES.♂

❖ Sun CHLORELLA 15-20 tabs daily,

   with

Twin Lab CITRUS BIOFLAVONOIDS 500MG. and MAGNESIUM 400MG.

❖ Rainbow Light CALCIUM PLUS CAPS 4, 3x daily.♀

HERBAL THERAPY

🌿 Ginkgo Biloba extract 3-4x daily under the tongue for several months.
   and
Evening Primrose oil caps 4 daily for 3 months.

🌿 Summer Savory and rose water tea. May be used internally and also as drops in the ear.

🌿 Other effective teas:
Yellow Dock
Yarrow Flwr.
Bayberry Bark

🌿 Effective ear extracts: (Dilute in water to use as drops).
◆ Lobelia
◆ Angelica ♀
◆ Peppermint

🌿 Mullein oil drops, 4-6 in each ear if there is pain.

BODYWORK

❖ Massage the ear; pull on the upper ear shell, the front of the ear and ear lobes.

❖ Acupressure: stroke gently downward from the top of the temple to the bottom of the cheek with the nails for 30 seconds on each side.

❖ REFLEXOLOGY POINT:

EAR POINTS

❖ Avoid continuous loud noise. (Listening to loud rock music through headphones on a regular basis is evidencing major ear problems.)

COMMON SYMPTOMS: Feeling of fullness and clogging in the ear; no pain, but extremely annoying ringing sound in the head; loss of good hearing.

COMMON CAUSES: Poor diet with too many mucous-forming foods; poor circulation; high blood pressure; imbalance in the inner ear; allergies; lowered immune defenses; raised copper levels; fluid congestion in the middle ear; hypoglycemia (raised blood insulin causing poor carbohydrate metabolism); metabolic imbalance; mastoid and sinus inflammation.

TONSILITIS

FOOD THERAPY

🐚 Go on a 24 hr. or 3 day liquid cleansing diet (pp. 25 and 27) to clear out body toxins.
Then, eat only fresh foods for the rest of the week during an attack. ◆ Have lemon juice and water each morning with plenty of other high vitamin C juices throughout the day, such as orange, pineapple, and grapefruit juice. ◆ Have a fresh carrot juice, and a potassium broth or essence (Pg. 33) once a day. ◆ Get plenty of vegetable protein for healing.

🐚 Have an Onion/Garlic broth each day. (Pg.36).

🐚 Avoid sugars, pasteurized dairy products, and all junk foods til condition clears.

🐚 Drink 6-8 glasses of bottled water daily to keep the body flushed.

VITAMINS/ MINERALS

✤ Zinc Gluconate throat lozenges as needed. ☺

✤ Liquid chlorophyll in water as a gargle.

✤ Nature's Plus ACEROLA C 500MG. CHEWABLES WITH BIOFLAVONOIDS 1-2 every hour during acute stages. and Beta Carotene 100,000IU daily as an anti-infective.

✤ Enzymatic Therapy VIRAPLEX CAPS 4 daily, with ORAL-ZYME LOZENGES as needed.

✤ Raw Thymus extract for more immune strength.

✤ Solaray pantothenic acid 1500Mg. with B 250Mg. to take down swelling. ♀

HERBAL THERAPY

🐚 Crystal Star ANTI-BIO CAPS 4-6 daily to flush lymph glands and clear infection.
with
CRISIS CAPS, 4-6 daily during the acute phase.

🐚 Crystal Satr COFEX TEA as a soothing throat coat; ASPIRSOURCE CAPS to relieve headache and throat pain. ☺

🐚 Effective extracts & drops:
◆ Echinacea to clear lymph
◆ Licorice for sore throat
◆ Crystal Star SUPER LICORICE EXTRACT
◆ Garlic oil
◆ Lobelia if there is fever ☺
◆ Mullein ☺

🐚 Use Mullein or Lobelia tea as a throat compress.

🐚 Sip Aloe Vera juice as needed.

🐚 Propolis lozenges as needed. ♂

BODYWORK

✤ Take a garlic or catnip enema during an attack to clear body poisons.

✤ Ice the throat with a towel wrapped over crushed ice.

✤ Gargle with a weak Tea Tree oil solution in water, every 2-3 hours.

✤ Take hot mineral salts baths frequently.

✤ Other effective gargles:
◆ Slippery Elm tea
◆ Golden Seal/ Myrrh solution.

✤ REFLEXOLOGY POINT:

TONSILS

COMMON SYMPTOMS: Swollen tonsils and lymph glands; difficulty swallowing; fever, chills, and tender sore throat; bad breath because of the infection; hearing difficulty because of infection.

COMMON CAUSES: Poor diet that aggravates the infection, with too many starches, sugars, and pasteurized dairy foods; not enough green vegetables and soluble fiber foods; constipation causing toxic build-up; food allergies, particularly to wheat and dairy; poor digestion, and non-assimilation of nutrients.

TOOTH TARTER ✧ PLAQUE ON THE TEETH

FOOD THERAPY

- Eat crunchy teeth-cleaning fresh vegetables; celery, carrots, broccoli, cauliflower, etc.

- Eat lots of green leafy vegetables. Have a large fresh salad every day.

- Avoid soft and gooey foods, and dairy products that leave a film on the teeth.

- Rub strawberry halves on the teeth. Leave on 1/2 hour. Rinse and brush.

- Chew all food well for jaw growth and prevention of corrosion.

VITAMINS/ MINERALS

- Enzymatic Therapy ACID-A-CAL CAPS 4 daily.

- Alta Health SIL-X SILICA CAPS 2-3 daily.

- Cal/Mag/Zinc 4 daily.

- Ascorbate vitamin C crystals with Bioflavs. and Rutin 1/4t. 4 x daily in water. Swish and hold in mouth before swallowing for best results.

- Use papain powder as a tooth powder.

- DynoMins Cal/Mag 500/500Mg. with vitamin D 1000IU for tooth strength.

- Massage gums with vitamin E oil, and take. Niacinamide 500Mg. 2x daily.

- FOR SALIVARY STONES:
  ◆ Potassium Iodide drops for 1-3 months.
  ◆ Ascorbate vitamin C 3000Mg. daily.

HERBAL THERAPY

- Twin Lab propolis tincture. Take under the tongue and hold as long as possible.

- Dissolve 1T. of food grade 3% H_2O_2 in an 8oz. glass of water, and use as a mouthwash daily for a month.

- Add 3 drops Tea Tree oil to water and use as a mouthwash.

- Solaray ALFAJUICE CAPSULES 4 daily
  or
  Sun CHLORELLA 1 packet daily, for concentrated green food.

- Crystal Star MEGA-MINERAL CAPS 4 daily for a month to build tooth enamel.♀

- Effective teas:
  Dandelion Root
  White Sage
  Parsley

BODYWORK

- Floss daily, and brush well after every meal if you have a tendency to tartar build-up.

- Mix equal parts of cream of tarter and sea salt, or baking soda and sea salt. Brush teeth to remove tarter.

- Wash and rinse the mouth often with cider vinegar or lemon juice. Scrub teeth with lemon rind.

COMMON SYMPTOMS: Bad breath; noticeable sticky film on the teeth; bad mouth taste.

COMMON CAUSES: Too many refined carbohydrates and sugars; excess red meat, caffeine and soft drinks that cause constipation and acid in the system; vitamin and fresh food deficiency.

271

TOOTHACHE
WISDOM TOOTH INFECTION

FOOD THERAPY

❧ Eat primarily fresh foods during acute stages to speed healing, with plenty of leafy greens and green drinks (Pg. 34).

❧ Then, to prevent tooth problems, eat lots of crunchy, crisp foods, such as celery, and other raw vegetables, nuts and seeds, and whole grain crackers.
◆ Eat calcium-rich foods: greens and shellfish.

❧ Ice the jaw for pain. Take a little wine or brandy and hold on the aching area as long as possible.

❧ Avoid soft, gooey foods. No sweets, soft drinks or sodas, if your teeth are not strong. ◆ Go light on acid citrus juices. (They are great for your insides, but not for your teeth).

❧ Chew food very well. Brush and floss well. All are exercise for the teeth and gums.

VITAMINS/ MINERALS

✢ Liquid chlorophyll in a small amount of water. Swish and hold in mouth as long as possible.♂

✢ DynaMins Cal/Mag 500Mg. each, 4 daily, **with Boron for better tooth growth.**
or
Nature's Life LIQUID CALCIUM PHOS. FREE WITH VITAMIN D

✢ Solaray DENTALIFE PACKETS 1 daily.

✢ B Complex 100Mg. with extra B₆ 100Mg. and Niacin 100Mg.

✢ Enzymatic Therapy ORALZYME LOZENGES as needed.

✢ DLPA 500Mg. or **Tryptophan 500Mg. as needed for pain.** ♀

✢ NatraBio TEETH & GUMS TINCTURE.

HERBAL THERAPY

❧ **Apply Clove oil directly to area as needed.**

❧ Take and apply directly:
◆ Valerian & Wild Lettuce extract.
◆ Black Walnut extract

❧ Crystal Star ANTI-BIO CAPS **or** EXTRACT during inflamed infection period.

❧ Crystal Star ASPIRSOURCE CAPSULES for nerve pain.
and
CALCIUM SOURCE and SILICA SOURCE CAPS for **building strong teeth.**

❧ **Solaray Turmeric capsules 4 as needed for pain.**

❧ Other effective capsules:
◆ Kava Kava
◆ Cayenne / Ginger
◆ Echinacea / Myrrh

❧ Effective teas:
◆ Sassafras
◆ Hops/Chamomile
◆ Slippery Elm

❧ **Alta Health SIL-X SILICA CAPS 4 daily.**

BODYWORK

✤ ACUPRESSURE: Squeeze the sides of each index finger at the end. Hold hard for 30 seconds.

✤ **Effective compresses:**
◆ **Hot comfrey**
◆ **Ginger**

✤ REFLEXOLOGY POINT:

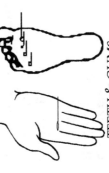

TEETH & GUMS

✤ **Rinse the mouth with a solution of equal parts Golden Seal and White Oak Bark tea to take down pain and swelling.**

✤ Effective applications:
◆ Lobelia tincture ☺
◆ White Flower oil
◆ Propolis tincture
◆ Eucalyptus oil

COMMON SYMPTOMS: Sore jaw and/or gums; dull or shooting pains; tooth or root nerve pain from a cavity; tooth and jaw crowding from wisdom teeth coming in to big, misaligned, etc.; pain from bruxism (tooth grinding at night); gum disease, or bleeding gums.

COMMON CAUSES: Too many refined sugars and red meats, producing acids; too many soft drinks; vitamin and mineral deficiency; diabetes; poor mouth hygiene.

TOXIC SHOCK

TOXIC SHOCK IS A VIRULENT STAPHYLOCOCCAL INFECTION THAT TAKES OVER THE BODY INCREDIBLY QUICKLY WHEN IMMUNITY IS DEPRESSED. A STRONG IMMUNE SYSTEM IS THE BEST AND ONLY DEFENSE.

FOOD THERAPY	VITAMINS/ MINERALS	HERBAL THERAPY	BODYWORK
❦ ALL OF THE FOLLOWING RECOMMENDATIONS ARE TO PREVENT RECURRENCE, AND TO STRENGTHEN THE IMMUNE SYSTEM AFTER EMERGENCY TREATMENT AND THE HOSPITAL STAY.	✤ Germanium 100-150Mg. daily (or dissolve 1gm. in 1qt. water, and take 1/4 cup daily).	❧ Crystal Star rebuilding formulas: 2 of each daily: ◆ ADRN ALIVE with BODY REBUILDER CAPS ◆ SUPERMAX CAPS ◆ POTASSIUM SOURCE CAPS ◆ SILICA SOURCE EXTRACT ◆ CARDI-STRENGTH CAPS ◆ ANEMI-GIZE CAPS ◆ HAWTHORNE EXTRACT ◆ ENERGY GREEN DRINK ◆ MIN-ZYME-MINOSDRINK	✤ Get emergency medical help immediately if you suspect toxic shock. It is rapidly life-threatening. Emergency help can often keep the victim alive if received in time. Natural therapies can help bring them back to health.
❦ Optimum and concentrated nutrition must be followed for recovery. Make sure you are including several fresh vegetable juices and green drinks every day (Pg. 33-34).	✤ CO Q 10 30Mg. daily, with Bromelain 1000Mg. daily. ✤ Vitamin C or Ester C powder with bioflavonoids and rutin, 1/2t. every 2 hours to bowel tolerance all during the healing period for collagen and interstitial tissue regrowth.	❧ Garlic/Parsley caps 6 daily.	✤ Apply alternating hot and cold compresses to collapsed veins or numb extremeties. Cayenne/ Ginger compresses for the hot application; plain ice water for the cold.
❦ Take 2T. each daily: Wheat germ Brewer's yeast	✤ Biotec EXTRA ENERGY ENZYMES 6 daily. with Highest potency YS or Premier 1 ROYAL JELLY 3t. daily.	❧ Solaray ALFAJUICE CAPS. ❧ Sun CHLORELLA or BARLEY GREEN MAGMA 2 packets daily.	✤ Change tampons frequently, or avoid them altogether. ◆ No super absorbent tampons at all.
❦ Eat high vegetable proteins for faster recovery; plenty of whole grains, soy foods, sprouts and sea foods; complex carbohydrates for strength, and cultured foods for G.I. flora.	✤ Alta Health SIL-X SILICA TABS for collagen and tissue formation. ✤ Unsulphured molasses 2T. with PABA 1000Mg. and Pantothenic acid 1000Mg. for hair regrowth.	❧ Mezotrace SEA MINERAL COMPLEX 4 daily. ❧ Floradix herbal iron liquid. 3x daily. ❧ Bancha or Kukicha twig tea for circulation.	✤ Avoid all pleasure drugs; self-injected, snorted, free-based, smoked, etc. The immune system is affected first.

COMMON SYMPTOMS: The symptoms happen so fast and are so extreme, the victim has almost no time to examine or judge them. Only someone close to the victim can see the virulence and react.

COMMON CAUSES: Pleasure drug use, debilitating in their own right, and with the chance of harmful poisons in the processing techniques; "New Age" eating on a long-term basis - low protein, primarily fruits and cleansing foods, no substance to grow or live on; vitamin B depletion and deficiency; malnutrition, leaving the body with lowered immunity, and wide open for a virulent virus to take over. See BUILDING & STRENTHENING IMMUNITY PAGES in this book for more information.

TUMORS
MALIGNANT

FOOD THERAPY	VITAMINS/ MINERALS	HERBAL THERAPY	BODYWORK
Keep the system very clean and clear with a diet high in greens, and low in dairy products and saturated fats.	Ascorbate vitamin C with bioflavonoids, 1/2t. every 2-3 hours to bowel tolerance during healing. **with** Marine carotene 100,000IU	Iodine Therapy: Crystal Star IODINE THERAPY CAPS or EXTRACT 3-4x daily, with Nature's Plus vitamin E 800IU. **or** Atomodine or Miodin drops 3-4x daily.	Apply green clay poultices.
Avoid heavy starches, refined sugars, and fried foods.	Germanium with Suma 50Mg. daily. ♀ **or** Solaray TRI O₂, 2 daily. ♂	Crystal Star ANTI-BIO CAPS if there is inflammation and infection, **with** Evening Primrose oil caps 6 daily for prostaglandin formation.	Apply calendula gel. Drink 4-5 cups daily calendula tea, when the tumor is too large, or too far advanced for an operation.
Drink only distilled bottled water - 6-8 glasses daily to keep toxic wastes quickly clear of the body.	Sun CHLORELLA or BARLEY GREEN MAGMA, 2 packets in water daily.	Siberian Ginseng extract 3-4x daily to retard growth.	Apply H₂O₂ PEROXY GEL for 1-2 months twice daily. A difference is noticeable in 3-4 weeks.
Begin with a short liquid cleansing diet (Pg. 25). During the first month of healing have at least one each of the following juices daily: Potassium broth (Pg. 33) A green drink (Pg. 34) Cranberry juice Pineapple juice Then, eat primarily fresh foods for a month.	Natren LIFE START #2, 1/2t. with meals. ♀	Comfrey tea 4-5 cups daily. ♂	Effective packs: Blue Violet Mullein/Lobelia Fresh Comfrey
	Phosphatidyl Choline (PC 55) 4 daily.	Other effective teas: Pau de Arco ♀ Red Clover ♂ Chamomile Chaparral	See CANCER PAGES in this book for more information.
Add whole grains, high fiber foods and steamed vegetables during the 4th week.	B Complex 150Mg. daily, with extra B₆ 250Mg. and pantothenic acid 500Mg.	Kelp tabs 8-10 daily.	

COMMON SYMPTOMS: Growing and mutating lumps and nodules internally or externally, that are often inflamed, weeping and painful; many times with adhesions to other tissue.

COMMON CAUSES: Poor diet with years of excess acid and mucous-forming foods; environmental , heavy metal , or radiation poisoning; X-rays and low grade radiation tests, such as mammograms causing iodine deficiency and thyroid malfunction..

FOOD THERAPY

❧ Follow a low fat, fresh foods vegetarian diet. High fats mean high estrogen production. (too much estrogen is a common cause of cysts and fibroids)

◆ Get adequate high quality protein daily (about 60-70 grams) from largely vegetable sources to avoid saturated fats: whole grains, sprouts, tofu, sea foods, low fat dairy, etc.

◆ Increase intake of B vitamin foods, such as brown rice, wheat germ and brewer's yeast. Avoid red meat, caffeine and refined sugars that can cause iodine deficiency.

◆ Add miso, sea vegetables, and leafy greens to alkalize the system.

◆ Avoid fried and salty foods, especially during menses.
◆ Avoid concentrated starches, full fat dairy products, and hard liquor on a continuing basis.

❧ Keep the diet high in fresh foods (about 50-60%).

❧ Take 4t. wheat germ oil daily for tissue oxygen.

❧ Have some fresh apple or carrot juice every day.

VITAMINS/ MINERALS

✤ Nature's Plus Vitamin E 800IU during healing.
with
Twin Lab MARINE CAROTENE 100,000IU daily.

✤ High Omega 3 oils or Shark Liver oil as an anti-infective.

✤ Ascorbate Vitamin C, Ester C with Bioflavonoids, 5000Mg. or Quercitin Plus, daily.
with
Alta Health SIL-X SILICA for collagen regrowth.

✤ Esteem Plus capsules 1 daily for 3 months to help thyroid balance.

✤ Sun CHLORELLA 20 daily and Germanium 100Mg. daily as antioxidants.

✤ Enzymatic Therapy RAW MAMMARY CAPS or RAW OVARY CAPS, or NUCLEOPROF CAPS.

HERBAL THERAPY

❧ Crystal Star WOMAN'S BEST FRIEND CAPSULES, 4 daily for 3 months.
with
Evening Primrose oil caps 4-6 daily for 3 months.
then

❧ Crystal Star LIV-ALIVE CAPSULES 2 daily as a mild liver cleanse.

❧ Iodine Therapy: often effective in 3-4 months. ATOMODINE or MIODIN DROPS 2-3x daily.
and/or
Crystal Star IODINE THERAPY CAPS/ EXTRACT. (Take with vit.E for best results)

❧ Effective extracts:
Echinacea
Sarsaparilla (as a source of progesterone)
Dong Quai/Damiana
C.Star SILICA SOURCE

❧ Crystal Star ANTI-SPAZ CAPS or CRAMP CONTROL EXTRACT for cramping.

BODYWORK

✤ Be careful of jumping into surgery. Many of these cysts/fibroids are not cancer, will not become cancer, and will disappear by themselves.

◆ Pain and excessive bleeding have disappeared within a matter of weeks with the change to a low fat, vegetarian diet.

✤ Avoid IUDs and X-rays as causes of fibroid tumors.

✤ Remember that synthetic estrogen increases the risk of uterine, ovarian and breast cancer.

✤ REFLEXOLOGY POINT:

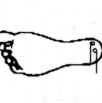

UTERUS & OVARIES

✤ See ENDOMETRIOSIS and OVARIAN FIBROIDS pages in this book for more information.

COMMON SYMPTOMS: Acute or chronic pain in the fallopian tubes or ovaries; disturbance in the normal menstrual cycle, with unfamiliar pain and discomfort in the lower abdomen; intermenstrual bleeding; painful intercourse; infertility; inability to sustain pregnancy; fever and coated tongue.

COMMON CAUSES: IUDs and/or radiation and X-rays that change cell function and structure; underactive Thyroid; prostaglandin and EFA deficiency; too much caffeine and saturated fats in the diet; high dose birth control pills and synthetic estrogen; obesity; hypertension; diabetes; high stress lifestyle and over-acid diet producing acid wastes in the body that are poorly eliminated due to chronic constipation.

VAGINITIS

FOOD THERAPY	VITAMINS/ MINERALS	HERBAL THERAPY	BODYWORK
Make sure the diet is primarily fresh foods during healing. Have a large green salad with sprouts every day. Keep meals very light, without heavy starches, sugars, or dairy products.	Beta Carotene 100,000IU daily, with Vitamin E 400IU 2x daily.	Effective extracts: (both as douches in water, and under the tongue internally) ◆ Black Walnut leaf ◆ Pau de Arco ◆ Garlic ◆ Ginkgo Biloba extract	Effective douches: (Add 1 oz.herbs to 1 qt. water. Steep and strain) ◆ Calendula flowers ◆ Crystal Star WHITES OUT DOUCHE for 3 days. ◆ Tea Tree oil ◆ White Oak bark ◆ Squaw Vine ◆ Cider vinegar/water ◆ Pau de Arco ◆ Witch Hazel herb
Drink 3-4 glasses of cranberry juice from concentrate daily.	Vitamin C (ascorbic acid), crystals, 1/2t. every 2 hours during healing, up to 5000Mg. daily. A weak solution in water may be used as a douche.	Other effective douches in water: ◆ Cayenne/Vinegar ◆ Chlorophyll ◆ Cayenne	
Avoid red meats, hard liquor, and caffeine while clearing a yeast infection.	B Complex 100Mg. daily, with extra B6 100Mg.	Crystal Star WHITES OUT # 1 and #2 CAPSULES, especially for more severe problems. with Garlic/Onion caps 6 daily.	Avoid contraceptive creams, suppositories and anti-biotics while getting rid of a yeast infection.
Eat plenty of fermented foods, such as yogurt and kefir, for friendly G.I. flora, especially if you have been taking medical anti-biotics for the problem.	Nutrition Resource NUTRIBIOTIC LIQUID CONCENTRATE, 1-2 drops in 8oz. water as a douche.		Apply cottage cheese, yogurt or acidolphilus powder to a sanitary napkin, or to a tampon, and insert to rebalance vaginal pH.
	Natren MEGA-DOLPHILUS, 1/2t. 4-6x daily in water. Also an excellent douche solution.	Crystal Star WOMAN'S BEST FRIEND CAPS 6 daily, with a sage/vinegar/water douche 2x daily.	
Effective douches: ◆ Basic vinegar (2T to 1qt. water) ◆ Diluted Mineral water ◆ Baking soda 2tsp./ honey 1tsp. in 1qt. water	Enzymatic Therapy HERPILYN CAPS 4 daily.	Sun CHLORELLA 1 packet daily. Also effective as a douche solution.	Use Tea Tree oil suppositories.
	Vitamin K 100Mg. 3x daily.		Apply Probiologics CERVAGYN.

COMMON SYMPTOMS & CAUSES: Often a condition, not a disease, where the vaginal pH is imbalanced. In general, there is itching, irritation, and inflammation of the vaginal tissues; foul odor, "cottage cheese" discharge; painful sex. Specifically, problems range from a low grade Vaginitis, or Candida fungal infection, to Gardnerella and severe Trichomonas, with symptoms increasing in severity, length of time and lack of response to conventional treatment.
See CANDIDA ALBICANS DIET AND HEALING SUGGESTIONS in this book for more information.

VARICOSE VEINS ✧ SPIDER VEINS

FOOD THERAPY	VITAMINS/ MINERALS	HERBAL THERAPY	BODYWORK
❧ Go on a short 24 Hr. (Pg. 27) liquid diet to clear circulation.◆ Then, eat only fresh foods for the rest of the week, with plenty of green salads and juices. Add a glass of cider vinegar and honey each morning.◆ Then follow a vegetarian diet for the rest of the month. Include sea foods, whole grains, brown rice, and steamed vegetables.	✤ Quercitin Plus with Brom-elain 500Mg. 4 daily. __or__ Pycnogenol caps 6 daily. ✤ Vitamin C crystals with bioflavonoids and rutin, 1/2t. every 2 hours to bowel tolerance daily for 1 month, for connective tissue and collagen formation. __and__ Vitamin E 400IU daily.	❦ Crystal Star VARI-TONE TEA, 2-3 cups daily. ❦ Effective extracts: ◆ Giukgo Biloba ◆ Hawthorne ◆ Bilberry ❦ Enzymatic Therapy HERBAL FLAVONOIDS CAPS 4 daily. ♀	✤ Walk every day, and swim as much as possible, for the best leg exercises. ◆ Elevate the legs when possible. ◆ Massage feet and legs every morning and night with diluted Myrrh oil. ◆ Go barefoot, or wear flat sandals. ◆ Walk in the ocean whenever possible for strengthening sea minerals.
❧ Have one of the follow-ing juices every day: Pineapple Carrot Citrus Green drink (Pg. 34)	✤ Nature's Plus vitamin E 800IU daily, __and__ Apply a mix of 1/4t vitamin E oil and 2T. liquid lecithin. (The feet and legs will tingle and feel hot as if thawing out).	❦ Butcher's Broom tea for circulation increase. ♂ ❦ BioForce VARICOSE VEINS TINCTURE.	◆ Walk in the early morning dew-covered grass. ✤ Take mineral or epsom salts baths.
❧ Take 2T. each daily: Lecithin' Brewer's yeast Wheat germ	✤ Enzymatic Therapy HEMTONE CAPS 3 daily, and Raw Adrenal complex capsules.	❦ Crystal Star HEMRR-EZE or CARDI-STRENGTH CAPS 3 daily.	✤ Use alternating hot and cold hydrotherapy (Pg. 31).
❧ Decrease dairy products, fried foods, prepared meats and red meats, and saturated fats.	✤ B₁₅ DMG sublingual daily.	❦ Effective compresses: ◆ White Oak bark.(Also take 8 white oak capsules daily) ◆ B&T CALIFLORA GEL ◆ Witch Hazel ◆ Plantain	❖ Apply H₂O₂ 3% PEROXY GEL to the legs and feet, 2x daily for 2 months.
❧ Avoid salty, sugary and caffeine-containing foods.	✤ Sun CHLORELLA 1 packet daily. ♂	❦ Apply calendula lotion or gel. Elevate legs while it soaks in to do its work.	◆ Effective compresses: ◆ Cider Vinegar ◆ Fresh Comfrey Lf. ◆ Calendula tea

COMMON SYMPTOMS: Dilated, swollen, painful, bulging leg veins; muscle cramps, and leg fatigue.

COMMON CAUSES: Poor diet with too many refined foods; vitamin E, C, and A deficiency; Essential fatty acid deficiency; constipation; pressure on the veins from overweight or pregnancy; poor posture; liver malfunction; poor circulation; hormone formation changes.

VENEREAL DISEASE

SYPHILIS ✦ GONORRHEA ✦ HPV

FOOD THERAPY	VITAMINS/ MINERALS	HERBAL THERAPY	BODYWORK

FOOD THERAPY

🍲 Follow a very cleansing liquid diet for 3-7 days (Pg. 26) during acute stages.

🍲 Take one <u>each</u> of the following juices daily:
◆ potassium broth or essence (Pg. 33).
◆ fresh carrot juice
◆ a green drink (Pg.34)
◆ Apple/Parsley juice

🍲 Then continue with a cleansing fresh foods diet. Include <u>several bunches of green grapes daily</u>, (an old remedy that still works).

🍲 Avoid refined, starchy, fried and saturated fat foods. Avoid red meats, pasteurized dairy products, and caffeine during healing.

VITAMINS/ MINERALS

✥ Beta Carotene 150,000IU as an anti-infective daily, with Vitamin C crystals 1/2t. every hour to bowel tolerance during acute phase, reduced to 5000Mg. daily for a month.

✥ Liquid Chlorophyll 3t. daily before meals, with Echinacea extract drops.
<u>or</u>
Sun CHLORELLA 1 packet daily.

✥ Natren MEGA-DOLPHILUS POWDER, 1/2t. 6x daily.

✥ Vitamin E 400IU 2x daily.

HERBAL THERAPY

🐾 Crystal Star ANTI-BIO CAPS or EXTRACT 4-6 x daily.
with
Crystal Star WHITES OUT #1 & #2 CAPSULES alternately as needed.

🐾 Effective extracts; may be applied locally and taken internally:
◆ Lobelia
◆ White Oak Bark ♂
◆ Sarsaparilla ♂
◆ Black Walnut.
◆ Burdock

🐾 Crystal Star DETOX CAPSULES for 1 month, 2-4 daily. May also be opened and applied to sores.

🐾 Bathe sores several times daily in a Golden Seal/Myrrh solution.

🐾 Effective teas:
◆ Pau de Arco
◆ Red Clover
◆ Oregon Grape
◆ Calendula

BODYWORK

✤ For HPV: The following natural therapies have been effective as an alternative to massive doses of medical anti-biotics which end up destroying much of the immune balance in the G.I. and genito-urinary tract:
◆ Food grade H$_2$O$_2$ 3% dilute solution (1T. in an 8oz. glass) daily for 1 month.
◆ Shark Liver oil
◆ Calendula tea
◆ Lysine cream and Lysine caps 1000Mg.
◆ Germanium 100Mg.
◆ Aloe Vera gel locally. Aloe vera juice internally.
◆ Enzymatic Therapy ACID-A-CAL CAPSULES.

✤ See VIRAL WARTS PAGE in this book for more information.

✤ If sores are also in the mouth, treat as for Thrush. See THRUSH FUNGAL INFECTION PAGE in this book.

COMMON SYMPTOMS: Painful, infected and often bloody sores in the genital area; heavy pus-filled discharge; high fever when infected, often leading to brain damage.
COMMON CAUSES: Sexual transmission from infected partner.

VERTIGO ✧ DIZZINESS
INNER EAR MALFUNCTION

FOOD THERAPY	VITAMINS/ MINERALS	HERBAL THERAPY	BODYWORK
☙ The diet should be low in saturated fats and cholesterol, and high in vegetable proteins and B vitamin foods, such as brown rice, broccoli, tofu, sea foods, and sprouts.	✤ B Complex 100Mg. with extra B6 100Mg., B12 2000Mcg. and panto-thenic acid 500Mg.	❧ Crystal Star GINKGO BILOBA EXTRACT DROPS as needed for balance RELAX CAPS for nerve rebuilding, and MEDITATION TEA.	✤ Acupressure point: pinch between the eyebrows 3x for 10 seconds each time during an attack.
☙ Take 2T. each daily: Brewer's yeast Wheat germ (or 2t. wheat germ oil)	✤ Rose Hips vitamin C or Ester C with bioflav-onoids and rutin, up to 5000Mg. daily.	❧ Crystal Star MEGA-MINERAL CAPS, with ADRN ALIVE and POTASSIUM SOURCE CAPS, 2 each daily.	✤ Press top of the arm, just above the wrist line for 15 seconds at a time.
☙ Avoid chemical-con-taining foods and preserved foods.	✤ Vitamin E 800IU daily.	❧ Effective teas: Catnip St. John's Wort Peppermint Hops/Blessed Thistle	✤ Chiropractic adjustment and shiatzu massage have shown effective improvement.
☙ Avoid all alcohol, marijuana, cocaine and balance-changing drugs.	✤ Glutamine 500Mg. daily	❧ Superior ROYAL JELLY/ GINSENG VIALS daily. ♂	✤ Attain ideal body weight for better body balance.
☙ Have a potassium broth or essence once a week for better body balance.	✤ DMG B15 sublingual daily.	❧ Butcher's Broom capsules if circulation is sluggish.	✤ REFLEXOLOGY POINTS:
	✤ Niacin Therapy to clear circulation, 250Mg. 3x daily.♂	❧ High potency YS or Premier One ROYAL JELLY 2t. daily, or GINSENG/ HONEY in water as a daily drink.♀	
	✤ Rainbow Light FOOD SENSITIVITY SYSTEM CAPSULES with meals, and CALCIUM PLUS CAPSULES with high magnesium 4 daily.		
	✤ Twin Lab Choline 600Mg. 2-3x daily.♂		
	✤ Enzymatic Therapy RAW ADRENAL COMPLEX CAPS.		

EAR POINTS

COMMON SYMPTOMS: A feeling of falling and lack of steadiness; lightheadedness upon standing quickly; off-balance feeling.

COMMON CAUSES: Poor circulation; lack of tissue oxygen; chronic anxiety; hypoglycemia; B vitamin deficiency.

279

VIRUS INFECTION ✧ STAPH INFECTION
VIRAL WARTS ◆ HPV

FOOD THERAPY	VITAMINS/ MINERALS	HERBAL THERAPY	BODYWORK
❦ Eat only fresh foods for three days during acute stages to keep the body alkaline and free flowing.	❖ Flush any open wound with food grade H_2O_2 3% solution, or Tea Tree oil.	❧ Herbs are well suited to management of viral conditions that are often resistant to medical treatment	❖ Overheating therapy is extremely effective in controlling virus multiplication. Even slight temperature increases can lead to considerable reduction of infection. See Airola "How To Get Well" for the proper technique.
❦ Take a glass of lemon juice and water each morning to stimulate kidney filtering.	❖ Vitamin C crystals with bioflavonoids, 1/2t. in water every hour during acute stages, reducing to about 5000Mg.daily.	❧ Step 1) Destroy the active virus. Use Crystal Star ANTI-VI or ANTI-BIO EXTRACTS or CAPS, or Lomatium, Golden Seal, or St. John's Wort extract; or shark liver oil or Astragalus capsules.	
❦ Take vegetable juices frequently during healing, with a potassium broth (Pg.33), or Vital Health WHITE BIRCH MINERAL WATER daily.	❖ Hylands HYLAVIR TABLETS as needed.	❧ Step 2) Limit harmful bacterial involvement.	❖ Blood temperature may also be raised by taking a hot sauna, and by hot parsley or ginger/ cayenne compresses applied to the affected area.
	❖ Country Life ENERGIX VIALS to restore energy.♂	❧ Use Echinacea/Myrrh,♀ Garlic or Chaparral caps.	
❦ Then include plenty of vegetable source proteins for faster healing; sea vegetables and sea foods, whole grains, sprouts, and soy foods.	❖ Beta Carotene 100,000IU daily, with vitamin E 400IU 2x daily, for 2 weeks.	❧ Step 3) Raise immunity. Use Source Naturals Shiitake mushroom capsules, Calendula tea, and Echinacea extract.	❖ Get some early morning sunlight on the body every day possible.
	❖ Raw Thymus drops 3-4x daily to restore immune defenses.		❖ Activate Kidney cleansing with a catnip or chlorophyll enema.
❦ Avoid all sugars, refined foods, caffeine, tobacco and alcohol (except for a little wine) during healing.	❖ Kal PYCNOGENOL CAPS as a source of super bioflavonoids.♂	❧ For children: use Osha root or horsetail/ oatstraw teas.☺	❖ See FLU PROFILE PAGE in this book for more information.
	❖ Natren LIFE START #2, 1/2t. 3x daily before meals.	❧ To restore body balance and alkalinity, use senna tea and Sun CHLORELLA.	

COMMON SYMPTOMS: Inflammation, boils, sores, and abscesses; breakdown of tissue into waste matter and pus; sore throat; high temperature and fever; reduced vitality; chronic fatigue and lethargy.

COMMON CAUSES: Lowered immunity; over-use of anti-biotics; too many refined foods and green vegetable deficiency; food or environmental allergies.

WARTS ✧ MOLES

FOOD THERAPY	VITAMINS/ MINERALS	HERBAL THERAPY	BODYWORK
❧ Add vitamin A rich foods to the diet, such as yellow and green fruits and vegetables, eggs, and cold water fish.	✣ The high dosage recommended here should be used for no longer than 2 -3 months at a time.	❧ Crystal Star ANTI-BIO CAPS or EXTRACT if there is inflammation or bacterial infection.	✣ For plantar warts: soak foot in the hottest water you can stand about 30 minutes daily for a month.
❧ Add yogurt and other cultured foods to the diet.	✣ Beta Carotene or Emulsified A 100,000-150,000IU as an anti-infective. (Nothing seems to happen for 1-2 months, then, they seem to disappear in a week or so all at once).	❧ Apply Tea Tree Oil religiously for 1-2 months, 3-4 times daily. Wonderful results. ☺	✣ H₂O₂ 3% PEROXY GEL. Rough up the wart with the smooth side of an emery board, and apply 2-3x daily. Wart or mole will slowly shrink and slough off. Do not squeeze or pick.
❧ Include asparagus, fresh figs, alfalfa sprouts and high vitamin C foods in the diet.		❧ Enzymatic Therapy VIRAPLEX CAPS.	✣ Hypnosis therapy has been successful in controlling warts and moles.
❧ Take a green drink (Pg. 34) or Crystal Star ENERGY GREEN DRINK with sea vegetables, every day for a month.	✣ Vitamin C crystals with bioflavonoids in water. Take internally, 1/2t. every 4 hours daily. Apply locally to affected area.	❧ Alta Health SIL-X SILICA CAPS 3-4 daily.	✣ Make a paste of charcoal and water and apply.
❧ Effective applications: ◆ Mixture of lemon juice, sea salt, onion juice and vitamin E oil. ◆ Garlic oil 2x daily ◆ Papaya skins ◆ Wheat germ oil ◆ Raw potato ◆ Castor oil 2x daily.	✣ Nature's Plus Vitamin E 800IU daily.(Also prick a capsule and apply) with Zinc 100IU daily.	❧ Effective applications: ◆ B&T CALIFLORA OINT. ◆ Aloe Vera gel ◆ Jojoba oil ◆ Wintergreen oil ◆ Swedish Bitters ◆ Cinnamon oil drops ◆ Crystal Star CALENDULA GEL	✣ Avoid smoking. It cuts off oxygen to the tissues.
	✣ Lysine cream applications, with Lysine capsules 500Mg. 3-4x daily.	❧ Garlic/Parsley caps 6 daily.	
	✣ B Complex up to 200Mg. daily, with extra B₆ 250Mg. daily.	❧ Apply Nutrition Resource NUTRI-BIOTIC SPRAY 2-3x daily.	

COMMON SYMPTOMS: Flat or raised nodules on the skin surface, sometimes causing pain and discomfort when rubbed or chafed; if virally caused, they can be contagious.

COMMON CAUSES: Vitamin A and mineral deficiencies; viral infection; widespread use of anti-biotics and vaccinations that depress normal immunity.

281

VIRAL & VENEREAL WARTS

HPV (HUMAN PAPILLO-VIRUS) ◆ PID (PELVIC INFLAMMATORY DISEASE)

Genital warts (HPV) are sexually transmitted from an infected person, either man or woman, and are extremely contagious. Symptoms can be latent and unknown by the infected party. The warts are usually evidenced on the genitalia and vagina, but can infect the ovaries, fallopian tubes, cervix, and uterus. They have been linked to cervical cancer, and often seem to be triggered by the co-factors of birth control pills, smoking, herpes and other venereal disease.

PID microorganisms are also sexually transmitted, but infection can also enter the body during miscarriage treatment, childbirth, surgery, or endometrial biopsy. The disease affects one or more of the reproductive organs, and symptoms can extend from a chronic dull ache in the lower abdomen, to strong pain felt in the middle and both sides of the abdomen.

Strong doses of anti-biotics are the usual medical treatment, but the most recent outbreaks (especially in teenagers) are showing resistance and non-response to these drugs.

Successful natural therapies are still in the experimental stages, but the following program has been effective.

1) Food grade H_2O_2 3% dilute solution, (1 tablespoon in an 8oz. glass of water) daily for a month; then rest for a month, and resume if necessary. If noticeable improvement has occurred in this first month, we have found that returning to this treatment may not be necessary. The body's defense forces will have taken over and can better continue on its own.

2) Crystal Star ANTI-VI CAPSULES 4 daily, with CRISIS CAPS to raise body temperature during acute stages; one week off and one week on til improvement is felt.

3) Shark Liver oil capsules 2-4 daily as an anti-viral agent.

4) Germanium 30-100Mg. as an effective wound-healing antioxidant.

5) Overheating therapy is very effective in controlling virus multiplication. Even slight body temperature increases can lead to considerable reduction of infection. See Airola "How To Get Well" for the effective technique.

6) Calendula tea, 3-4 cups daily.

As with other modern opportunistic diseases, a strong immune system is the best treatment and the only defense.

See HERPES GENITALIS, VIRAL & STAPH INFECTION, and ENDOMETRIOSIS PAGES in this book for more information and treatment suggestions.

WATER RETENTION ✧ BLOATING ✧ EDEMA

FOOD THERAPY	VITAMINS/ MINERALS	HERBAL THERAPY	BODYWORK
Water retention is often a problem of not enough water. Dieting can take away foods that previously provided water. Medical diuretics and other drugs can dehydrate. You may just not be drinking enough. If the body does not have sufficient water, fluid levels go out of balance, and it begins to retain more water in an effort to compensate.	Vitamin C crystals with bioflavs. and rutin, 1/2 t. in water or juice every 2-3 hours until relief. Then 3-5000Mg daily for prevention.	Crystal Star BLDR-K CAPS or DIURCAPS, 4-6 daily and/or BLDR-K FLUSH tea. and CEL-U-LITE CAPS 3-4 daily for 1-3 months for enhanced liver function.	Don't overuse chemical/medical diuretics. They cause potassium and mineral loss, and eventually fatigue and muscle weakness.
	B Complex 100Mg. daily with extra B₆ 250Mg. 2x daily. with Twin Lab LIQUID K 2-4t. daily.	Hawthorne extract as needed. ♀	Take hot 20 minutes saunas, often.
Drink at least 6-8 glasses of bottled water daily for free flowing functions, waste removal, and appetite suppression.	Bromelain 500Mg. daily.	Effective diuretic teas: Cornsilk/Dandelion ♀ Juniper/Uva Ursi ♂ Parsley Cleavors Fenugreek	Crystal Star POUNDS OFF BATH as a strong diaphoretic.
	Enzymatic Therapy ACID-A-CAL CAPS 3 daily. with Betaine HCl 3x daily.		Crystal Star DRAWING & SWEATING HERBAL WRAP.
Eat largely fresh foods for 3 days to increase the body's food water content without density. Have a leafy green salad every day with plenty of cucumbers, parsley, and celery.	Lecithin 1900Gr. 4 daily.	Crystal Star TINKLE TEA as needed.	Exercise every day to keep circulation and body metabolism free-flowing.
	N.F. ALL LIVER GLANDULAR tabs. ♀	Raw Lymph or Echinacea extract with Burdock tea.	Elevate head and shoulders for sleeping.
Avoid starchy, sugary, and salty foods. Reduce meats and dairy foods that demand more water to dissolve.			

COMMON SYMPTOMS: Swelling of hands, feet, ankles and stomach; PMS symptoms; headache and bloating.

COMMON CAUSES: Too much salt, red meat or MSG; kidney or bladder infection; oral contraceptives reaction; hypothyroidism; PMS symptoms; adrenal exhaustion; protein and B Complex deficiency; hormonal changes, especially estrogen output; climate changes; ; allergies; poor circulation; potassium depletion; corticosteroid drug reaction; obesity; constipation; lack of exercise.

283

WEIGHT LOSS ✧ EXCESS FAT RETENTION

There are often several reasons you may not be losing the excess body fat you want to. Weight problems are as varied as the individuals who have them. **The first step is to take a look at your diet problem.** It it a sluggish Thyroid? A lazy metabolic rate? Glandular malfunction causing a pear shaped figure? Habit hunger? Stress eating? Brown fat? Cellulite? Poor liver function? Bloating and puffiness from excess fluid retention? Hyperinsulinism? An undeniable sweet tooth? Poor circulation? Constipation? Poor assimilation of certain foods, such as dairy or wheat products? Lack of exercise? **Identifying the real problem with some concentrated attention on true self-knowledge is sometimes half the battle. Only then can you choose the right solutions, the right products, and the right diet system. Weight loss is not easy in today's life style, but it can be accomplished on a long term basis, and without side effects. So go for it! You will like your looks and your life better. Permanent weight control is a real achievement.**

FOOD THERAPY

- The 4 keys to an effective weight control diet: *low fats, high soluble fiber from complex carbo-hydrates, regular exer-cise, plenty of water.*

- No fast, fatty, fried, or junk foods.

- One Tblsp. each before meals to suppress appetite: ◆ Wheat germ ◆ Brewer's yeast.

- Water can get you over weight loss plateaus. Drink it, and all liquids before eating to suppress appetite.

- To achieve ideal weight, keep calories between 800-1500 per day, depending on body frame.

- Small amounts of caffeine after a meal can raise thermogenesis (calorie burning) and increase metabolic rate. Liver/fat meta-bolism must be considered with this knowledge.

VITAMINS/ MINERALS

- ❖ **Enzymatic Therapy** THYROID/ TYROSINE CAPS **with CARNITINE 500Mg.** for metabolic increase.

- ❖ **Enzymatic Therapy** RAW PITUITARY, RAW MAM-MARY and THYROID/ TYROSINE for glandular/pear-shaped problems.

- ❖ **Source Naturals** SUPER AMINO NIGHT CAPS ♂ or **Quantum** NIGHT TRIM ♀

- ❖ **Lewis Labs** WEIGH DOWN **with Chromium picolinate** for appetite control and retaining muscle while losing fat.

- ❖ STOP DROPS for appetite control.

- ❖ **Solaray** SUPER SLIM CAPS a KLAB₆ formula.

- ❖ **Mexican Wild Yam** caps for highest natural DHEA, for appetite suppression.

HERBAL THERAPY

- ❧ **Rainbow Light** SPIRULINA HERBAL DIET COMPLEX CAPS for appetite control.

- ❧ **Esteem Plus** DAYTIME, and **TRIM & FIRM** NIGHTIME CAPS for metabolic increase.

- ❧ **Gymnema Sylvestre** caps to reduce sugar cravings.

- ❧ **Laci LeBeau** SUPER DIETERS TEA, or DIETER'S TREAS-URE TEA for effective flushing.

- ❧ **BioSource** guar gum caps before meals for a full feeling.

- ❧ **Spirulina, Chlorella, and Bee Pollen** for high proteins, energy and balance.

- ❧ See Crystal Star WEIGHT LOSS PRODUCTS on the next page.

BODYWORK

- ❖ **Exercise for 5 minutes, or take a short walk, before eating to raise blood sugar levels, and decrease appetite.**

- ❖ Take regular, daily exer-cise: pleasant and non-strenuous is the key; per-serverance is the secret.

- ❖ Take a short brisk walk after dinner to increase metabolic rate during the night.

- ❖ Do not try to lose more than 1% of your body weight per week. The body does not adjust properly, and you end up re-gaining the weight.

- ❖ Eat smaller, more frequent meals.

- ❖ Take all regular supplements after meals to avoid appetite stimulation.

284

CRYSTAL STAR WEIGHT LOSS COMBINATIONS

Crystal Star has a wide range of natural dieting aids that can address diverse weight loss problems with fresh-dried herb strength, and many years of success behind them. Once you can identify your own weight control difficulty, Crystal Star products can often help with the solution.

APPE-TIGHT DIET CAPS: a mild, subtle formula to help keep you from overeating. It allows the body to alert you when it needs nutrients for fuel, instead of "habit eating;", or psychological need. May be used successfully with <u>THY-METABS CAPS</u> when the weight loss problem is a sluggish thyroid.

THY-METABS: full of natural iodine and other minerals to strengthen and balance the thyroid gland. Helps regulate metabolism, so that food and nutrients are put to better use, and don't just "sit there" in the system unavailable for fuel or nutrition.

CEL-U-LIGHT DIET SUPPORT CAPSULES: basically a liver cleansing and support formula, to help the liver better do its fat metabolizing job. Cellulite fat is often a result of a partially exhausted or poorly functioning liver, and many people develop "brown fat" globules around the hips, abdomen, and thighs as youthful metabolic rates slow down.

LEAN AND CLEAN DIET CAPSULES: have two-pronged activity; as a mild body flush during dieting, and concentrated nutrients for energy and sugar balance to quell cravings.

LEAN AND CLEAN DIET TEA: is effective alone or with other diet formulas to increase body flushing activity as fats are dissolved and released .

SCALE DOWN DIET EXTRACT: a strong chickweed and spirulina combination for convenient appetite suppression, available protein and balance.

CLEANSING & FASTING TEA: an excellent adjunct to a weight loss program incorporating short or moderate fasting. These herbs support nutrition, strengthen circulation, and help accumulated waste release from the fasting process.

DIURCAPS: a mild flushing combination to strengthen kidney/urethral activity.

ZING!: an herbal energizer containing natural caffeine. May be used as a short-term appetite suppressant, or after a meal to stimulate metabolic activity.

POUNDS OFF BATH: a strong diaphoretic for <u>external use only:</u> to help the body sweat out excess fluids and waste through the skin.

TIGHTENING & TONING HERBAL BODY WRAP: a European spa kit to help in cellulite release and improvement in muscle, vein and skin tone.

◆ See the back of this book for formula ingredients.

285

THE MODERATE FASTING DIET

Fasting sounds like a good fast way to lose weight, and sometimes it is; when you are getting enough nutrients from fresh fruit and vegetable juices. Unfortunately, there are three inherent problem conditions with a fast for weight loss. **1)** The body tends to form more fat at first, when you are not eating at all. It feels threatened by the lack of nutrients, and tries to protect itself by retaining fats for survival. **2)** Fasting can be dangerous unless you are taking in organically grown foods. The DDT and other pesticides on commercially grown foods are very quickly absorbed into the bloodstream when there is no solid food to slow them down. They can lodge in the bones, and often cause a toxic reaction. **3)** A fast means that the body is cleansing and discarding wastes more rapidly than new tissue is being made. A temporary degree of discomfort may be felt in terms of headache, bowel looseness, or loss of energy. These symptoms are usually just initial detoxification signs, that are gone within a few days. They are a small price to pay for getting rid of long-accumulated fat cells. **Weight loss cannot occur until these cells are reduced.**

If you do decide to fast for short periods of intense weight loss, here is a good modified way to do it, with plenty of nutrition. **As with all effective diets, water is a key to the success of this fasting diet. Drink 6-8 glasses a day of bottled water to flush out released fats and body wastes, and to avoid the problems of sagging skin, lost muscle tone, and constipation.** This diet is most effective when used from 1-3 weeks at a time with a week of light eating in between.

ON RISING: take a glass of lemon juice and water to cleanse the blood and kidneys of toxins released during the night.

BREAKFAST: have some fresh fruit, **and** a glass of apple or pineapple/papaya juice, with 1T. psyllium powder or liquid bentonite added to provide fiber, and bowel flushing; **or** a glass of aloe vera juice.

MID-MORNING: have a glass of fresh carrot juice, **or** an herbal dieting tea, such as Crystal Star CLEANSING & FASTING TEA, or LEAN.N' CLEAN DIET TEA.

LUNCH: have a meal replacement drink, such as Nature's Plus SPIRUTEIN, or Lewis Labs WEIGH DOWN; or a meal replacement supplement such as Rainbow Light SPIRULINA HERBAL DIET COMPLEX, or Esteem Plus capsules.

MID-AFTERNOON: have some crunchy raw vegies with a kefir cheese or all vegetable puree dip, **with** a small bottle of mineral water, or a cup of herb tea, such as peppermint or licorice root, or Crystal Star HIGH ENERGY TEA.

DINNER: have a fresh green leafy salad with lots of cucumbers, celery, carrots, sprouts, and a lemon/oil dressing, **and** a cup of miso or clear broth soup; **or** a cup of Vegex YEAST PASTE BROTH for high B Vitamins.

BEFORE BED: have a cranberry or apple juice with 1T. psyllium powder, or liquid bentonite; **or** a glass of aloe vera juice. Take a walk around the block before bed, to stimulate good metabolic activity during the night.

Remember the effective rules for quicker weight loss:
1) Fresh fruit or juice in the morning to use up your own glycogen reserves, and set up good metabolic balance.
2) A good, balanced meal replacement drink, wafers or supplement at midday.
3) A short brisk walk after dinner.
4) Small meals whenever you eat.

EATING RIGHT, LIGHT & LOW FAT

For permanent weight loss and weight control, a biochemical change is necessary. This is achieved through regular **daily** exercise, and eating right and light. Eat only whole foods. Avoid all junk and processed foods that can destroy the new fat-metabolizing body system you have encouraged. Poor nutrition causes constant hunger, and the predictable desire to eat the wrong foods and "empty calories". Reduce caffeine, carbonated sodas, and acid-forming foods, such as red meats and full fat dairy products. They too, can keep the liver from metabolizing fats correctly. Fat is not all bad. It is essential in small amounts, for good body function and readily available fuel. (The average overweight person has too high blood sugar, and low, poorly metabolized fat levels.) Use vitamins, herbs and other diet supplements as aids for your diet, not agents.
THERE ARE 4 KEYS TO PERMANENT WEIGHT CONTROL: 1)LOW FATS 2)SOLUBLE FIBER FROM COMPLEX CARBOHYDRATES 3)REGULAR EXERCISE 4)PLENTY OF WATER . (Thirst is often mistaken for hunger. Drinking water will save many calories throughout the day).

The following diet should be used for at least three months to insure that your body and metabolism have re-aligned and stabilized in the new way of eating, and to guard against re-gaining the weight As your weight loss progresses, modify your favorite recipes to use less fat, no chemical foods, and baking instead of frying. This way, you can continue to have your favorite things without feeling deprived or guilty, and the weight won't come back.

ON RISING: take 2 lemons squeezed in a glass of water, to flush fats and clean the kidneys.

BREAKFAST: have a cleansing/building protein drink for energy without muscle wasting, such as Nature's Plus SPIRUTEIN, Nutri-Tech ALL 1, or Crystal Star MIN-ZYME-MINOS DRINK, **and** some fresh fruits.

MID-MORNING: have some yogurt with more fresh fruit; **or** a small bottle of mineral water, or a cup of herb tea, such as Crystal Star LEAN 'N' CLEAN DIET TEA, or HIGH ENERGY TEA, or a mint tea with lemon.

LUNCH: have a fresh leafy green salad, with some baked tofu, a baked potato, or brown rice, with low fat dressing or sauce; **or** a light vegetable, black bean, lentil, or miso soup, and some steamed vegetables with a light soy/ginger sauce; **or** a whole grain or vegetable pasta salad, with seafood, salad vegies, and a light sauce.

MID-AFTERNOON: have some crunchy raw vegies, with a kefir or yogurt cheese dip, and some whole grain crackers; **and** a green drink (Pg. 34), Sun CHLORELLA DRINK, a bottle of mineral water, or refreshing herb tea; **and/or** a hard boiled egg with a little sesame salt, and rice cakes or whole grain crackers with kefir cheese.

DINNER: have a large dinner salad with seafood or chicken, vegetables and nuts or seeds, **and** a cup of soup; **or** a chinese vegetable stir fry with brown rice and a light clear soup; **or** baked or broiled fish or seafood, with some steamed vegetables and a whole grain, such as brown rice, bulgur, or millet; **or** a whole grain or vegetable pasta casserole, with a cup of soup or small salad; **or** roast turkey with light cornbread, and a leafy green salad with poppyseed dressing.

T.V./EVENING SNACK: have some un-buttered popcorn, with an herbal seasoning. (It's good for you, and the airiness will fill you up, and keep you from wanting heavier or "habit" foods.

BEFORE BED: have a cup of Vegex YEAST PASTE BROTH, or a glass of apple or papaya juice, **or** a cup of mint tea.

287

MORE WEIGHT LOSS WATCHWORDS & OTHER EFFECTIVE PRODUCTS

◆ **Water can get you over the dieting "plateau problem".** Most dieters have experienced the phenomenon of initial weight loss and results from a good program, and then the slowing or stopping of weight loss, no matter how much exercise or calorie restriction they did. **The problem is often not enough water.** Dieting takes away foods that previously provided water. If that water isn't replaced, the body's fluid levels go out of balance and the body retains water which is perceived as weight. When the system gets enough water, the liver breaks down and releases more fat, and hunger is curtailed.

◆ **Changing your diet composition is a key to weight control.** You can eat **two to three times more volume of low fat foods** than high fatty foods, and still lose weight.

◆ For gland imbalance and a pear shaped figure, follow the Enzymatic Therapy "Pear shaped Program", and add daily for best results; 2T. lecithin granules, vitamin E 400IU, Choline/Inositol, B Complex 100Mg., and a low carbohydrate diet.

◆ Living the **thin life** is not a lifelong deprivation sentence. Once your basic metabolism processes have re-aligned and stabilized, and desired weight is regularly maintained, you can have overeating days without losing weight control. Balance these with undereating days, such as when you will be eating out, or with company, so that ideal weight can be maintained.

◆ For carbohydrate metabolism, take B Complex vitamins while dieting.
◆ For compulsive eating, take Tyrosine 500Mg. 2-3x daily.
◆ For better thermogenesis of fat calories, take Carnitine 500Mg. 2x daily and Argenine/Ornithine 1000Mg. at bedtime.
◆ For effective appetite suppression, take phenalalanine 500Mg. before meals. (do not take if sensitive to phenalalanine)
◆ For metabolic and circulation sluggishness, take CO Q 10 30Mg. daily.

KIDS ☺ OBESITY & FITNESS

Until the nineteen sixties, overweight and weight control wasn't very much of a problem with kids. But ever since the fifties, over-refined and junk foods have changed parents' metabolism and cell structure. Many times, as with the immune defense system, hereditary factors from the parents of the fifties and sixties have passed the food assimilation problems and deficiencies to the kids of today. **And that's in addition to the wide variety of junk and non-food foods, peer pressure, lack of exercise, and T.V. advertising that the kids themselves are exposed to every day.** Weight problems are mushrooming with American children. For all the current adult consciousness and attention to diet, recent statistics show that our children and teenagers are the fattest they have ever been! Obesity rates for young children jumped 54% between 1960 and 1981, and 30% for teenagers They jumped another 50% between 1981 and 1988.
The 1985 study by the President's Council on Physical Fitness showed two very disconcerting facts: **that 85% of the children and teenagers tested failed the fitness tests, and that as many as 90 percent of our children already have at least one risk factor for a degenerating disease.**
Poor lifestyle eating habits, and lack of exercise are at the base of this poor performance. Your kids need you for good information, and as good diet role models to help them establish positive lifelong healthy eating habits.

See "COOKING FOR HEALTHY HEALING" by Linda Rector-Page for complete weight loss diets for both kids and adults.

FOOD THERAPY	VITAMINS/ MINERALS	HERBAL THERAPY	BODYWORK
The diet should consciously include plenty of vegetable protein, such as whole grains, seafoods, sprouts and soy foods; mineral-rich foods, such as leafy greens, as foods, vegetables and molasses; and vitamin A foods, such as carrots, greens, and broccoli.	Natural products with Retin A effects: ◆ Zia PAPAYA PEEL ◆ 1 teasp. aloe vera gel mixed with 1 pricked vitamin E 400IU capsule. ◆ Jason COLLAGEN AMPULES ◆ Reviva LIGHT SKIN PEEL applied high potency royal jelly ampules ◆ Reviva NIGHT CREAM & DAY CREAM ◆ Biotec AGELESS BEAUTY CAPSULES 6 daily.	Apply a facial mix: 1t. Vegetable Glycerine, 1t. Rosewater, 1t. Witch Hazel, 3T. Honey. Leave on 15-20 minutes.	Avoid smoking and all forms of tobacco. Tar and nicotine deprive the skin of oxygen, causing shriveling/wrinkles.
Avoid refined sugars, oxalic-acid forming foods, red meats, and caffeine containing foods. All are very drying to the skin.		Iodine Therapy: Atomodine or Miodin drops in water daily with vitamin E 400IU. or Crystal Star IODINE THERAPY CAPS or EXTRACT DROPS, or MINZYME-MINOS DRINK.	Apply food grade H_2O_2 PEROXY GEL to wrinkles before bed as a source of absorbable oxygen.
Take 2T. each daily: Lecithin granules Wheat germ Brewer's yeast Molasses	Free radical scavengers for wrinkling caused by environmental pollutants: ◆ Twin Lab SUPER GERMANIUM WITH SUMA ◆ Biotec AGELESS BEAUTY ◆ Vitamin E w/ selenium ◆ Ginkgo Biloba extract	Evening Primrose oil caps 4 daily for prostaglandin production.	Zia PAPAYA PEEL, ESSENTIAL HYDRATING EXTRACT, and SUPER HYDRATING MASK are all effective for wrinkles.
Rub fresh papaya skins on the face. for retin A effect.	Bromelain 500Mg. daily.	Apply aloe vera gel mixed with a pricked vitamin E 400IU capsule.	Effective softening massages for wrinkles: ◆ Jojoba oil ◆ Sesame oil ◆ Wheat germ oil ◆ Vitamin E oil ◆ Aloe Vera gel
Mix 1 whipped egg white and 2T. cream. Pat on face; let dry 20 minutes. Rinse off.	Vitamin C with bioflavs and rutin 3000-5000Mg. daily for collagen and interstitial production.	Steam face with hydrating/toning herbs: ◆ Chamomile flowers ◆ Eucalyptus leaves ◆ Rosemary leaves	Use a gentle balancing mask once a week, such as Crystal Star HERBAL TONING MASK. ◆ Follow with a blend of aloe vera gel and vitamin E oil.
	B Complex 100Mg. daily with extra PABA 1000Mg.	Apply a mix of tincture of benzoin, vegetable glycerine, honey and cologne drops. Leave on 15 min. Rinse off.	FACIAL EXERCISES REALLY HELP SKIN ELASTICITY AND TONE.

COMMON CAUSES: Skin dehydration often caused by hormone (Estrogen depletion); poot diet with too much tobacco, fried foods, caffeine, and alcohol; broken capillaries; weak vein walls.

289

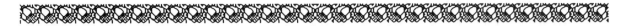

Crystal Star is a small personal company without a large staff, marketing division or advertising program. The extra money we spend goes toward herbal education and research, and the quality of our ingredients. We feel that our product results speak for Crystal Star Herbs better than any advertising campaign we might devise.

ABOUT CRYSTAL STAR HERBAL COMBINATIONS

Natural medicines that work, for health that lasts.

Crystal Star Herbal Combinations are essentially body balancers - especially formulated to bring specific areas of the body back into balance so it can heal and regulate itself.
Herbs are synergistic in combination. They work far better combined with other herbs than alone.

Quality is the **most important** element in any herbal formula. **Crystal Star** uses the finest quality herbs that we can find and afford. (Our Ginseng, for instance costs over $100 a pound).
Many of our herbs are organically grown or wildcrafted in the fresh air of the California and Oregon foothills, and on coastal botanical farms. Most others come from the Orient, where herb quality is much prized. All of our combinations are formulated and filled in small batches to assure you of freshness and the most potent product you can buy.

Crystal Star Herbs is a complete line of herbal preparations, including extracts, capsules, teas, baths, douches, gels, European Spa products, pot pourris and natural florals.

In response to those of you who have expressed a wish for more information about the products recommended in this book, the formulations are listed on the following pages so you will have a basis for judgement in relation to your own healing program

If you have questions about formula ingredients, would like a catalogue, or wish to place an order, you may call or write:

CRYSTAL STAR HERBS
20065 B HIGHWAY 108
SONORA, CA. 95370
(209)- 532-6474

NOTE: Crystal Star buys herbs every week to keep our stock fresh and at the peak of potency. We can generally absorb small cost fluctuations to keep our prices stable. But because the world herb market is extremely volatile, and the current supply of organic herbs very limited, and much in demand, the prices quoted must be subject to change without notice.

CRYSTAL STAR HERBAL COMBINATIONS

CAPSULES
Each capsule contains 550-600Mg. of high quality ingredients. Mineral and Amino Acid amounts are approximate since many capsules are hand packed.

ADRN-ALIVE™

A Licorice/Sarsaparilla combination to support an exhausted system and increase energy.

THE INGREDIENTS:

Licorice Rt.	Ascorbate Vit. C
Sarsaparilla	Ginger Rt.
Bladderwrack	Capsicum
Irish Moss	Panto. Acid 50Mg.
Uva Ursi	Betaine HCl 20Mg.
	Vit. B$_6$ 15Mg.

Available sizes: 60 count

ALRG CAPS™

A cleansing and balancing Mullein combination for pollen sensivities.

THE INGREDIENTS:

Marshmallow	Golden Seal Rt.
Mullein	ParsleyRt.
Ma Huang	Rose Hips
Burdock Rt.	Capsicum
Chaparral	Panto.Acid 30Mg.

Available sizes: 60 count and120 count

ANEMI-GIZE™

A Beet Root, Dandelion, Alfalfa combination providing highly absorbable Iron and trace minerals necessary for health and energy.

THE INGREDIENTS:

Beet Rt.	Nettles
Alfalfa	Burdock
Dandelion Rt.	Dulse
Yellow Dock Rt.	Comfrey Rt.
Parsley Rt	Capsicum

Available sizes: 90 count

ANTI-BIO™

An Echinacea, Golden Seal and Myrrh combination.

The Ingredients:
Echinacea Augustifolia Rt. and Lf.

Purpurea Rt. & Lf.	Marshmallow
Golden Seal Rt.	Turmeric
Myrrh Gum	Elecampane
Chaparral	Yarrow
Capsicum	Potass.Chl. 20Mg.

Available sizes: 30 count and 60 count

ANTI-HST™

A balancing, clearing combination with unsprayed High Desert Bee Pollen.

The Ingredients:

Bee Pollen	Juniper Berry
Chaparral	Rose Hips
Ma Huang	Parsley Rt.
Marshmallow	Capsicum
Golden Seal Rt,	Panto.Acid 50Mg.
Burdock Rt	Vit. B$_6$ 25Mg.

Available sizes: 60 count

ANTI-SPAZ™

A relaxing Cramp Bark combination.

The Ingredients:

Cramp Bark	Eur. Mistletoe
Black Haw	Kava Kava
Rosemary	Peony Rt.
St. John's Wort	Wild Yam
Red Raspberry	Passion Flower
	Kelp

Available Sizes: 60 count

APPE-TIGHT DIET CAPS™

A Chickweed, Gotu Kola diet support combination.

THE INGREDIENTS:
Gotu Kola	Black Walnut
Chickweed	Licorice
Fennel	Guar Gum
Ephedra	Papain
Kelp	Echinacea Pur. Rt.
Safflower	Lecithin
Hawthorne Berry	Ornithine 50Mg.
	Vit.B6 25Mg.

Available sizes: 60 count and 120 count

ASPIR-SOURCE ™

A soothing, relieving White Willow combination.

THE INGREDIENTS:
White Willow	Valerian
Rosemary	Scullcap
Wood Betony	Raspberry
Blue Violet	Ginger
	Blue Vervain

Available sizes: 90 count

BLDR-K CAPS™

A Golden Seal / Juniper combination to help cleanse and flush the system.

THE INGREDIENTS:
Juniper Berry	Ginger
Parsley Rt.	Mullein
Golden Seal Rt.	Vit. B6 50Mg.
Uva Ursi	Pot. Chl.15Mg.
Marshmallow	

Available sizes: 60 count and 120 count

BODY RE-BUILDER

Effective herbal nutrients to build a healthy body. Rich in absorbable minerals for strength and energy.

THE INGREDIENTS:
Spirulina	Golden Seal Rt
Unsprayed Bee Pollen	Sib. Ginseng
Ascorbate Vit. C	Kelp
Desiccated Liver	Wild Cherry
Alfalfa	Rose Hips
Hawthorne Lf. & Bry.	Parsley Rt.
Amino Acid Cmpd.50Mg.	Zinc 30Mg.
Carrot calcium 30Mg.	

Available sizes: 60 count

BONZ™

A Comfrey Rt. and Horsetail combination with highly absorbable minerals for strength and re-building.

THE INGREDIENTS:
Carrot Calcium	Chaparral
Comfrey Rt.	Shavegrass
Black Cohosh	Dulse
St. John's Wort	Licorice
Parsley Rt.	Burdock
White Oak Bk.	Marshmallow
Plantain Lf.	Slippery Elm
Oatstraw	Nettles
	Zinc 15Mg.

Available sizes: 60 count and 120 count

BWL-TONE™

A soothing, cleansing Peppermint Oil combination.

THE INGREDIENTS:
Peppermint & Peppermint Oil	
Comfrey Rt.	Pau de Arco
Marshmallow Rt.	Ginger
Slippery Elm	Wild Yam

Available sizes: 60 count and 120 count

CALCIUM SOURCE CAPS™

Highly absorbable Calcium and trace minerals from herbs. Especially rich in Silica for bone, hair and nail strength.

THE INGREDIENTS:
Org. Carrot Pwr. 150Mg.   Borage Seed
Oatstraw   Shavegrass
Comfrey Rt.

Available sizes 60 count

CANDIDEX™

Gentle, effective herbal nutritional support.

THE INGREDIENTS:
Pau de Arco   Licorice Rt.
Black Walnut   Burdock Rt.
Lactobac. & Bifidus   Thyme
Garlic   Sarsaparilla
Barberry Bk.   Rosemary
Sodium Caprylate   Dong Quai
Spirulina   Damiana
Echinacea Aug. & Pur.   DLPA 25Mg.
Ascorbate Vit. C 45Mg. Calc.Cit.25Mg.
Cranberry powder   Zinc 15Mg.

Available sizes: 100 count

CARDI-STRENGTH

A Hawthorne, Ginkgo Biloba, Vitamin E combination for strength and stability.

THE IMGREDIENTS:
Hawthorne Leaf, Berry & Flower
Siberian Ginseng
Motherwort   Comfrey Rt.
Gingko Biloba   Lecithin
D-Alpha Vit. E 25IU   Choline 20Mg.
                         Niacin 15Mg.

Available sizes: 75 count

CEL-U-LIGHT DIET SUPPORT™

An effective cleansing aid to good metabolism.

THE INGREDIENTS:
Fenugreek Seed   Golden Seal Rt.
Gotu Kola   Lecithin
Garlic   Milk Thistle Seed
Quassia   Choline 25Mg.
Black Cohosh   Fennel Seed
Chaparral   Kola Nut
Red Sage   Vit. B$_6$ 15Mg.

Available sizes: 60 count and 120 count

CHOL-EX™

An effective fiber and herb combination.

THE INGREDIENTS:
Guar Gum   Black Cohosh
Apple Pectin   Spirulina
Lecithin   Fenugreek Seed
Hawthorne Berry   Capsicum
Veg. Acidolphilus   Panto. Acid 25Mg
Siberian Ginseng   Vit. B$_6$ 25Mg.

Available sizes: 90 count

CHOL-LO FIBER TONE™

The ultimate fiber product. A delicious, all natural blend of nature's most complete fiber to help keep your system clean and healthy.
Now in 2 tasty flavors: Essential Orange, and Acerola Cherry.

THE INGREDIENTS:
Organic Oat Bran   Apple Pectin
Organic Flax Seed   Acerola Fiber
(High Omega 3 Oils)   Org.Fennel
Psyllium Husks   Sweet Herb
Vegetable Acidolphilus
Guar Gum   Orange/Cherry oil

Available sizes: 12 oz. package

COLD SEASON DEFENSE

A Garlic and Rose Hips Vit. C combination.

THE INGREDIENTS:

Garlic	Parsley Rt.
Rose Hips	Ginger
Ascorbate Vit. C	Rosemary
Bayberry	Boneset
Unsprd. Bee Pollen	Capsicum
Veget. Acidolphilus	Potass. Chl.15Mg.
St. John's Wort	Zinc 15Mg.

Available sizes: 60 count

CRISIS CAPS™

Rose Hips, Vitamin C and herbs for first stage prevention and defense.

THE INGREDIENTS:

Bayberry	White Willow
Rose Hips	Cloves
Ascorbate Vit. C	White Pine
Ginger	Capsicum

Available sizes: 60 count

DETOX!

A strong combination for fasting support, oxygenation and cleansing.

THE INGREDIENTS:

Red Clover	Alfalfa
Licorice	Milk Thistle
Chaparral	Sarsaparilla
Burdock	Astragalus
Pau de Arco	Yellow Dock
Echinacea Purpurea	Ginger
Asscorbate Vit. C	Prickly Ash
Garlic	Buckthorne
Kelp	Potass. Chl.15Mg.

Available sizes: 60 count and 100 count

DIUR-CAPS™

A gentle Cornsilk combination .

THE INGREDIENTS:

Uva Ursi	Cleavors
Cornsilk	Ginger
Parsley Lf.	Kelp
Juniper Berry	Dandelion Rt.
Marshmallow	Vit. B_6 50Mg.
	Potass. Chl.15Mg.

Available sizes: 60 count and 120 count

EASY CHANGE™

A Black Cohosh, Dong Quai and Cramp Bark combination to encourage normality and balance in the female system.

THE INGREDIENTS:

Black Cohosh	Squaw Vine
Dong Quai	Blue Cohosh
Cramp Bark	Uva Ursi
False Unicorn	Red Raspberry
Damiana	Bayberry
Lady Slipper	Pennyroyal
Sarsaparilla	Ginger
Carrot Calcium	

Available sizes: 60 count and 120 count

ENERGY GREEN DRINK MIX

A body building concentrated green drink for highly absorbable complete minerals, trace minerals and proteins.

THE INGREDIENTS:

Brown Rice Protein	Sarsaparilla
Spirulina	RoseHips
Alfalfa	Wakame
Unsprayed Bee Pollen	Dulse
Oats	Licorice
Siberian Ginseng Rt.	Gotu Kola
Roasted Dandelion Rt.	Lemon juice

Available sizes: 8 ounces.

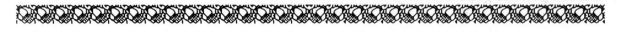

ESTR-AID™

Herbal nutrients to encourage female balance.

THE INGREDIENTS:

Black Cohosh   Licorice
Sarsaparilla   False Unicorn
Dong Quai   Squaw Vine
Damiana   Wild Yam

Available sizes: 90 count

ENDOCRINE BALANCE
(special order only)

Herbal nutrients to balance, nourish, regulate and extend gland and cell life.

THE INGREDIENTS:

Sarsaparilla   Gotu Kola
Irish Moss   Saw Palmetto
Licorice   Kelp
Siberian Ginseng   Black Cohosh
Fo-Ti-Tieng   Alfalfa
Spirulina   Ginger
Dong Quai   Glutamine 20Mg.

Available sizes: 60 count

FEEL GREAT™

A whole body tonic, containing the true heavy-weights of the herbal kingdom, to enhance daily rejuvenation of the body's vital substances. The longer the use, the greater the benefits in strength, stamina and balance.

THE INGREDIENTS:

Korean White Ginseng   Hawthorne Lf.
Siberian Ginseng   Ginkgo Biloba
Unsprayed Bee Pollen   Kelp
Golden Seat Rt.   Saw Palmetto
Spirulina   Schizandra
Sarsaparilla   Alfalfa
Gotu Kola   Yeast 500
Dong Quai   Capsicum
Suma   Choline 20Mg.
Black Cohosh   Zinc 15Mg.
                        Amino Acids

Available sizes: 75 count

FEMALE HARMONY™

Herbal nutrients to balance, tone and regulate the female system. An aid to relief of PMS symptoms.

THE INGREDIENTS:

Dong Quai   Fennel
Damiana   Angelica
Sarsaparilla   Yellow Dock
Burdock   Peony Rt.
Rosemary   Golden Seal
Nettles   Ephedra
Licorice   Red Clover
Rehmannia   Eur. Mistletoe
Dandelion   Chamomile
Oatstraw   Ginger
Hawthorne Lf. & Bry. Cinnamon

Available sizes: 75 count

FIBER & HERBS COLON CLEANSE

Herbs to help clean, clear, tone and strengthen the elimination system.

THE INGREDIENTS:

Butternut Bark   Fennel Seed
Cascara   Licorice
Rhubarb Rt.   Ginger
Psyllium Husk   Irish Moss
                      Barberry Bk.

Available sizes: 60 count and 120 count.

FIVE WEEK FORMULA
(Special order only)

Prepeares and strengthens the body in the 5 weeks prior to birth.

THE INGREDIENTS:

Red Raspberry   Blessed Thistle
Squaw Vine   Black Cohosh
False Unicorn
Available sizes: 100 count

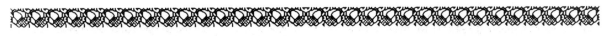

HEAVY METAL
(Special order only)

Herbs to help neutralize and remove the effects of heavy metals taken into the body from environmental pollutants.

THE INGREDIENTS:

Ascorbate Vit. C	Astragalus
Kelp	Licorice
Bladderwrack	Parsley Rt.
Bugleweed	Prickly Ash
	Potass Chl. 30Mg.

Available sizes: 100 count

HEMRR-EZE

A Stone Root, Slippery Elm soothing combination.

THE INGREDIENTS:

Stone Rt.	Mullein
Slippery Elm	Heal All
Golden Seal Rt.	Cranesbill
Witch Hazel	Rose Hips

Available sizes: 90 count

HERBAL DEFENSE CAPS™

An Echinacea, Pau de Arco protection formula.

THE INGREDIENTS:

Echinacea Angust	Spirulina
Pau de Arco	Golden Seal Rt.
Siberian Ginseng	Schizandra
Garlic	Bayberry
Ascorbate Vit C 50Mg.	Yarrow
Burdock	Rose Hips
Astragalus	Elecampane
Chaparral	Red Sage
Unsprayed Bee Pollen	Kelp
Hawthorne Lf. & Bry.	Capsicum
Suma	Potass Chl. 20Mg.
	Zinc 15Mg.

Available sizes: 90 count

HERBAL ENZYMES™

A Ginger/Mint combination to aid in acid-alkaline balance.

THE INGREDIENTS:

Ginger	Peppermint
Fennel	Spearmint
Vegetable Acidolph.	Catnip
Cramp Bark	Papaya Pwd.
	Turmeric

Available sizes: 90 count

HERPEACE™

An Astragalus and L-Lysine combination to restore body Amino Acid balance.

THE INGREDIENTS:

Astragalus	Red Sage
L-Lysine	Oregon Grape
Chaparral	Myrrh Gum
Yellow Dock	Marshmallow
Echinacea	Wild Yam
Sarsaparilla	

Available sizes: 90 count

HIGH PERFORMANCE

Herbs for zest, energy, stamina and physical endurance.

THE INGREDIENTS:

Siberian Ginseng	Schizandra
Unsprd.Bee Pollen	Ephedra
Sarsaparilla	Yarrow
Gotu Kola	Ginger
Spirulina	Capsicum
Licorice	Carrot Cal. 20Mg.
Dandelion	Argenine-20Mg.
Wild Yam	Ornithine-20Mg.
	Zinc-20Mg.

Available sizes: 75 count

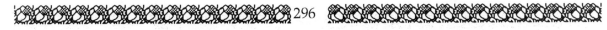

HI-PRESSURE CARE

A Garlic, Hawthorne, Ginger combination.

THE INGREDIENTS

Garlic	Ginger
Hawthorne Lf & Flwr.	Parsley Rt.
Siberian Ginseng	Dandelion
Guar Gum	Golden Seal
Hawthorne Berry	Capsicum
	Vit. B$_6$ 15Mg.

Available sizes: 90 count

HYPO-BLUES CAPS

A Spirulina, Licorice combination to help build a strong protein base, and encourage a feeling of well-being in the body.

THE INGREDIENTS:

Licorice	Wild Yam
Spirulina	Gotu Kola
Dandelion Rt	Amino Acid Cpd.
Cedar Berries	Guar Gum
Alfalfa	Horseradish

Available sizes: 90 count

INSUL FORM CAPS

A natural tonic to encourage balance and regulation.

THE INGREDIENTS:

Cedar Berries	Uva Ursi
Dandelion Rt.	Bilberry
WildYam	Horseradish
Licorice	Capsicum
Guar Gum	Pant. Acid 25Mg.
Elecampane	Glutamine 25Mg.
Mullein	Zinc-10Mg.
Kelp	Manganese10Mg.

Available sizes: 75 count

IODINE THERAPY™

A sea greens complex for highly absorbable potassium and iodine.

THE INGREDIENTS:

Kelp	Watercress
Kombu	Irish Moss
Dulse	Spirulina
Alfalfa	Borage Seed
	Nettles

Available sizes: 60 count.

IRON SOURCE CAPS

Highly absorbable, non-constipating herbal Iron and Trace Minerals.

THE INGREDIENTS:

Beet Rt	Watercress
Yellow Dock	Parsley Lf.
Nettles	Dulse
Dandelion Rt.	Gentian

Available sizes: 60 count

LEAN 'N' CLEAN DIET CAPS™

Herbal nutritional support for effective energy and cleansing while dieting.

THE INGREDIENTS:

Spirulina	Fennel
Unsprd. Bee Pollen	Lecithin
Senna	Ginger
Dulse	Phenalal. 20Mg.
Guar Gum	Vit. B$_6$ 25Mg.
Alfalfa	Potass. Chl.15Mg.

Available sizes: 60 count and 120 count

LIV-ALIVE™

A Beet Root, Milk Thistle cleansing combination

THE INGREDIENTS:
Beet Rt
Milk Thistle seed
Oregon Grape Rt
Dandelion Rt.
Wild Yam
Yellow Dock Rt
Licorice
Fennel Sd.
Barberry
Cascara Sagrada
Ginger
Golden Seal Rt.
Choline-15Mg.
Inositol-15Mg.

Available sizes: 60 count and 120 count

LOVE CAPS FEMALE

Herbs to turn her attention to a loving mood.

THE INGREDIENTS:
Dong Quai
Damiana
Sarsaparilla
Licorice
Gotu Kola
Burdock
Parsley Lf.
Ginger
Guaraña
Ephedra
Yohimbe Bk.

Available sizes: 60 count

LOVE CAPS MALE

Herbs to turn his attention to a loving mood.

THE INGREDIENTS:
Sarsaparilla
Damiana
Siberian Ginseng
Kava Kava
Yohimbe Bk.
Saw Palmetto
Wild Yam
Ephedra
Muira Pauma
Gotu Kola
Capsicum
Ginger
Guaraña
Niacin 25Mg.
Zinc-20Mg.

Available sizes: 60 count

MALE CAPS
(special order only)

Herbs to rebalance, revitalize and regulate the male system.

THE INGREDIENTS:
Sarsaparilla
Siberian Ginseng
Licorice
Saw Palmetto
Gotu Kola
DandelionRt,
Fo-Ti-Tieng
Yellow Dock
Oats
Unspryd Bee Pollen
Burdock Rt.
Kelp
Schizandra Bry.
Hawthorne Lf.
Alfalfa
Ginger
Ornithine 30Mg.
Argenine 30Mg.
Zinc 20Mg.

Available sizes: 75 count

MEGA MINERAL

Highly absorbable herbs supplying the necessary minerals, trace minerals, and building blocks for health. Excellent for hair, skin, nails and digestive well-being.

THE INGREDIENTS:
Alfalfa
Nettles
Irish Moss
Yellow Dock
Watercress
Parsley Rt.
Spirulina
Kelp
Comfrey Rt.
Parsley Lf.
Borage Sd.
Dulse
Glutamine 20Mg.

Available sizes: 60 count

MENTAL CLARITY™

A Ginseng combination encouraging recall and alertness.

THE INGREDIENTS:
Korean Wht. Ginseng
Gotu Kola
Fo-Ti-Tieng
Siberian Ginseng
Ginkgo Biloba
Gotu Kola
Rosemary
Lecithin
Prickly Ash
Kelp
Capsicum
Phenalal. 50Mg.
Glutamine 25Mg.
Potass. Chl.20Mg.
Choline 15Mg.

Available sizes: 75 count

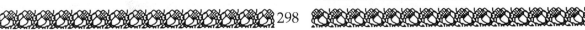

MASTER BUILDER CAPS

Effective herbal nutirents for enhanced body development.

THE INGREDIENTS:
Gotu Kola	Kelp
Rosemary	Capsicum
Prickly Ash	Glutamine 50Mg.

Available sizes: 60 count

MIN-ZYME-MINOS™ DRINK MIX

A vigorous drink mix, rich in proteins, minerals, trace minerals, alkalizing enzymes and full spectrum amino acids.

THE INGREDIENTS:
The Sea Vegetable Blend:
Dulse	Hijiki
Wakame	Sea Palm
Kombu	Spirulina

The Herbal Blend:
Alfalfa	Watercress
Oatstraw	Horsetail
Borage	Raspberry
Dandelion	Siberian Ginseng
Licorice	Parsley Rt. & Lf.
Comfrey Rt.	Rosemary
Yellow Dock	Red Sage
Nettles	

The Food Blend:
Miso Broth Powder	Brewer's Yst. 500
Soy Protein Powder	Veg. Acidolphilus
Cranberries	

Available sizes: 8 ounces

MIGRAID

Herbal nutrients and support for better body balance and prevention.

THE INGREDIENTS:
Wild Lettuce	Catnip
Feverfew	Rosemary
Licorice	Gentian
Valerian	DLPA-25Mg.

Available sizes: 90 count

NIGHT CAPS™

Herbs to encourage a natural, better quality of rest and sleep.

THE INGREDIENTS:
Valerian	Carrot Cal. 15Mg.
Scullcap	GABA 30Mg.
Passion Flower	Vit. B$_6$ 20Mg.
Kava Kava	Taurine 20Mg.
Hops	Niacin 15Mg.

Available sizes: 60 count

PANEX™

A Valerian/Wild lettuce combination.

THE INGREDIENTS:
Valerian	White Willow Bk
Wild Lettuce	DLPA- 30Mg.
St. John's Wort	Capsicum
	Magnesium 25Mg.

Available sizes: 100 count

PANCRAID
(special order only)

Regulates body activity to process sugars normally, and encourage healthy hormone and enzyme secretions.

The Ingredients:
Saw Palmetto	Vegetable Acid.
Licorice	Golden Seal Rt.
Juniper Bry	Mullein
Barberry	Bladderwrack
Prickly Ash Bk.	Capsicum

Available sizes: 60 count

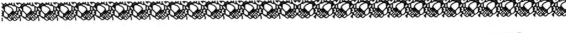

P.O. #1

Cleansing alkalizing herbs.

THE INGREDIENTS:

Echinacea Angust.	Yellow Dock
Echinacea Purp.	Capsicum
Chaparral	L-Lysine 50Mg.

Available sizes: 60 count Use alternately with P.O. #2 for best results.

P.O. #2

Calming soothing herbs.

THE INGREDIENTS:

Jewel Weed	Fresh Mugwort
Comfrey Lf	Black Cohosh
Red Raspberry Lf.	Kava Kava

Available sizes: 60 count Use alternately with P.O. #1 for best results.

POTASSIUM SOURCE CAPS

Concentrated sea vegetables and green herbs for optimum metabolic activity. Each capsule contains 95Mg. of Potassium, and 400Mg. Iodine from herbal and sea plant sources.

THE INGREDIENTS:

Norwegian Kelp	Watercress
Dulse	Alfalfa
Spirulina	Parsley Rt. & Lf.
Dandelion Rt	Glutamine 25Mg.

Available sizes: 60 count

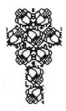

PRE-NATAL HERBS

High assimilation, easily absorbed, non-constipating herbal nutrients, to provide gentle, quickly utilized micro-nutrients and minerals.

THE INGREDIENTS:

Red Raspberry Lf.	Fennel
Nettles	Rosemary
Yellow Dock Rt.	Veg. Acidolph.
Oatstraw	Blessed Thistle
Alfalfa	Vit. B_6 25Mg.
Ascorbate C 50Mg.	Dry Vit. E 20IU

Available sizes: 100 count

PROS-CAPS

A Saw Palmetto, Golden Seal Root combination to cleanse and soothe inflammation.

THE INGREDIENTS:

Licorice	Uva Ursi
Golden Seal Rt.	Marshmallow
Saw Palmetto	Carrot Cal. 15Mg.
Parsley Rt.	Ginger
Juniper Bry.	Capsicum
Gravel Rt.	Zinc-30Mg.
	Dry Vit. E 20IU

Available sizes: 60 count and 120 count

RELAX CAPS™

High quality nutrients to help restore and soothe exhausted nerves.

The Ingredients:

Black Cohosh	Wood Betony
Lady Slipper(Dom.)	Oatstraw
Black Haw	Eur. Mistletoe
Valerian	Scullcap
Kava Kava	Carrot Cal. 15Mg.

Available sizes: 50 count and 90 count

RESPIRCAPS™

An anti-oxidant balancing combination.

THE INGREDIENTS:
Mullein	Slippery Elm
Wild Cherry Bk.	Marshmallow
Pleurisy Rt.	Licorice
Plantain	Chickweed
Comfrey Rt.	Kelp
Horehound	Capsicum
Rose Hips	Cinnamon

Available sizes: 60 count and 120 count

RTH EASE™

A Yucca, Alfalfa, Devils Claw combination.

THE INGREDIENTS:
Yucca	Yarrow
Chaparral	Licorice
Alfalfa Seed	Hydrangea
Devil's Claw Rt.	Parsley Rt.
Comfrey Rt	Rose Hips
Buckthorne	St. John's Wort
Black Cohosh	Turmeric
Slippery Elm	Hawthorne Bry.
Burdock	Pant. Acid 25Mg.
Dandelion	DLPA 25Mg.
Bilberry	Vit. B_6 25Mg.

Available sizes: 75 count and 140 count

SKIN THERAPY #1

A Dandelion and Burdock cleansing combination.

THE INGREDIENTS:
Dandelion Rt.	Licorice
Burdock	Yellow Dock Rt.
Echinacea Purp.	Chamomile
Chapparal	Glutamine 25Mg.
Red Clover	Vit. B_6 25Mg.

Available sizes: 90 count

SKIN THERAPY #2

A Chickweed and Licorice smoothing combination.

THE INGREDIENTS:
Chickweed	Sarsaparilla
Licorice	Chamomile
Dandelion	Rosemary
Burdock	Rose Hips
Alfalfa	Wild Yam
Yellow Dock	Glutamine 25Mg.
Chaparral	Zinc 15Mg.

Available sizes: 90 count

STONES AWAY

Herbal nutrients to aid in flushing out inorganic mineral wastes that contribute to sediment formation.

THE INGREDIENTS:
Dandelion Rt.	Milk Thistle Seed
Parsley Rt.	Licorice
Hydrangea	Marshmallow
Gravel Rt.	Lemon Balm
Wild Yam	Lecithin
Ginger	

Available sizes: 60 count and 120 count

SUPERMAX™

Highly absorbable herbal nutrition for maximum energy, endurance and vitality. Nourishes without stimulants. Provides energy without exciting the nervous system.

THE INGREDIENTS:
Chinese Red Ginseng	Gotu Kola
Spirulina	Liverall
Unsprd Bee Pollen	Alfalfa
Siberian Ginseng	Kelp
Suma	Pant. Acid 20Mg.
Amino Acid Cmpd. 50Mg.	

Available sizes: 50 count and 75 count

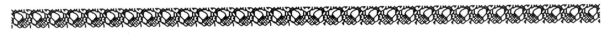

THERADERM CAPS™

An excellent source of absorbable minerals for building healthy skin.

THE INGREDIENTS:
Dandelion Rt.	Licorice
Chaparral	Kelp
Burdock	Nettles
Yellow Dock Rt.	St. John's Wort
Echinacea	L-Lysine 40Mg.
Turmeric	

Available sizes: 90 count

THYMETABS™

Herbs rich in natural Iodine and minerals to promote energy and vitality.

THE INGREDIENTS:
Irish Moss	Mullein
Kelp	Parsley Lf.
Parsley Rt	Carrot Cal 15Mg.
Watercress	Glutamine 25Mg.
Sarsaparilla	

Available sizes: 60 count

ULCR COMPLEX

A soothing Licorice combination.

THE INGREDIENTS:
Golden Seal	Licorice Rt.
Slippery Elm	Comfrey Rt.
Myrrh	Capsicum

Available sizes: 90 count.

VERMEX™

A Black Walnut and Pumpkin Seed cleansing combination.

THE INGREDIENTS:
Black Walnut Hull	Comfrey Rt.
Garlic	Gentian
Pumpkin Seed	Slippery Elm
Butternut Bark	Wormwood
Cascara Sagrada	Fennel Sd.

Available Sizes: 100 count

VISI-CARE™

An Eyebright and Bilberry combination.

THE INGREDIENTS:
Eyebright	Ginkgo Biloba
Bilberry	Red Raspberry
Parsley Rt.	Bayberry
Golden Seal Rt.	Capsicum
Passion Flower	Angelica
Hawthorne Lf.	

Available sizes: 60 count and 120 count

WHITES OUT #1

A Golden Seal & Myrrh combination for the female system.

THE INGREDIENTS:
Golden Seal Rt	Echinacea Rt.
Myrrh Gum	Chaparral
Pau de Arco	Veg. Acidolph.

Available sizes: 60 count Take with Whites Out # 2 for best results.

WHITES OUT # 2

A Comfrey Root and Burdock combination for the female system.

THE INGREDIENTS:

Comfrey Rt.	Squaw Vine
Juniper Bry.	Dandelion Rt.
Burdock Rt.	Uva Ursi
Parsley Rt.	

Available sizes: 60 count Take with Whites Out # 1 for best results.

WOMAN'S BEST FRIEND

An elasticizing, strengthening, toning combination for a woman's balance.

THE INGREDIENTS:

Cramp Bark	Uva Ursi
Squaw Vine	Rose Hips
Sarsaparilla	Red Raspberry
Golden Seal	Capsicum
Peony Rt.	False Unicorn
Rehmannia	Ginger
Dong Quai	Blessed Thistle

Available sizes: 90 count

ZING!

An herbal energizer containing natural caffeine.

THE INGREDIENTS:

Guaraña Sd.	Capsicum
Kola Nut	Phenalala. 50Mg.
Ephedra	Ginger
Astragalus	

Available sizes: 75 count

HEALTHY LIFE ANIMAL MIX™

A wonderful combination for a pet's health and well-being. Helps control fleas, ticks and mites. Improves skin and coat health. Aids digestion, circulation and regularity.

THE INGREDIENTS:

Brewer's Yeast	Garlic
Kelp	Dandelion Rt.
Spirulina	Comfrey Lf.
Alfalfa Lf.	Wheat Germ
Bran	Sod. Asc. C
Lecithin	Soy Protein

Available sizes: 8 oz. glassine-lined bag.

MOTH FREE™
MOTH REPELLENT

All natural. Allergy Free. Repels moths, not you.

THE INGREDIENTS:

Cedarwood Chips	Basil
Rosemary Lf.	Bay Lf.
Lemon Grass	Rosemary Oil
Natural Cellulose	Eucalyptus Oil
Lavender	Cedar Oil

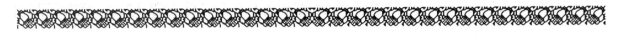

EXTRACTS

Crystal Star extracts are all packaged in easy-to-take 1oz. dropper bottles. The herbs are in low-alcohol extractions of 40-60% alcohol, dependeng on the particular herb. They may be used with confidence by those who react poorly to high pharmaceutical alcohol levels.

To enjoy these extract without alcohol, simply put the desired amount of drops into a cup of warm water, and allow the alcohol to evaporate for 5 minutes before drinking.

BILBERRY LEAF
Vaccinium Myrtillus

A strong extract of this highly acclaimed herb, potent with active flavonoids.

DONG QUAI/DAMIANA: 50%/50%

A combination for female balance and well-being.

ECHINACEA:

Angustifolia and Purpurea 50%/50%

A superior combination that encompasses root, leaf and flower of both powerful species of the herb, Angustifolia and Purpurea, in one convenient liquid. A gentle, non-toxic but effective herbal tonic, that may be taken every 3-4 hours during high risk seasons.

GINKGO BILOBA LEAF

A potent extract of an amazing plant with a long list of myriad benefits. It may be used 2-3 times daily or as needed.

HAWTHORNE LEAF & BERRY:
50%/50%
Crataegus Oxyacanthus

All parts of the English Hawthorne are biologically active. Crystal Star recognizes this fact by including the leaf and flower as well as the berry in this extract. It has a very high bioflavonoid content, providing a tonic quality and feeling of balanced well-being.

MILK THISTLE SEED
Silybum Marianum

Milk Thistle is a potent herb, high in anti-oxidant properties that prevent free-radical damage.

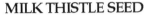

SIBERIAN GINSENG
Eleutheroccocus Senticosus

A superior adaptogen to increase physical energy and combat fatigue.

SUPER LICORICE
Glycyrrhiza Glabra

This extract is made from one of the few known organic sources of Licorice in the world. The very small yearly crop comes from Australia.

VALERIAN & WILD LETTUCE:
50%/50%
Valeriana Officinalis/Lactuca Elongata

The roots and leaves for this combination are organically grown and extracted from the fresh picked plant. Their volatile oils are very high, for gentle but effective relaxation.

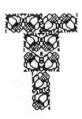

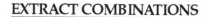

EXTRACT COMBINATIONS

ADRN

A tonic and toning formula for increased and better energy use.

THE HERBS:

Licorice
Sarsaparilla

Bladderwrack
rish Moss

ALRG/HST

Herbal support to help overcome environmental sensitivities.

THE HERBS:

Ephedra
Chapparal
Marshmallow

Golden Seal Rt.
Burdock Rt.
Wild Cherry Bk.

ANTI-BIO™

A double Echinacea/Golden Seal combination.

THE HERBS:

Echinacea Angustifolia
Echinacea Purpurea
Golden Seal Rt.

Myrrh Gum
Chapparal

ANTI-VI™
Lomatium & St. John's Wort 50%/50%

A combination for high risk seasons with anti-viral properties.

BLDR-K FLUSH

Relieving herbs to clear and flush.

THE HERBS:

Cornsilk
Juniper Bry.
Uva Ursi
Parsley Rt. & Lf.

Dandelion Rt.
Golden Seal Rt.
Marshmallow
Ginger rt.

CIRCU-EXTRA

Quickly absorbable herbs to put pep into a sluggish system, and counteract fatigue.

THE HERBS:

Siberian Ginseng
Gotu Kola
Ginkgo Biloba

Cayenne
Ginger Rt.

CRAMP CONTROL

A Cramp Bark combination for gentle soothing relief.

THE HERBS:

Black Haw
Cramp Bark

Kava Kava
Rosemary

ESTRO-MONE'™

A tonic and toner for the female system.

THE HERBS:

Black Cohosh
Dong Quai
Damiana
Licorice
Sarsaparilla

Peony Rt.
Oatstraw
Red Raspberry
Rosemary

HEADACHE DEFENSE

A Feverfew / Ginkgo Biloba extract combination.

THE HERBS:
Feverfew
Siberian Ginseng
Gingko Biloba Lf.
Cayenne

HERBAL DEFENSE TEAM™

A formula high in herbal oxygenators, minerals and restoratives.

THE HERBS:
Garlic
Echinacea Rt.
Pau de Arco
Hawthorne Lf. & Fl.
Astragalus
Siberian Ginseng
Golden Seal Rt.
Rose Hip Vit. C
Elecampane
Chaparral

HIGHLY ABSORBABLE HERBAL CALCIUM

Calcium, Magnesium and trace elements from herbs. Especially rich in Silica extract which the body uses to form healthy tissue and bone.

THE HERBS:
Horsetail
Oatstraw
Comfrey Rt.
Borage

HIGHLY ABSORBABLE HERBAL IRON

Iron and trace mineral extracts from herbs. Rich, absorbable, non-constipating.

THE HERBS:
Yellow Dock
Nettles
Watercress
Dandelion Rt.

HIGHLY ABSORBABLE MINERAL COMPLEX

A complete mineral and trace mineral extract complex from herbs, providing the building blocks of health.

THE HERBS:
Horsetail
Yellow Dock
Nettles
Alfalfa
Watercress
Irish Moss
Parsley Rt. & Lf.
Comfrey Rt. & Lf.

IODINE THERAPY

A sea greens complex for absorbable potassium and iodine.

THE HERBS:
Kelp
Kombu
Dulse
Alfalfa
Irish Moss
Horsetail
Watercress
Wakame

LIV TONIC™

Effective herbal nutrients to cleanse and restore.

THE HERBS:
Oregon Grape
Milk Thistle Seed
Dandelion Rt.
Yellow Dock Rt.
Ginkgo Biloba Lf.
Red`Sage
Licorice Rt.
Wild Yam
Fennel Sd.
Cascara Sag.

LOVING MOOD EXTRACT FOR MEN

A Ginseng, Oats and Damiana combination.

THE HERBS:
Siberian Ginseng
Damiana
Oats
Dandelion Rt.
Cayenne
Licorice

RTH TONE

A highly absorbable Devil's Claw/Yucca combination.

THE HERBS:

Devil's Claw · White Willow
Yucca Echinacea
Siberian Ginseng Capsicum

SCALE DOWN DIET EXTRACT™

A strong Chickweed and Spirulina combination.

THE HERBS:

Chickweed Lemon Peel
Spirulina Fennel
Licorice Senna Lf.
Dulse Ephedra
Gotu Kola

SLEEP EASE™

A calming Valerian and Wild Lettuce combination to encourage sweet sleep.

THE HERBS:

Valerian Hops
Scullcap Wild Lettuce
Passion Flower

STRESS RELIEF

Calming, soothing, restorative herbs.

THE HERBS:

Black Cohosh Wood Betony
Black Haw Kava Kava
Scullcap Carrot Calcium

ULCR COMPLEX

A soothing licorice combination.

THE HERBS:

Licorice Comfrey Rt.
Golden Seal Myrrh
Slippery Elm Capsicum

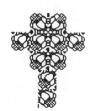

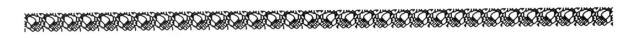

MEDICINAL TEAS

BEAUTIFUL SKIN TEA

A cleansing purifying drink. May also be used as a facial wash; simply soak cotton balls in the strong tea and apply.

THE HERBS:
Licorice	Parsley
Burdock Rt.	Comfrey Lf.
Rosemary	Comfrey Rt.
Rose Hips	Sage
Dandelion Rt.	Fennel Sd.
Sarsaparilla	Thyme

BLDR-K FLUSH

Herbal nutrients for fluid ease.

THE HERBS:
Juniper Bry.	Parsley Lf.
Cornsilk	Cleavors
Buchu	Comfrey Lf.
Uva Ursi	Ginger
Plantain	Marshmallow Rt.

BONZ TEA™

A strengthening, high mineral tea.

THE HERBS:
Horsetail	Alfalfa
Comfrey Rt	Licorice
Oatstraw	Marshmallow
Burdock	Dulse
Nettles	

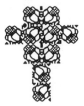

CHILL CARE™

A warming cozy tea.

THE HERBS:
Peppermint	Safflowers
Elder Flwr. & Bry.	Cloves
Coltsfoot	Rose Hips
Hyssop	Cinnamon
Licorice	Ginger
Yarrow	Boneset
	Sweet Herb

CHINESE ROYAL MU TEA

A traditional Chinese blend, used as a strong regenerative tonic for the whole body. An excellent addition to a macrobiotic diet.

THE HERBS:
Chinese Ginseng	Sassafras
Sarsaparilla	Ginger
Licorice	Star Anise
Marshmallow	Cloves
Dandelion Rt. Roasted	Orange Peel
Burdock	Cinnamon

CLEANSING & FASTING TEA™

Beneficial, strengthening herbal support for a successful cleanse.

THE HERBS:
Red Clover	Milk Thistle Seed
Hawthorne Lf	Echinacea Purpurea
Pau de Arco	Blue Malva
Nettles	Shavegrass
Sage	Yerba Santa
Alfalfa	Lemon Grass
Gotu Kola	

COFEX TEA™

To soothe and quiet the tickle.

THE HERBS:

Wild Cherry
Licorice
Cinnamon
Slippery Elm

Sarsaparilla
Orange Peel
Fennel

CRAN-DIDA™

A gentle, effective alkalizing tea to neutralize intolerances, and set up an environment for better body balance.

THE HERBS:

Pau de Arco
Cranberry Juice Pwr.
Rosehips
Licorice
Damiana

Echinacea Rt.
Burdock
Myrrh
Hibiscus
Lemon Balm
Cinnamon

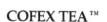

CREATIVI-TEA™

Herbal nourishment for the memory and alertness centers of the body.

THE HERBS:

Siberian Ginseng
Damiana
Juniper Bry.
Gotu Kola
Kava Kava

Licorice
Cloves
Muira Pauma
Spearmint

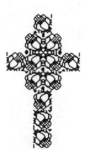

CUPID'S FLAME™

An herbal tea to encourage a loving mood.

THE HERBS:

Damiana
Prince Ginseng
Sarsaparilla
Licorice
Fo-Ti-Tieng
Gotu Kola

Saw Palmetto
Kava Kava
Angelica
Ginger
Muira Pauma
Allspice

DEEP BREATHING TEA

Herbal nutrients to increase oxygen use.

THE HERBS:

Wild Cherry
Safflowers
Mullein
Parsley
Sage

Thyme
Blackberry Lf.
Ginger
Pleurisy Rt.
Sweet Herb

EYELIGHT TEA

A soothing, brightening Bilberry and Eyebright blend. May be used internally or externally.

THE HERBS:

Eyebright
Bilberry
Passion Flower
Plantain

Elder Flr.
Rosemary
Golden Seal Rt
Red Raspberry

FEEL GREAT™

A delicious all-over body tonic.

THE HERBS:

Red Clover
Alfalfa
Hawthorne Lf. & Flr.
Spearmint
Sage

Comfrey Lf.
Dandelion
Lemon Grass
Dulse
Sweet Herb

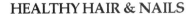

FEMALE HARMONY™

Herbal nutrients to balance, tone and regulate the female system.

THE HERBS:
Red Raspberry	Rose Buds
Licorice	Lemon Grass
Nettles	Spearmint
Sarsaparilla	Strawberry
Rose Hips	Sweet Herb

FLOW EASE

Herbs to relieve and relax the female system.

THE HERBS:
Cramp Bark	Ginger
Chamomile	Sarsaparilla
Angelica	Spearmint
Squaw Vine	Sweet Herb

FLOW ON TEA™

An herbal solution for women.

THE HERBS:
Pennyroyal	Blue Cohosh
Motherwort	Lovage
Juniper Bry.	Canada Snake Rt.
Angelica	Tansy

GOOD NIGHT TEA

Sweet, deep, better quality sleep.

THE HERBS:
Chamomile	Orange Buds
Spearmint	Rosebuds
Scullcap	Lemon Grass
Passion Flower	Blackberry
Hops	Rosemary
Elder Flower	Sweet Herb

HEALTHY HAIR & NAILS

Herbs with highly absorbable minerals and proteins to strengthen hair and nails. May also be used externally as a conditioning rinse.

THE HERBS:
Horsetail	Lemon Grass
Dandelion	Parsley Lf.
Alfalfa	Fenugreek Sd.
Rosemary	Peppermint
Coltsfoot	Nettles
Comfrey Lf.	Sweet Herb

HEMA-CLEANSE™

A Gingko Biloba, Pau de Arco cleansing combination.

THE HERBS:
Pau de Arco	Ginger
KukichaTwig	Calendula
Ginkgo Biloba	Yellow Dock
Hawthorne Lf & Flr.	Peppermint
Sage	Butcher's Broom
Sassafras	Blackberry

HERBAL DEFENSE TEA™

A Red Clover/Astragalus protection formula.

THE HERBS:
Red Clover	St. John's Wort
Burdock Rt.	Schizandra Bry.
Hawthorne Lf. & Flr.	Sage
Astragalus	Marshmallow
Prince Ginseng	Suma
Licorice Rt.	Lemon Grass
Boneset	

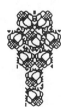

HIGH ENERGY TEA™

Herbs to energize.

THE HERBS:
Gotu Kola	Peppermint
Red Clover	Kava Kava
Red Raspberry	Prince Ginseng
Damiana	Cloves

HIGH PRESSURE TONIC

A potent combination to lower pressure and increase system energy.

THE HERBS:
Hawthorne Lf. & Flr.	Ginger Rt.
Scullcap	Valerian
Dandelion Rt. & Lf.	Rose Hips
Siberian Ginseng	Hibiscus

HYPO BLUES TEA

An herbal tonic and balancing blend providing easily absorbable protein and minerals.

THE HERBS:
Siberian Ginseng	Gotu Kola
Peppermint	Nettles
Alfalfa	Dandelion Rt.
Licorice Rt.	

INCREDIBLE DREAMS™

Herbs to help remember your dreams.

THE HERBS:
Fresh Mugwort	Red Raspberry
Kava Kava	Spearmint
Rosemary	Alfalfa
Lemon Balm	Sweet Herb

LAXA-TEA

A gentle cleansing, regulating blend.

THE HERBS:
Senna	Turkey Rhubarb
Fennel	Peppermint
Ginger	Parsley Lf.
Papaya	Calendula
Hibiscus	Lemon Balm

LEAN 'N CLEAN DIET TEA™

Herbal nutritional support for your diet. A flushing Senna and Uva Ursi combination.

THE HERBS:
Fennel	Buchu Lf
Uva Ursi	Burdock Rt.
Senna Lf & Pod	Cleavors
Red Clover	Flax Seed
Hibiscus	Parsley Lf.
Lemon Peel	Sassafras

LIV-FLUSH™

A liver and gallbladder cleansing combination with Pau de Arco and Milk Thistle Seed.

THE HERBS:
Dandelion Rt.	Oregon Grape Rt.
Watercress	Red Sage
Yellow Dock	Licorice
Pau de Arco	Milk Thistle Seed
Hyssop	Hibiscus
Parsley Lf.	

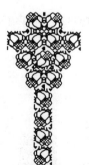

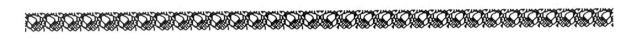

MEALS END™

For minty fresh breath, and a comfortable ending to a meal.

THE HERBS:

Hibiscus   Papaya
Rosemary   Peppermint

MEDITATION TEA™

A warming tonic for mind and body. Herbs for mellow inner awareness and energy.

THE HERBS:

Cardamom   Ginger
Cinnamon   Peppercorns
Cloves   Fennel

MOTHERING TEA™

Herbal nutrition for a mother's dramatic body changes and adjustments.

THE HERBS:

Red Raspberry   Alfalfa
Nettles   Lemon Grass
Comfrey Lf.   Strawberry Lf.
Spearmint   Fennel Sd.
Ginger   Sweet Herb

NICO-STOP™

Diet support for your efforts to kick the habit.

THE HERBS:

Licorice Rt.   Dulse
Gentian Rt.   Sassafras
Chamomile   Sweet Herb
Peppermint

OPEN UP TEA

Expectorant herbs to clear the clog.

THE HERBS:

Mullein   Fennel
Pleurisy Rt.   Marshmallow
Comfrey Rt.   Calendula
Ma Huang   Boneset
Rose Hips   Ginger
Peppermint   Sweet Herb

POLLEN-EX TEA™

Herbs to help overcome pollen allergy symptoms.

THE HERBS:

Comfrey Rt   Ginger
Horehound   Orange Peel
Peppermint   Burdock Rt.
Rosebuds   Ephedra
Rosehips   Cloves
Anise Seed   Sweet Herb

RELAX TEA

Herbs to soothe, and relax the mind, and restore mental energy.

THE HERBS:

Lemon Balm   Rosebuds
Spearmint   Cinnamon
Licorice   Rosemary
Yerba Santa   Orange Peel
Lemon Grass   Sweet Herb

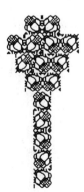

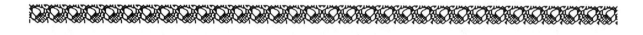

RESPIR-TEA™

Herbal support for cleansed breathing, high in aromatic oils.

THE HERBS:
Fenugreek Sd.	Anise Seed
Hyssop	Sassafras
Horehound	Marshmallow
Rose Hips	Boneset
Slippery Elm	Peppermint
Comfrey Rt	Sweet Herb

R^TH EASE TEA

A Devil's Claw combination to relieve and relax.

THE HERBS:
Oregon Grape	Gravel Rt.
Chaparral	Cleavors
Devil's Claw	Sasssfras
Red Clover	Prickly Ash
Ginger	Slippery Elm

"STRESSED OUT" TEA

Calming, soothing, relaxing herbs.

THE HERBS:
Catnip	Wood Betony
Rosemary	Gotu Kola
Blue Violet	Peppermint
Feverfew	Blessed Thistle
Chamomile	Sweet Herb
White Willow	

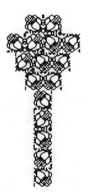

THERADERM TEA™

Soothing herbs for the skin. Use internally, or externally as a wash. Simply soak cotton balls in strong tea and pat on.

THE HERBS:
Burdock	Calendula
St. John's Wort	Licorice
Chamomile	Borage Seed
Dandelion Rt.	Blue Vervain
Comfrey Lf. & Rt.	Sage

TINKLE TEA

A Fennel and Parsley combination for release and relief.

THE HERBS:
Uva Ursi	Sassafras
Fennel	Lemon Peel
Parsley Lf.	Dulse
Senna	Ginger

VARI-TONE

Herbs high in strengthening, toning Bio-flavonoids.

THE HERBS:
Hawthorne Lf. , Flwr. & Bry.	
Bilberry Lf.	Myrrh Gum
Ginkgo Biloba	Eucalyptus
Gotu Kola	Comfrey Rt.
White Oak Bk.	Lemon Peel
Rose Hips	Senna

SPECIAL NOTE
The cutting of herbs for tea bags creates facets on the herb structure causing the loss of the essential volatile oils. **Crystal Star** herbs are very high in these oils. Therefore, we package our teas only in bulk, and we blend our teas fresh every week. Keep teas covered while brewing to hold in these oils.

RESOURCES

❖ Best Ways Magazine

❖ Better Health Through Natural Healing: Dr. Ross Trattler, D.C.

❖ Cooking For Healthy Healing: Linda Rector-Page, N.D., Ph. D

❖ Country Life: Nutritional Literature, by Marcia Zimmerman

❖ Dr. Pitcairn's Complete Guide To Natural Health For Dogs & Cats: Dr. R.H. Pitcairn, DVM

❖ Enzymatic Therapy: Nutritional Formulas For The Right Body Chemistry

❖ Everybody's Guide To Homeopathic Medicines: S. Cummings & Dana Ullman

❖ The Healing Nutrients Within: E.R. Braverman, M.D. & Carl C. Pfeiffer, M.D., Ph. D.

❖ The Holistic Herbal: David Hoffman

❖ How To Get Well: Paavo Airola

❖ The How To Herb Book: V.J. Keith & Monteen Gordon

❖ Lets Live Magazine

❖ Nutrition Almanac: Lavon J. Dunne

❖ Nutrition News: Riverside, Calif.

❖ Stories The Feet Have Told Through Reflexology: Eunice D. Ingham

❖ The Way Of Herbs: Michael Tierra

❖ The staff and clients of Country Store Natural Foods, whose self-healing efforts and accomplishments have contributed invaluable concrete information and evidence.

❖ Whole Foods Magazine

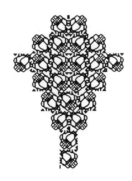

INDEX

A

B

SPINAL MENINGITIS, 258
SPLEEN, 259
SPORTS INJURIES, 49-52, 260
SPORTS MEDICINE, 49-52, 261
SPOTS BEFORE THE EYES, 149
SPRAINS , 260
STAMINA, 146
STAPH INFECTION, 280
STERILITY, 192
Steroids, 51; Natural Replacements, 261
STOMACH & DUODENAL ULCERS, 262
STOMACH UPSET, 124
STREP INFECTION, 243, 257
STREP THROAT, 257
STRESS, 263
STRETCH MARKS, 56, 245
STROKE , 172
Sulphur, 12
SUNBURN , 264
SURGERY, RECOVERY, 46-47
SWOLLEN BREASTS , 231
SWOLLEN GLANDS, 257
SYPHILIS, 278

T

T.B., 206
TOOTHACHE, 271
TACHYCARDIA, 171
TASTE & SMELL LOSS, 265
Taurine, 16
TEETHING, 58, 266
TENDONITIS, 267
Threonine, 16
THROMBOSIS, 236
THRUSH, 58, 154
THRUSH FUNGAL INFECTION, 58
THYROID HEALTH, 268
TINNITUS , 269
TONSILITIS, 270
TOOTHACHE AND INFECTION, 272
TOOTH TARTER, 271
TORN LIGAMENTS, 260
TOXEMIA, 56
TOXIC SHOCK, 273
TRIGLYGERIDES, 113
TUMORS, MALIGNANT, 274; BENIGN, 131
Tryptophane, 16
Tyrosine, 16

U

UFAs - Unsaturated Fatty Acids, 14
ULCERATIONS, 65, 254
ULCERS, 137, 262
UPSET STOMACH, 124

UTERINE FIBROIDS AND CYSTS, 230, 275
UTERINE HEMORRHAGING, 56

V

VAGINAL YEAST INFECTION, 276
VAGINITIS, 276
VARICOSE VEINS, 56, 277
VASCULAR HEADACHES, 214
VENEREAL DISEASE, 278
VENEREAL WARTS, 282
VERTIGO, 277
VIRAL WARTS, 280, 282
VIRUS INFECTION, 122, 280
ABOUT VITAMINS, 13, 14
Vitamin A, 13,
Vitamin B_1 - Thiamine, 13
Vitamin B_2 - Riboflavin, 13
Vitamin B_3 - Niacin, 13
Vitamin B_5- Pantothenic Acid, 14
Vitamin B_6- Pyridoxine, 14
Vitamin B_{12}- Cobalamin, 14
Vitamin B_{15}-Pangamic Acid, 14
Vitamin C, 14
Vitamin D, 14
Vitamin E, 14
Vitamin K, 14
VITILIGO (depletion and lack of skin pigmentation), 253
VOMITING, 217

W

WARTS, 280, 281
WASP STINGS, 194
ABOUT WATER, 41
WATER RETENTION, 280, 283
WEAK SYSTEM, 58
WEIGHT LOSS, 284-288
WENS, 131
WHOOPING COUGH, 58
ABOUT NATURAL WINES, 40
Women after hysterectomy, childbirth, D & C, or suction curretage, 183
WORMS & PARASITES, 58, 234
WOUNDS, 130
WRINKLING AND DRY CRACKED SKIN, 253
WRINKLES,289

Y

Yogurt, 40

Z

Zinc, 12